T0296792

Neurodegenerative Disorders

Orla Hardiman • Colin P. Doherty
Editors

Marwa Elamin • Peter Bede
Associate Editors

Neurodegenerative Disorders

A Clinical Guide

Second Edition

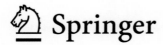 Springer

Editors
Orla Hardiman
Academic Unit of Neurology
Trinity Biomedical Sciences Institute
Dublin
Ireland

Colin P. Doherty
Academic Unit of Neurology
Trinity Biomedical Sciences Institute
Dublin
Ireland

Associate Editors
Marwa Elamin
Academic Unit of Neurology
Trinity Biomedical Sciences Institute
Dublin
Ireland

Peter Bede
Academic Unit of Neurology
Trinity Biomedical Sciences Institute
Dublin
Ireland

ISBN 978-3-319-23308-6   ISBN 978-3-319-23309-3   (eBook)
DOI 10.1007/978-3-319-23309-3

Library of Congress Control Number: 2015958656

Springer Cham Heidelberg New York Dordrecht London
© Springer International Publishing Switzerland 2016

Printed on acid-free paper

Springer International Publishing AG Switzerland is part of Springer Science+Business Media
(www.springer.com)

Contents

Contributors

Sharon Abrahams Human Cognitive Neuroscience-Psychology, Euan MacDonald Centre for Motor Neurone Disease Research, Centre for Cognitive Aging and Epidemiology, University of Edinburgh, Edinburgh, UK

Thomas H. Bak The Anne Rowling Regenerative Neurology Clinic, Centre for Clinical Brain Sciences (CCBS), University of Edinburgh, Edinburgh, UK

Centre for Cognitive Ageing and Cognitive Epidemiology , University of Edinburgh, Edinburgh, UK

Peter Bede Academic Unit of Neurology, Trinity Biomedical Sciences Institute, Dublin, Ireland

Leonard H. van den Berg Department of Neurology, University Medical Center Utrecht, Utrecht, The Netherlands

Colm Bergin Department of Infectious Diseases, St. James's Hospital, Dublin, Ireland

Department of Clinical Medicine, Trinity College, Dublin, Ireland

David Bradley Department of Neurology, St. Jame's Hospital, Dublin, Ireland

Tom Burke Academic Unit of Neurology, Trinity Biomedical Sciences Institute, Dublin, Ireland

Zeina Chemali Departments of Neurology and Psychiatry, Massachusetts General Hospital, Massachusetts Eye and Ear Infirmary, Harvard Medical School, Boston, MA, USA

Robert F. Coen Memory Clinic, Mercer's Institute For Research on Aging, St. James's Hospital, Dublin, Ireland

Department of Gerontology, Trinity College Dublin, Dublin, Ireland

Lisa Costelloe Department of Neurology, Beaumont Hospital, Dublin, Ireland

Kirk R. Daffner Center for Brain/Mind Medicine, Department of Neurology, Brigham and Women's Hospital, Harvard Medical School, Boston, MA, USA

Colin P. Doherty Academic Unit of Neurology, Trinity Biomedical Sciences Institute, Dublin, Ireland

Department of Neurology, St. James's Hospital, Dublin, Ireland

Marwa Elamin Academic Unit of Neurology, Trinity Biomedical Sciences Institute, Dublin, Ireland

Stanley Fahn Department of Neurology, Columbia University Medical Center, New York, NY, USA

Denise Fitzgerald Queens University, Belfast, Ireland

Jean Fletcher Schools of Medicine and Biochemistry and Immunology, Trinity College Dublin, Dublin, Ireland

Damien Gallagher Geriatric Psychiatry, Sunnybrook Health Sciences Centre, University of Toronto, Toronto, ON, Canada

Joseph Harbison Department of Medical Gerontology, Mercer's Institute for Successful Ageing, St James's Hospital, Dublin, Ireland

Department of Medical Gerontology, Trinity College, Dublin, Dublin, Ireland

Orla Hardiman Academic Unit of Neurology, Trinity Biomedical Sciences Institute, Dublin, Ireland

Daniel Healy Department of Neurology, St. James's Hospital, Dublin, Ireland

Royal College of Surgeons in Ireland, Dublin, Ireland

Siobhan Hutchinson Cognitive Neurology Clinic, St. James's Hospital, Dublin, Ireland

Parameswaran Mahadeva Iyer Academic Unit of Neurology, Trinity Biomedical Sciences Institute, Dublin, Ireland

Julie A. Kelly The Academic Unit of Neurology, Trinity Biomedical Sciences Institute, Trinity College Dublin, Dublin, Ireland

Sean P. Kennelly Medical Gerontology, Trinity College, Dublin, Dublin, Ireland

Acute Medical Unit, Tallaght Hospital, Dublin, Ireland

Rose Ann Kenny Department of Medical Gerontology, Mercer's Institute for Successful Ageing, St James's Hospital, Dublin, Ireland

Department of Medical Gerontology, Trinity College, Dublin 2, Dublin, Ireland

Matthew C. Kiernan Brain and Mind Centre, Sydney Medical School, University of Sydnes, Royal Prince Alfred Hospital, Camperdown, NSW, Australia

Janine Kirby Department Neurology, Sheffield Institute of Translational Neuroscience, Sheffield University, Sheffield, UK

Walter Koroshetz Neurological Disorders and Stroke Institute, National Institutes of Health, Bethesda, MD, USA

Brian A. Lawlor Department of Psychiatry, Trinity College Dublin, Dublin, Ireland

Marina A. Lynch Trinity College Institute of Neuroscience, Lloyd Building, Trinity College, Dublin, Ireland

Tim Lynch Department of Neurology, Dublin Neurological Institute, Mater Misericordiae University Hospital, Dublin, Ireland

Sinead Maguire Academic Unit of Neurology, Trinity Biomedical Sciences Institute, Dublin, Ireland

Patricia McNamara Academic Unit of Neurology, Trinity Biomedical Sciences Institute, Dublin, Ireland

Simon Mead MRC Prion Unit, Department of Neurodegenerative Disease, UCL Institute of Neurology, Queen Square, London, UK

NHS National Prion Clinic, National Hospital for Neurology and Neurosurgery, University College London Hospitals NHS Foundation Trust, London, UK

Dragos L. Mihaila Department of Neurology, SUNY Upstate Medical University, Syracuse, New York, USA

Hiroshi Mitsumoto Department of Neurology, Columbia University Medical Center, New York, USA

Seán O'Dowd Department of Neurology, St. James's Hospital, Dublin, Ireland

Trinity College Medical School, Dublin, Ireland

David Oliver Wisdom Hospice, Consultant in Palliative Medicine, High Bank, Rochester, UK

University of Kent, Kent, UK

Diana A. Olszewska Department of Neurology, Dublin Neurological Institute, Mater Misericordiae University Hospital, Dublin, Ireland

Niall Pender Department of Neuropsychology, Beaumont Hospital, Dublin, Ireland

Academic Unit of Neurology, Trinity College Dublin, Dublin, Ireland

Lewis P. Rowland Department of Neurology, The Neurological Institute of New York, Columbia University Medical Center, New York, USA

Peter Rudge MRC Prion Unit, Department of Neurodegenerative Disease, UCL Institute of Neurology, Queen Square, London, UK

NHS National Prion Clinic, National Hospital for Neurology and Neurosurgery, University College London Hospitals NHS Foundation Trust, London, UK

Pamela J. Shaw Sheffield Institute for Translational Neuroscience (SITraN), University of Sheffield, Sheffield, UK

Jeremy M. Shefner Barrow Neurological Institute, University of Arizona College of Medicine, Phoenix, AZ, USA

Joseph Trettel Department of Neurobehavioral Medicine, Gaylord Hospital, Wallingford, CT, USA

Richard A. Walsh Department of Neurology, Tallaght Hospital, Dublin, Ireland

Lilia Zaporojan Academic Unit of Neurology, Trinity College Dublin, Dublin, Ireland

Taha Omer Academic Unit of Neurology, Trinity Biomedical Sciences Institute, Dublin, Ireland

Common Themes in the Pathogenesis of Neurodegeneration

Marina A. Lynch, Orla Hardiman, Marwa Elamin, Janine Kirby, and Lewis P. Rowland

1.1 Introduction

As the population increases in size and life expectancies continue to rise, so do the number of people diagnosed with neurodegenerative diseases. This term refers to age-dependent progressive diseases, caused by degeneration of the central nervous system (CNS). Traditionally, these conditions were characterized clinically, but with advances in imaging, it has become possible to attribute specific clinical manifestations of disease to degeneration in specific anatomical regions of the CNS. Histopathological analysis, genetic studies, and proteomic interrogation have further refined the diagnosis of neurodegenerative diseases.

Neurodegenerative diseases share certain common features including histopathology, clinical course, and molecular mechanisms of pathogenesis. Comparing two different diseases, there may be both overlap with regard to some features and divergence of other aspects. As new categories of disease emerge, some are seen to share common pathogenic features and genetic origins.

The aim of this chapter is to describe the common themes that underlie the major neurodegenerative diseases, and to draw biochemical, histopathological, and molecular genetic parallels across the different disease categories that are outlined in the remainder of this book.

M.A. Lynch (✉)
Trinity College Institute of Neuroscience, Lloyd Building, Trinity College Dublin, Ireland
e-mail: lynchma@tcd.ie

O. Hardiman • M. Elamin
Academic Unit of Neurology,
Trinity Biomedical Sciences Institute,
Dublin, Ireland
e-mail: orla@hardiman.net;
marwaelamin08@gmail.com

J. Kirby
Department Neurology, Sheffield Institute of Translational Neuroscience, Sheffield University, Sheffield, UK
e-mail: J.Kirby@sheffield.ac.uk

L.P. Rowland
Department Neurology, New York Institute of Neurology, Columbia University Medical Center, New York, NY, USA
e-mail: lpr1@mail.cumc.columbia.edu

1.2 Common Clinical Features of Neurodegenerative Diseases

In 2003, Przedborski and colleagues recognized the clinical and pathological manifestations of neurodegenerative diseases, which:

- Affect "specific subsets of neurons"
- Arise without clear explanation and could be either inherited or acquired
- "Progress relentlessly"
- Are often age-related, increasing in frequency with advancing age

© Springer International Publishing Switzerland 2016
O. Hardiman, C.P. Doherty (eds.), *Neurodegenerative Disorders: A Clinical Guide*,
DOI 10.1007/978-3-319-23309-3_1

- Are often accompanied by microscopic signs of four stages of disorder:
  - Neuronal pathology
  - Neuronal cell death
  - Disappearance of neuronal cell bodies
  - Glial proliferation

The following may serve as a brief overview of common clinical features of neurodegenerative diseases:

The chronic clinical course is relentlessly progressive until death.

The disorder is not reversible by any known therapy although drug therapy or gene therapy generally give marginal and temporary improvement.

Phenotypic variability is commonly seen.

Cognitive impairment and dementia are common manifestations in neurodegenerative disorders but are not seen in all forms. The diagnosis of dementia has been formalized so that cognitive changes in frontotemporal dementia (FTD) and Alzheimer disease can generally be differentiated by formal neuropsychological tests.

The major risk factor is advancing age. The term age-related neurodegenerative disease is commonly used.

The condition appears to be heritable in a small percentage of cases.

In the familial form of the disease, the onset occurs up to a decade before onset of the sporadic form of the disease.

Different clinical manifestations are mediated by dysfunction of different anatomical regions of degeneration.

Advances in genetics of neurodegenerative diseases have demonstrated that diverse clinical phenotypes may share similar genotypes, and that clinically similar phenotypes may be associated with a wide variety of genotypes.

Several different neurodegenerative diseases may appear together within a family even though they carry the same underlying genetic mutation.

Features of more than one neurodegenerative diseases can coexist in one patient. There are clinical, pathological and genetic commonalities between amyotrophic lateral sclerosis (ALS) and FTD, such that these diseases are thought to represent a spectrum of disease rather than distinct disease entites. For example, In the ALS–parkinsonism–dementia complex of Guam, patients have evidence of two motor diseases as well as dementia.

1.3 Classification of Neurodegenerative Diseases

Neurodegenerative diseases are diagnosed primarily on the basis of history and clinical examination (Fig. 1.1). Diagnostic criteria, based primarily on clinical findings, have been generated for most of the common neurodegenerative diseases. The suspected diagnosis is then confirmed by carrying out directed tests in the fields of neurophysiology, neuropsychology, neuroimaging, or genetic analysis. These are sometimes used to rule out disease mimics, such as in the case of motor neuron disease where there is in diagnostic test in the form of an electromyogram (EMG). Often, the best diagnostic tool is the observation of the patient over the course of time; antemortem tissue analysis usually does not play a role in diagnosis.

Eponymous classifications (e.g., Alzheimer disease, Parkinson disease, and Huntington disease) remain useful in a clinical setting, as the diagnosis generates a framework for clinical discussion, prognostication, and disease management.

However, it is increasingly recognized that neurodegenerative diseases can also be subdivided into categories based on pathological or genetic characteristics, as outlined in Fig. 1.1, and as the field advances, diagnostic categories for some diseases will accordingly require some adjustment.

A number of common themes have emerged in the pathogenesis of various neurodegenerative diseases. Whether these commonalities are simply secondary processes, which reflect the fact that neurons have a limited repertoire by which to die, or whether they reveal important initiating upstream mechanisms remains unclear.

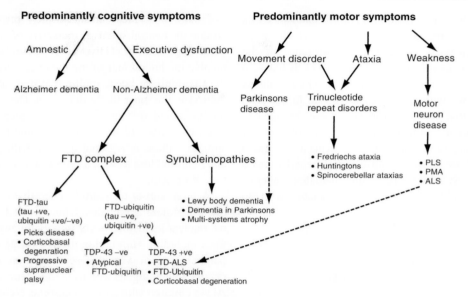

Fig. 1.1 Clinical Classification of Neurodegenerative conditions

In the following section, some putative common pathogenic molecular mechanisms will be discussed, but it is worth bearing in mind that it is not currently possible to distinguish between mechanisms that initiate disease and those that contribute to disease progression. Both may yield targets suitable for therapeutic intervention, but only the former can yield knowledge that will lead to disease prevention.

1.4   Common Themes in Genetics

Familial aggregation of specific neurodegenerative diseases is well recognized, with both autosomal dominant and autosomal recessive inheritance observed. Excepting the trinucleotide repeat disorders, which exhibit Mendelian inheritance often with full penetrance and anticipation, neurodegenerative disorders have a small percentage of familial cases and a large percentage of apparently sporadic cases. Sporadic and familial cases are usually phenotypically and histologically indistinguishable, although the onset of familial cases tends be earlier. This suggests that genetic mutations accelerate the molecular processes that lead to late-onset sporadic disease.

A number of causative genes have been discovered for specific neurodegenerative diseases. An understanding of gene function has helped to elaborate mechanisms of disease, as well as providing a platform for research into similar mechanisms in other neurodegenerative diseases. For example, mutations in APP, Presenilin 1, and Presenilin 2, which occur in early onset alzheimer disease (AD), and ADAM10 in late-onset AD, cause altered protein production and increased aggregation of β-amyloid protein (Aβ). Similarly, mutation of α-synuclein leads to aggregation of the protein in Lewy bodies, a feature also seen in the most common cause of inherited PD, caused by mutation of LRRK2. Mutations in genes associated with oxidative stress pathways, SOD1 and DJ1, have been implicated in familial amyotrophic lateral sclerosis (ALS) and PD, respectively. The discovery of TARBDP, FUS and an intronic repeat in C9ORF72 in both ALS and frontotemporal dementia (FTD)-ALS has established a role for RNA dysfunction in several neurodegenerative diseases.

Genome-wide association studies and high-throughput sequencing have identified susceptibility genes in many neurodegenerative conditions. Moreover, overlap between susceptibility genes has been reported. APOE4 is well established as a risk factor for early and late-onset AD. However, meta-analysis has shown that presence of the allele is also linked to PD and FTD. It has also been shown that the number of APOE4 alleles correlates with age of disease onset. In addition, genes that cause neurodegenerative disease can also act as susceptibility factors in others. For example, more than 34 CAG repeats in the ataxin gene 2 are known to cause spinocerebellar ataxia type 2 (SCA2), whilst an intermediate number of repeats (27–33) have been associated with an increased risk for ALS.

1.5   Common Themes in Neuropathology

Thorough pathological diagnosis depends on the pathologist having access to accurate clinical information as well as tissue analysis. Pathological diagnostic criteria presume that phenomena involved in degeneration tend to occur together, but invariably they are evident at different time points during the disease. Thus, interpretation of the neuropathological data must take into account when in the clinical course of the disease the pathological assessment has been performed.

Both gross and microscopic tissue examination can help to identify pathological processes and can also differentiate features that are purely degenerative, and those that emerge from the innate responses to protect and repair. Finding the site of the earliest visible alteration helps in establishing the diagnosis. For example, degeneration in the hippocampal and frontal lobe pyramidal neurons is associated with AD, in the dopaminergic neurons of the substantia nigra with PD, in the upper and lower motor neurons of the pyramidal system with ALS and in the medium-sized spiny GABAergic neurons of the striatum with HD.

Dementia coupled with mainly limbic atrophy suggests Alzheimer disease (AD), while mild atrophy implies Lewy body disease. Moderate cognition decline in the setting of asymmetric, motor and sensory impairment, with reduced

metabolic activities, and atrophy prevailing around the central sulcus is indicative of corticobasal degeneration. However, if these changes involve the lateral half of the putamen, caudal to the mammillary body, multiple system atrophy (MSA) is the most likely diagnosis. Despite the topographical differences in neurodegenerative diseases, gross histopathological findings are similar – there is regional atrophy with gliosis and neuronal loss as well as abnormal accumulation of protein.

A large subset of neurodegenerative diseases display protein aggregates. Ubiquitinated neuronal nuclear inclusions occur in polyglutaminopathies including Huntington disease (HD). Either parenchymal or vascular accumulation of Ab occurs with aging, as well as in the occurrence of AD in children with Down syndrome. Neostriatal large neurons are rather resistant compared to medium size neurons in HD, but they degenerate in progressive supranuclear palsy and in AD. Loss of spinal motor neurons is typical in amyotrophic lateral sclerosis (ALS), whereas glial cells degenerate in MSA. TDP-43-positive neuronal cytoplasmic inclusions, originally thought to be characteristic of ALS and subsequently FTD, are also detected in AD, PD HD and SCA2, though the location of the inclusions varies with disease. Lewy bodies are a hallmark of Parkinson disease with or without dementia and involve many classes of neurons.

In summary, the three practical steps that are useful while appraising the pathologic phenotypes of neurodegenerative diseases are:

1. Identifying the sites or systems where the brunt of the tissue loss occurs, which might be revealed on neuroimaging at some time points during the disease, or eventually on postmortem examination. However, also consider other regions which may allow subclassification of the disease, such as the characteristic extra motor pathology in the hippocampus, associated specifically with C9ORF72 repeat expansion.
2. Cataloging the cells undergoing degeneration.
3. Identifying the abnormal aggregates, their cellular (neuronal vs. glial cells) and topographic

propensities (extracellular, cytoplasmic, or nuclear).

General experience confirms that these steps are crucial for assigning the most appropriate diagnosis to most of the currently classifiable neurodegenerative diseases.

1.6   Selective Vulnerabilities

Cells are constantly placed under stress because of intrinsic metabolic processes and also because of a number of extrinsic factors. Neurons are even more vulnerable as they facilitate neurotransmission and maintain the metabolic needs required for long axonal projections. Larger neurons with myelinated axons extending long distances appear to be most vulnerable. These neurons have high energy requirements, are especially reliant on axonal transport, and have a larger surface area for exposure to environmental toxins. Coupled with the fact that once damaged they cannot regenerate, neurons in general represent a vulnerable group of cells.

Why are certain subgroups of neurons more susceptible than others?

A number of hypotheses have been proposed to account for specific selective susceptibility of certain neurons to specific pathological processes (Table 1.1). Neuroblasts arise from the neuroectoderm at 8 weeks of fetal life and then proceed to differentiate into highly specialized neurons. Even though all neurons of an individual have the same genes, it is the gene expression profile that determines the highly specialized function of a specific neuron. This degree of specialization is

Table. 1.1 Neurologic diseases and selectively vulnerable cells

Disease	Vulnerable neuron
Parkinson disease	Dopaminergic neurons
Alzheimer disease	Cholinergic neurons
Amyotrophic lateral sclerosis	Upper and lower motor neurons
Frontotemporal dementia	Frontotemporal cortical neurons
Huntington disease	GABAinergic neurons

thought to render individual neurons more susceptible to anoxia and oxidative stress, and factors that lead to selective vulnerability include the type of neuron and the neuronal microenvironment.

The dopaminergic neurons located in the substantia nigra in PD are particularly prone to reactive oxygen species (ROS)-induced injury. This selective vulnerability is believed to derive from the fact that neurons in the substantia nigra have very high levels of iron and copper, both of which are capable of catalysing ROS formation. Additional evidence suggests that the substantia nigra may have low stores of antioxidant molecules such as glutathione, thereby increasing neuronal susceptibility to the damaging effects of ROS. However, this does not explain the vulnerability of neurons associated with PD in other regions of the brain such as autonomic ganglia, brainstem, and spinal cord.

In ALS, motor neurons are affected primarily, although it is now recognized that non-motor neurons are involved in cognitive dysfunction. Motor neurons are large cells and often have long axonal fibers. In lower motor neurons, these fibers may stretch over a meter in order to supply distal muscles. They require a strong cytoskeleton, neurofilament network, and efficient axonal transport system. Motor neurons are highly metabolic and exquisitely sensitive to energy demands. Any one or a multitude of these factors makes motor neurons vulnerable. As is the case in the substantia nigra, deficiencies of protective agents such as glutathione and cytosolic calcium-binding proteins can add to neuronal stress.

The different phenotypic characteristics of individual diseases remain difficult to explain. In Mendelian diseases, differences can be evident within families with the same mutation. For example, a proband with familial ALS may present with flail arm and slow progression, while another family member may present with rapidly progressive bulbar onset disease. Similarly, some patients with AD may have executive or visuospatial deficits, while others have an amnestic syndrome. In kindreds with triplication of APP, the clinical disease segregates into two distinct phenotypes: those with classical AD indistinguishable from idiopathic AD and those with vascular dementia and a stroke-like syndrome. The causes of these phenotypic variations remain to be determined.

1.7   Aberrant Protein Structure

The formation of aberrant structures by more than 20 different proteins appears to underlie a large disease group, many of which afflict the CNS (Table 1.2). Indeed, deposits of protein aggregates are histological hallmarks of many neurodegenerative diseases and consequently, the proteins involved and the mechanism of their aggregation is under intense scrutiny.

The mechanism by which the attainment of an aberrant protein structure causes disease is still unclear and may involve both the loss of a vital physiological function, and the acquisition of toxic properties.

While loss of function can be harmful, toxic gain of function is invariably pathogenic. Toxicity may be direct or indirect. For instance, an aberrant protein structure might bind to a specific receptor directly, causing an inappropriate activation of a cascade that initiates cellular changes, which in turn lead to compromise of cellular function. Alternatively, aberrant structures might acquire properties that allow them to interact with and destabilize cellular membranes or other proteins, thus causing a secondary toxicity. Moreover, accumulation of aberrant proteins may strain the normal mechanisms responsible for controlling protein folding and degradation, resulting in a generalized loss of protein homeostasis and consequent toxicity. In the cases where there are large repeat expansions within the noncoding region of the gene, these can act as templates for repeat associated non-ATG (RAN) translation, generating aberrant repeat peptides which also accumulate in the cell.

Oligomerization or polymerization of aberrantly folded proteins is concentration dependent. Changes in production, degradation, or clearance of native protein are hypothesized to underlie the assembly of aberrantly folded protein. Once formed, such structures are thought to be the primary event driving pathogenesis (Fig. 1.2). Consequently, many of the therapies under development are designed either to: (1) decrease the

Table. 1.2 Neurologic diseases associated with aberrant protein structure

Disease	Protein deposited	Site of deposition
Parkinson disease	a-synuclein	Intracellular (Lewy neuritis and Lewy bodies)
Multiple systems atrophy	a-synuclein	Intracellular argyrophilic inclusions in both oligodendroglia and neurons
Hereditary cerebral amyloid angiopathy	Cystatin C	Extracellular
Congophilic amyloid angiopathy	b-amyloid	Extracellular
Alzheimer disease	b-amyloid	Extracellular (amyloid plaques)
Alzheimer disease	Tau	Intracellular (paired helical filaments)
Frontotemporal dementia	Tau	Intracellular inclusions (paired helical filaments and Pick bodies)
Frontotemporal dementia	TDP43-ubiquitin	Cytoplasmic inclusions
Familial British dementia	ABri	Extracellular (amyloid plaques)
Familial British dementia	ADan	Extracellular (amyloid plaques)
Transmissible spongiform encephalopathies	Prion protein	Extracellular amyloid plaques and/or diffuse deposits
Amyotrophic lateral sclerosis	TDP43-ubiquitin	Cytoplasmic inclusions and ubiquitin-positive neuronal threads
Huntington disease	Mutant huntingtin	Nuclear and cytoplasmic inclusions
Inherited spinocerebellar ataxias	Various proteins with polyglutamine expansions	Nuclear and cytoplasmic inclusions

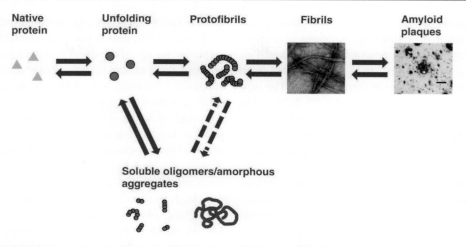

Fig. 1.2 Pathways to aberrant protein structure and aggregation in amyloid related diseases: The process is initiated by denaturation, unfolding, or misfolding (indicated by the transition from blue triangle to red circle). Proteins can form oligomers or amorphous aggregates or small, structured polymers known as protofibrils. Protofibrils mature into amyloid fibrils and then into aggregates of amyloid fibrils. Current data indicate that all aberrant protein structures (i.e., all structures shown other than the native monomer) are toxic

quantity of soluble native protein, or (2) remove aberrant protein.

It has been suggested that a threshold of abnormal aggregation must be reached before clinical signs appear, but it is as yet unclear whether deposited protein aggregates or other smaller protein assemblies are the principle mediators of disease. Evidence against deposits of protein aggregates as mediators of disease comes from the finding that many aggregated proteins are found in brains of elderly individuals who die without clinical signs of disease.

1.8   Inclusion Bodies

Inclusion bodies are relatively large electron-dense structures that contain membrane-limited protein aggregates. Such deposits often contain ubiquitin-positive material, which is believed to accumulate due to impairment of the ubiquitin-proteasome system (UPS). Under normal conditions, cytoplasmic proteins are tagged for destruction by the enzymatic addition of four or more ubiquitin molecules, but build-up of substrate, decreased efficiency of ubiquitin conjugation, or impaired degradation of ubiquitinated protein can trigger accumulation of partially ubiquitinated protein aggregates. For instance, it is believed that impaired ubiquitination of α-synuclein may explain how mutations in the PARK2 gene cause early onset PD. PARK2 encodes an E3 ubiquitin ligase (Parkin), which when mutated appears less efficient at ubiquitinating α-synuclein and aggregates of partially ubiquitinated α-synuclein accumulate in cytoplasmic structures known as Lewy bodies.

Pathological inclusion bodies are also seen in ALS, FTD, and HD. However, it is not clear if inclusions are purely pathogenic since Marinesco bodies and Hirano bodies are also found in aged asymptomatic individuals. Moreover, several studies have documented the detection of inclusions in functional neurons, implying that these structures may be protective, sequestering the misfolded proteins in the cell, rather than pathogenic.

1.9   Altered RNA Metabolism

There is increasing interest in the role of aberrant RNA processing in the pathogenesis of neurodegenerative disease. Mutations in two important genes, FUS and TDP-43, identified in a small percentage of familial ALS and FTD cases, are associated with altered RNA processing. Similarly, loss of function mutations in another RNA regulator, progranulin, has been linked with FTD, which, in turn, may be associated with motor neuron disease in some families. The protein products of TDP-43 and FUS/TLS (FUsed in Sarcoma, Translocated in LipoSarcoma) are both structurally similar to heterogeneous ribonucleoproteins (hnRNP), which are involved in multiple aspects of RNA processing.

Mutations in the TAR DNA binding protein, TDP-43, and the protein, FUS/TLS have widespread downstream effects on multiple differentially spliced mRNA species, as both proteins form cytoplasmic inclusions, thereby limiting their RNA binding function in the nucleus. Consequently, it is anticipated that quite diverse pathogenic pathways are triggered depending on the RNA binding protein and the type of neurons involved. The mutations in the TDP-43 gene are seen in some familial ALS cases, but cytoplasmic inclusions containing ubiquitinated and hyperphosphorylated forms of wild-type TDP-43 may be found in cases of sporadic ALS, as well as other neurodegenerative disorders.

Sequestration of RNA binding proteins and transcription factors are also thought to play a role in neurodegenerative diseases associated with repeat expansions, such as in HD, SCAs and ALS. This is particularly relevant to those where the expansion is in the non-protein coding region of the gene, such as in SCA10, SCA36 and C9ORF72-related ALS, where sequences of up to several thousand repeats bind hnRNPs and other splicing factors, thereby disrupting the splicing of many other messenger RNAs.

1.10 Oxidative Stress

In all cells, but particularly highly metabolically active cells such as neurons, there is a constant production and elimination of reactive oxygen species (ROS). At any time, the balance is such that an unusual increase in ROS or loss of antioxidant protection can lead to accumulation of ROS and ensuing cellular damage through oxidation of lipids and proteins. High levels of ROS can cause nuclear DNA and RNA oxidation and repairing such damage requires substantial expenditure of metabolic energy. If the damage is not adequately repaired, this can lead to cellular dysfunction and apoptosis. Accumulated oxidative damage of DNA and RNA has been observed in AD, PD, ALS and dementia with Lewy bodies. Calcium plays an integral role in signalling within the cell and also in maintenance of cellular homeostasis. As part of the role in signalling, ROS activate calcium channels and deactivate calcium pumps. This leads to abnormally high intracellular levels of calcium, which in turn may lead to cell death. Mitochondrial ROS also cause increased uptake of calcium ions with increased membrane permeability, resulting in the release of cytochrome-C, which initiates the apoptotic cascade.

In vivo and in vitro studies have shown that nicotinamide adenine dinucleotide phosphate (NADPH) oxidase derived from microglia play an important role in the generation of ROS. In PD, microglia-specific NADPH oxidases are involved in the production of ROS, which may contribute to the death of dopaminergic neurons. A similar process is seen in ALS, whereby oxygen radicals produced by microglial NADPH oxidase are believed to injure motor neurons. Evidence from the mutant SOD1 mouse model of ALS indicates that genes encoding NADPH oxidase are up-regulated in disease and this leads to an increased concentration of ROS in mouse spinal cord tissue. In addition, the PD and ALS genes, DJ-1 and SOD1 respectively, protect against oxidative stress. DJ-1 is a sensor of oxidative stress, inducing antioxidant genes, such as the transcription factor NRF2, whilst SOD1 is an antioxidant enzyme. However, mutation of SOD1 leads to reduced NRF2 levels, whilst DJ-1 mutations lead to a reduction in NRF2-induced antioxidant response genes. This has led to NRF2 being a major target for pharmacological manipulation.

1.11 Mitochondrial Dysfunction

Mitochondria play a crucial role in the production of cellular energy using the respiratory chain. Consequently, accumulated mitochondrial dysfunction is implicated in both normal aging and neurodegeneration. Proposed mechanisms of this effect include failure to meet the energy needs of the cell, calcium misregulation, leading to cell death, over production of ROS, and cytochrome C-induced apoptosis.

Well-documented incidents have shown that ingestion of certain neurotoxins can lead to the sudden onset of clinical syndromes identical to neurodegenerative diseases such as Parkinson disease or Huntington disease. Two such events led to the discovery that some neurotoxins are potent inhibitors of complexes within the mitochondrial respiratory chain. In 1982, seven young drug abusers injected intravenous forms of a synthetic heroin derivative, 1-methyl-4-phenyl-4-propionoxypiperidine (MPPP), and developed the signs and symptoms of PD. This was because of the presence of a contaminant, 1-methyl-4-phenyl-1,2,3,6-tetrahydropyridine (MPTP). When pure MPTP is injected into animals, it causes specific degenerative of dopaminergic neurons in the substantia nigra pars compacta and produces an irreversible and severe parkinsonism phenotype. After infusion, MPTP crosses the blood–brain barrier and is taken up by glia and serotonergic neurons and converted to MPDP+ and then to MPP+. Thereafter, MPP+ is released and specifically taken up by dopaminergic neurons and concentrated in mitochondria where it acts as a potent inhibitor of mitochondrial complex I. Similarly, expo-sure to 3- nitropropionic acid (3NPA) leads to rapid onset of a Huntington- type syndrome. It is now known that 3NPA is an inhibitor of mitochondrial complex II. Discovery that exogenous neurotoxins can inhibit mitochondrial complexes leading to rapid onset of neurological symptoms suggests that mitochondrial dysfunction plays a central role in these diseases.

1.12 Excitotoxicity

Glutamate is an important excitatory neurotransmitter in the CNS and its misregulation has been implicated in the development of neurodegenerative diseases. Glutamate has essential roles in synaptic transmission and plasticity, which are important in learning and memory as well and sensory and motor functions. Transmission of glutamate is mediated through three major receptors – N-methyl-d-aspartate receptors (NMDA), a-amino-3-hydroxy-5-methyl-4-isoxazoleproprionic acid (AMPA) receptors, and kainite receptors. The glutamate excitotoxicity hypothesis postulates that excessive synaptic glutamate causes over-activation of the postsynaptic NMDA and AMPA receptors resulting in neuronal death. High glutamate levels, which continuously activate postsynaptic receptors, may lead to increased intracellular calcium and catabolic enzyme activity. Downstream effects can include depolarization of mitochondrial membrane, activation of the caspase system, and production of reactive oxidation species, all of which culminate in cell death (Fig. 1.3). Excessive synaptic glutamate may be potentiated because of a fault in the cellular glutamate reuptake system. Excitatory amino-acid transporter 2 (EAAT2) is a glutamate transporter involved in cerebral glutamate transport. It has been postulated that some patients with ALS have decreased expression of this protein. Similar studies carried out in patients with AD have also shown a reduction in EAAT 2 expression. It has been shown that GLUR2, an AMPA glutamate receptor subtype responsible for calcium permeability into the postsynaptic cell, is not expressed in motor neurons affected by ALS because of a defect in the editing process for messenger RNA encoding the GLUR2 receptor. Absence of a functional GLUR2 subunit allows calcium influx into the postsynaptic cell and results in cellular damage.

Parkin, which is the gene product of PARK2, has regulator effects on excitatory glutaminergic synapese. Abnormalities in parkin production can lead to enhanced synaptic activity and may even trigger an increase in the number of glutamate receptors. Excessive glutaminergic activity may be responsible for nigral excitotoxicity.

Given this evidence, it would seem beneficial to down-regulate glutamate activity in patients affected by neurodegenerative disease. Riluzole has a direct and indirect blocking effect on glutamate receptor activation and is proven to slow the progression of ALS. Unfortunately, no other

Fig. 1.3 Proposed mechanisms of glutamate-induced excitotoxicity

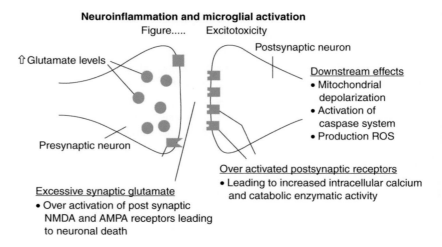

anti-glutamate agent has been successful in disease treatment.

1.13 Neuroinflammation and Microglial Activation

Neuroinflammation, which is a characteristic of many, if not all, neurodegenerative diseases, involves a complex interaction between all cells present in the CNS including infiltrating cells. The key change that typifies neuroinflammation is activation of microglia and, to a lesser extent, astrocytes and the associated increased expression of inflammatory molecules. An epidemiological study carried out in 1980s was the first to postulate an association between inflammation and neurodegeneration. The study demonstrated that the incidence of AD was lower in patients with rheumatoid arthritis (RA) who had been on long-term anti-inflammatory treatment compared to those who had not. Others suggested a similar decreased risk of developing PD though a recent meta-analysis suggests the risk reduction is slight.

Detailed descriptions of systemic and CNS specific proinflammatory cascades have fuelled the hypothesis that neuroinflammation plays an active role in the process of neurodegeneration. Microglia are CNS-specific cells that share many functions with macrophages, although we now know that microglia are an ontogenically distinct population of cells derived from primitive haematopoetic cells in the yolk sac.

In their resting state, microglia are in surveillance mode, and constantly sample the surrounding milieu to detect signals associated with injured brain tissue. However, since the primary function of microglia is to protect the brain from insult (e.g. infection, injury), they rapidly respond to stressors and adopt the so-called M1 inflammatory activation state. Having eliminated the threat or the consequences of the threat, the cells return to the resting state or adopt the M2, anti-inflammatory phenotype; M2 cells play a role in tissue repair. The evidence suggests that when the M1 activation state persists, damage to tissues of the CNS can occur.

The subdivision of microglia into M1 and M2 cells is undoubtedly an over-simplification and a number of M2 subtypes exist, as is the case for macrophages. This reflects the highly plastic nature of microglia, the array of receptors that are expressed on the cell surface and their ability to respond to numerous stimuli. At this time, however, the functions that are ascribed to phenotypes lack clarity. It remains unclear whether microglial activation contributes to the pathogenesis of neurodegenerative diseases like AD and PD or whether the changes that accompany the diseases induce cell activation. Although microglial activation may be a contributory factor, is unlikely to be the primary cause of any neurodegenerative process, but the initial challenge

Fig. 1.4 Schematic model of how mutant SOD1 aggregates lead to altered axonal transport in ALS

i) Toxicity at synapses
ii) Loss of positive feedback
iii) Mitochondrial disruption leading to decreased energy

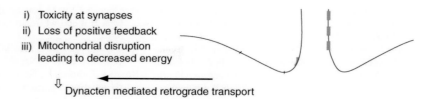

⇓ Dynacten mediated retrograde transport

probably induces an inflammatory cascade, which in turn initiates maladaptive processes and positive feedback loops that cause further pathological inflammation.

Postmortem examination of brain tissue from PD patients has demonstrated activated microglia in the substantia nigra pars compacta. In AD, microglial activation and neuroinflammatory changes are triggered by amyloid accumulation whereas inflammatory molecules can also increase amyloid precursor protein processing. This positive feedback loop results in a cascade that is ultimately damaging to neurons.

An analogy on the macroscopic scale can be drawn to acute brain injury such as a stroke, where reparative attempts by the brain tissue can cause oedema, which in turn leads to an increase in intracranial pressure and even death. In the same way, processes that set out to reverse neurodegeneration may actually contribute to secondary damage. Understanding the balance between protective and destructive capabilities of microglia has led to trials seeking to slow progression of neurodegenerative diseases by dampening down neuroinflammatory processes.

1.14   Disrupted Axonal Transport

In neurons, proteins and lipids are manufactured in the cell body and are transported along axonal projections, which can extend over a meter in length, to synaptic terminals. Conversely, neurotrophic factors transported from synaptic terminals help to regulate cellular function. This process is called fast axonal transport and is an essential part of cellular homeostasis.

Dysfunction in the axonal transport system was first studied in large motor neurons. A decreased level of kinesin-mediated anterograde

transport and retrograde dynein-mediated transport was observed in patients with ALS. Since then, research has shown that SOD1 aggregates interact with the retrograde transport system in a way that may lead to axonal dysfunction (Fig. 1.4). A decrease in retrograde transport could lead to toxicity at synaptic terminals as well as a loss of positive feedback from factors that stimulate neuronal survival. Mitochondrial distribution could be affected, resulting in a mismatch in energy provision. The accumulation of damaged mitochondria at synaptic terminals could cause increased terminal ROS production.

Conclusion

While arguments can be made regarding pathophysiological processes that make neurons vulnerable to degeneration, we still do not know fully why some people are physiologically more susceptible to specific neurodegenerative diseases, and why different neurodegenerative diseases cluster within some kindreds. It is clear that the common neurodegenerative conditions share similar processes. Increased understanding of the pathophysiologic processes for neurodegenerative diseases is likely to lead to disease-modifying therapeutic interventions that may be beneficial over a range of different clinical phenotypes.

Further Reading

Al-Chalabi A, Enayat ZE, Bakker MC, et al. Association of apolipoprotein E epsilon 4 allele with bulbar-onset motor neuron disease. Lancet. 1996;347:159–60.
Beetend K, Sleegers K, Van Broeckhoven C. Current status on Alzheimer disease molecular genetics: from past, to present to future. Hum Mol Genet. 2010 Apr 15;19(R1):R4–R11.

Boillee S, Cleveland DW. Revisiting oxidative damage in ALS: microglia, Nox and mutant SOD1. J Clin Invest. 2008;118:474–8.

Byrne S, Heverin M, Elamin M, Bede P, Lynch C, Kenna K, MacLaughlin R, Walsh C, Al Chalabi A, Hardiman O. Aggregation of neurologic and neuropsychiatric disease in amyotrophic lateral sclerosis kindreds: a population-based case-control cohort study of familial and sporadic amyotrophic lateral sclerosis. Ann Neurol. 2013;74((5):699–708.

Dickson DW. Linking selective vulnerability to cell death mechanisms in Parkinson's disease. Am J Pathol. 2007;170(1):16–9.

Gilbert RM, Fahn S, Mitsumoto H, Rowland LP. Parkinsonism and motor neuron diseases: twenty-seven patients with diverse overlap syndromes. Mov Disord. 2010 Sep 15;25(12):1868–75.

Heidler-Gary J, Hillis AE. Distinctions between the dementia in amyotrophic lateral sclerosis with frontotemporal dementia and the dementia of Alzheimer's disease. Amyotroph Lateral Scler. 2007;8(5):276–82.

Kawahara Y, Ito K, Sun H, Aizawa H, Kanazawa I, Kwak S. RNA editing and death of motor neurons. Nature. 2004;427:801.

Kumar V, Cotran RS, Robbin SJ. Robbins basic pathology. 7th ed. Philadelphia: Elsevier Science; 2003.

Lau A, Tymianski M. Glutamate receptors, neurotoxicity and neurodegeneration. European J Physiology. 2010;460:525–42.

Ling SC, Polymenidou M, Cleveland DW. Converging mechanisms in ALS and FTD: disrupted RNA and protein homeostasis. Neuron. 2013;79(3):416–38. doi:10.1016/j.neuron.2013.07.033.

Mattson MP, Magnus T. Ageing and neuronal vulnerability. Nat Rev Neuroscience. 2006;7:278–94.

Milani P, Ambrosi G, Gammoh O, Blandini F, Cereda C. SOD1 and DJ1 converge at Nrf2 pathway: a clue for antioxidant therapeutic potential in neurodegeneration. OxidMedCellLongev.2013.doi:10.1155/2013/836760.

Morfini GA, Burns M, Binder LI, et al. Axonal transport defects in neurodegenerative diseases. J Clin Neurosci. 2009;29(41):127776–12786.

Mosher KI, Wyss-Coray T. Microglial dysfunction in brain aging and Alzheimer's disease. Biochem Pharmacol. 2014;88(4):594–604. doi:10.1016/j.bcp.2014.01.008. Epub 2014 Jan 18. Review. PubMed PMID: 24445162;PubMed Central PMCID: PMC3972294.

Perry VH, Nicoll JA, Holmes C. Microglia in neurodegenerative disease. Nat Rev Neurol. 2010;6:193–201.

Polymenidou M, Cleveland DW. Prion-like spread of protein aggregates in neurodegeneration. J Exp Med. 2012;209(5):889–93.

Przedborski S, Vila M, Jackson-Lewis V. Neurodegeneration: what is it and where are we? J Clin Invest. 2003;111:3–10.

Ross CA, Porter MA. Protein aggregation and neurodegenerative disease. Nat Med. 2004 Jul;10 Suppl:S10–7.

Russo I, Bubacco L, Greggio E. LRRK2 and neuroinflammation: partners in crime in Parkinson's disease? J Neuroinflammation. 2014;11:52. doi:10.1186/1742-2094-11-52.

Sadler TW. Langman's medical embryology. 8th ed. Philadelphia: Lippincott Williams & Wilkins; 2000.

Schapansky J, Nardozzi JD, LaVoie MJ. The complex relationships between microglia, alpha-synuclein, and LRRK2 in Parkinson's disease. Neuroscience. 2015;302:74–88.

Schon EA, Manfredi G. Neuronal degeneration and mitochondrial dysfunction. J Clin Invest. 2003;111(3):303–12.

Skaper SD, Facci L, Giusti P. Mast cells, glia and neuroinflammation: partners in crime? Immunology. 2014;141(3):314–27. doi:10.1111/imm.12170. Review.

Spatola M, Wider C. Genetics of Parkinson's disease: the yield. Parkinsonism Relat Disord. 2014;20(S1):S35–8.

Sun S, Cleveland DW. TDP-43 toxicity and the usefulness of junk. Nat Genet. 2012;44(12):1289–91. doi:10.1038/ng.2473.

Todd PK, Paulson HL. RNA-mediated neurodegeneration in repeat expansion disorders. Ann Neurol. 2010;67:291–300.

Tovar-y-Roma LB, Santa-Cruz LD, Tapia R. Experimental models for the study of neurodegeneration in amyotrophic lateral sclerosis. Mol Neurodegener. 2009;4:31.

Van den Heuvel DMA, Harschnitz O, van den Berg LH, Pasterkamp RJ. Taking a risk: a therapeutic focus on ataxin-2 in amyotrophic lateral sclerosis? Trends Mol Med. 2014;20:25–35.

Walsh MJ, Cooper-Knock J, Dodd JE, Stopford MJ, Mihaylov SR, Kirby J, Shaw PJ, Hautbergue GM. Decoding the pathophysiological mechanisms that underlie RNA dysregulation in neurodegenerative disorders: a review of the current state of the art. Neuropathol Appl Neurobiol. 2015 Feb;41(2):109–34.

Wilhelmsen KC, Lynch T, Pavlou E, Higgins M, Nygaard TG. Localization of disinhibition-dementia-parkinsonism-amyotrophy complex to 17q21–22. Am J Hum Genet. 1994;55(6):1159–65.

Xinkum W, Michaelis EK. Selective neuronal vulnerability to oxidative stress in the brain. Front Aging Neurosci. 2010;2(12).

Imaging Biomarkers in Neurodegenerative Conditions

2

Parameswaran Mahadeva Iyer, Colin P. Doherty, and Peter Bede

2.1 Qualitative Imaging Signs and Semi-quantitative Rating Scales in Neurodegeneration

The role of conventional MR imaging in neuro-degeneration is relatively limited. MRI is routinely used in the initial, diagnostic phase of neurodegenerative conditions, primarily to rule out alternative diagnoses, such as extensive vascular changes, hydrocephalus or space occupying lesions. The qualitative interpretation of MRI scans in neurodegeneration is challenging and the ascertainment of pathological volume loss is particularly difficult. A number of disease-specific rating scales have been developed to aid

P.M. Iyer
Academic Unit of Neurology,
Trinity Biomedical Sciences Institute, Dublin, Ireland
e-mail: parames68@gmail.com

C.P. Doherty
Academic Unit of Neurology,
Trinity Biomedical Sciences Institute,
Dublin, Ireland

Department of Neurology, St. James's Hospital,
Dublin, Ireland
e-mail: colinpdoherty@gmail.com

P. Bede (✉)
Academic Unit of Neurology,
Trinity College, Dublin, Ireland
e-mail: bedep@tcd.ie

the identification of cortical atrophy, but visual inspection alone is often equivocal in early stage neurodegeneration. Quantitative MRI techniques such as voxel-based morphometry (VMB) or surface-based morphometry (SBM) are superior in identifying disease-specific atrophy patterns in comparison to age-matched controls. Despite the above limitations, standard clinical neuroimaging in neurodegeneration often provides subtle diagnostic clues, which may support a clinical diagnosis.

ALS is associated with high signal along the corticospinal tracts (CST), sometimes referred to as the "wine glass appearance" on coronal imaging. Bilateral CST signs in ALS are best appreciated on axial T2-weighted or Flair imaging in the posterior limb of the internal capsule. Similarly to other neurodegenerative conditions, thinning of the corpus callosum is also often observed in ALS and motor cortex atrophy may be noted on visual inspection. FTD exhibits genotype and phenotype specific atrophy patterns in conjunction with marked ventriculomegaly. Imaging in Semantic dementia (SD) shows a characteristic pattern of left temporal lobe atrophy whereas Progressive non-fluent aphasia (PNFA) is associated with striking left perisylvian atrophy. Patients with behavioural FTD often exhibit orbitofrontal volume loss and disproportionate caudate head atrophy. Progressive supranuclear palsy (PSP) is associated with significant midbrain atrophy, which may manifest in the "morning glory sign" on axial imaging due the loss of the lateral convexity of the tegmentum or the "mickey mouse appearance" due to antero-posterior midbrain reductions. Sagittal imaging in PSP may reveal the "hummingbird sign" or "penguin sign" due to disproportionate superior midbrain atrophy. T2-weighted and Flair hyperintensities are occasionally observed in the tectum of the midbrain and in the inferior olivary nucleus which often appear enlarged in PSP. T2-weighted imaging in Multiple system atrophy (MSA), especially in MSA-C often reveals hyperintensities in pontocerebellar tracts in the cerebellum, middle cerebellar peduncles and in the pons i.e.,: "hot cross bun sign". MSA-C is further associated with considerable atrophy of the olivary nuclei and the middle cerebellar peduncle. T2 weighted imaging in MSA-P (striatonigral degeneration) may reveal increased T2 signal around the lateral aspect of the putamen, called the "putaminal rim sign". Creutzfeldt-Jakob disease may have heterogeneous radiological presentations as varying degree of cortical, basal ganglia and thalamic T2 hyperintensities may be observed. The characteristic posterior thalamic involvement is called the "Pulvinar sign". The combination of symmetrical pulvinar and dorsomedial thalamic nuclear hyperintensity on T2-weighted or Flair imaging may manifest as the "Hockey-stick sign". Characteristically, axial DWI in CJD shows restricted diffusion in the same brain regions where T2 hyperintensities are observed. Significant caudate head atrophy is typically observed in Huntington disease (HD) resulting in "squaring" or "box-like" enlargement of the frontal horns. Putaminal volume reductions and signal hyperintensities may also be noted. Mesial temporal lobe and temporoparietal cortical atrophy are the hallmark features of Alzheimer's disease. The enlargement of the parahippocampal fissures on coronal imaging and the enlargement of the posterior cingulate and parieto-occipital sulci of sagittal imaging support the diagnosis. The Koedam score for Parietal Atrophy (Grade 0–3) is based on these observations. While the above qualitative radiological signs are often observed, they are poorly specific to a single neurodegenerative condition and are not sensitive for diagnostic or biomarker purposes. Semi-quantitative approaches include single plane measurements and ratios, such as the frontal horn width to intercaudate distance ratio (FH/CC) in HD, midbrain to pons area ratio (MB/P) in PSP or the Magnetic resonance parkinsonism index (MRPI). Other semi-quantitative methods rely on validated scoring systems such as the global cortical atrophy scale (GCA), posterior atrophy score of parietal atrophy (PA/Koedam score) or the medial temporal lobe atrophy score (MTA score).

2.2 Quantitative Neuroimaging: Grey Matter Techniques

Clinical MRI pulse sequences of busy medical centers are carefully optimized to acquire whole-brain imaging data in a relatively short time and frequently use slice gaps and relatively limited spatial resolution. Quantitative imaging pipelines on the other hand require high quality, high resolution 3 dimensional data sets without slice gaps. Surface based morphometry (SBM) and voxel based morphometry (VBM) are two most widely used techniques to measure group-level grey matter alterations Fig. 2.1. SBM is primarily used to highlight focal cortical thickness reductions while VBM measures relative T1-signal intensities as a proxy for volumetric changes. MRI based quantitative imaging requires purpose designed pulse-sequence to ensure high quality data. The digital data-sets are subsequently fed into analysis pipelines, which are essentially a series of mathematical steps, often referred to as "post-processing". The initial processing steps of both SBM and VBM require motion corrections and the digital removal of scalp and skull related data; i.e.,: brain extraction. Additionally, diffusion-based native MRI data undergo Eddy current corrections.

2.3 Voxel-Based Morphometry

VBM is one the most widely used grey matter techniques which enables the statistical comparison of study groups, correlations with

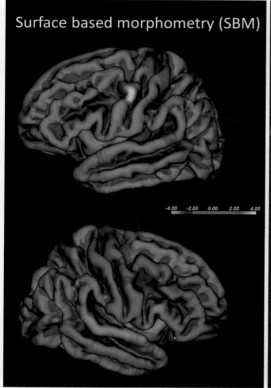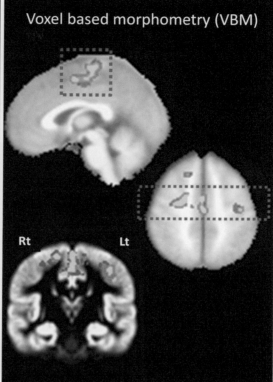

Fig. 2.1 Surface based morphometry (*SBM*) and voxel based morphometry (*VBM*) comparing cohorts of healthy controls and ALS patients. The analyses highlight motor cortex atrophy and additional grey matter changes in frontal and temporal brain regions of ALS patients compared to healthy controls

clinical parameters and retrieval of information from the individual patient data. The standard VBM pipeline begins with the tissue-type segmentation of three dimensional structural data into grey matter, white matter and CSF components. The resulting grey matter data is then registered to a standard anatomical reference system, such as the "MNI space", typically using non-linear registration. In order to equally represent the anatomical features of the various study groups a study-specific symmetrical grey matter template is created to which all native grey matter data is subsequently registered, modulated to correct for local expansion or contraction and finally smoothed. Statistical analyses are carried out following these preprocessing steps, applying general linear models and using permutation-based non-parametric testing.

2.4 Surface-Based Morphometry

The pre-processing steps of cortical thickness measurements include motion corrections, averaging of the structural T1-weighted data, removal of non-brain tissues, segmentation of the subcortical white matter and deep grey matter volumetric structures, intensity normalization, tessellation of the grey matter-white matter boundary, and automated topology corrections. Surface inflation and registration to a spherical atlas utilizes individual cortical folding patterns to match cortical geometry across subjects. Regions of significant cortical thickness differences are explored following these pre-processing steps separately in left and right hemispheres typically using False Discovery Rate (FDR) corrections to correct for multiple comparisons.

Fig. 2.2 Principles of diffusion tensor imaging and the most frequently utilized diffusivity measures

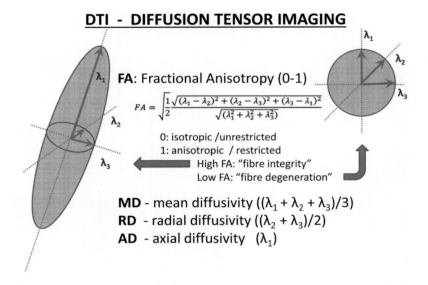

DTI - DIFFUSION TENSOR IMAGING

FA: Fractional Anisotropy (0-1)

$$FA = \sqrt{\frac{1}{2}\frac{\sqrt{(\lambda_1 - \lambda_2)^2 + (\lambda_2 - \lambda_3)^2 + (\lambda_3 - \lambda_1)^2}}{\sqrt{(\lambda_1^2 + \lambda_2^2 + \lambda_3^2)}}}$$

0: isotropic /unrestricted
1: anisotropic / restricted
High FA: "fibre integrity"
Low FA: "fibre degeneration"

MD - mean diffusivity $((\lambda_1 + \lambda_2 + \lambda_3)/3)$
RD - radial diffusivity $((\lambda_2 + \lambda_3)/2)$
AD - axial diffusivity (λ_1)

Fig. 2.2 Principles of diffusion tensor imaging and the most frequently utilized diffusivity measures

2.5 Quantitative Neuroimaging: Diffusion Tensor Imaging (DTI)

DTI is based on the principle that water molecules move freely and randomly in any direction in an unrestricted medium, their movement is "isotropic". In a biologic environment however, such movement is restricted by various membranes, fibers and macromolecules. Thus, at a tissue level the direction of movement of water molecules would be restricted in certain directions and less restricted in others. Relatively restricted movement, "anisotropy" suggests cellular integrity in the CNS, e.g., water movement is restricted perpendicular to the main axis of axon whereas water molecules move relatively freely along the main axis of the axon. A large number of DTI derived metrics is utilized to characterize white matter integrity at a voxel level, such as fractional Anisotropy (FA), mean diffusivity (MD), radial diffusivity (RD), or axial diffusivity (AD). Other indices include relative anisotropy, linear component, planar component, spherical component. The most frequently reported diffusivity parameter is fractional anisotropy (FA), where a high value close to 1 indicates fiber integrity (anisotropy) and a relatively lower value indicates pathological change. Axial diffusivity (AD) is generally regarded as a marker of axonal integrity and radial diffusivity (RD) is considered a marker of myelination Fig. 2.2. Based on these measures, a number of statistical methods have been devised to measure white matter alterations in specific white matter tracts, crossing-fibers, or to measure structural connectivity between brain regions. Tractography, high-angular-resolution diffusion imaging, Q-ball vector analysis and tract-based spatial statistics are just some of the many DTI-based imaging techniques Fig. 2.3.

2.6 MR Spectroscopy

Spectroscopy provides metabolic information on selected brain regions. MRS is most frequently based on proton, sodium, or phosphorous nuclei. Proton spectroscopy provides good signal to noise ratio enabling the reliable measurement of brain metabolites. MRS data may be collected from selected regions-of-interest (ROI), but more recently whole-brain MRS sequences have also been developed. Single Voxel Spectroscopy (SVS) is used where the study hypothesis is linked to a well-defined ROI. Multi-voxel techniques, such as Chemical Shift Imaging (CSI) is used when metabolic changes are mapped over larger brain regions. MRS data acquisition typically includes shimming of the magnetic field to correct for field inhomogeneity and the suppression of water signal in order to accurately detect metabolite peaks in the spectra. The most

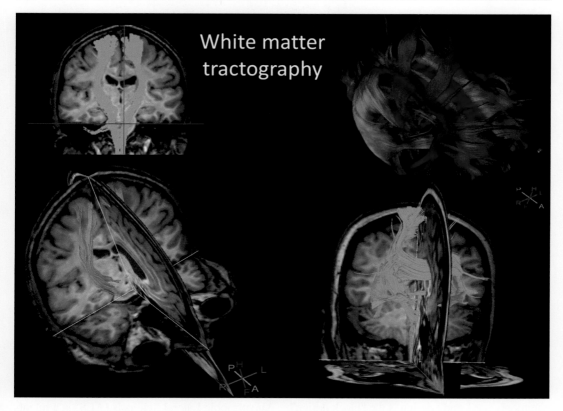

Fig. 2.3 Example of diffusivity based white matter tractography highlighting the corticospinal tracts and the commissural fibers of the corpus callosum

commonly measured metabolites include N-acetyl Aspartate (NAA), Choline (Cho), Creatine (Cr), Lactate, Myo-inositol, GABA, Glutamate (Glx). Choline is regarded as a marked of cell membrane turnover marker, and is associated with cell division and membrane breakdown such as demyelination. Creatinine is linked to metabolic activity and decreased creatine levels may be indicative of tissue necrosis secondary to hypoxia or neurodegenerative process. N-acetyl Aspartate (NAA) is generally regarded as a marker of neuronal integrity, and decreased NAA in comparative analyses is typically interpreted as a proxy for degenerative change. Lactate is a marker of anaerobic metabolism indicative of hypoxia, ischemia or mitochondrial pathology. Myo-inositol is generally regarded as a glial cell marker and increased levels have been associated with Alzheimer type and HIV-associated dementias. Increased Glutamate and Glutamine have been associated with hepatic encephalopathy.

2.7 Positron Emission Tomography (PET)

PET is one of the most versatile functional imaging techniques, which uses radioactive isotopes to assess metabolic changes in various brain regions. The most commonly used isotopes include 18-Fluorodeoxy-Glucose (FDG), 18F-6-flourodopa a dopamine precursor, C-PK11195 indicates neuroinflammation by binding to trans-locator proteins, 11C-Flumazenil which binds to GABA-A receptors, 11C-PMP measures acetyl-cholinesterase activity, WAY-100,635 binds to 5 – HT1a receptors, and C-L-Deprenyl which binds to MAO-B. Novel PET ligands contribute increasingly to our understanding of neurodegenerative changes by mapping selectively distinct physiological networks. In spite of its cost implications, requirement for a near-site cyclotron to produce short half-life isotopes and its limited availability, PET offers unrivalled sensitivity to highlight disease-specific pathology. Combined PET/MRI scanners are increasingly used in research institutions to capitalize on the high spatial resolution of MRI and the receptor-specificity of PET.

2.8   Functional MRI (fMRI)

FMRI is a non-invasive functional imaging technique which evolved from being a tool of experimental physiology and psychology into an instrument routinely used in epilepsy surgery planning and research studies of neurodegeneration. fMRI measures the blood oxygen dependent (BOLD) signal in the brain tissue to assess areas of metabolic activity either at rest or during specific tasks. Areas with higher metabolic activity utilize more oxygen leading to regional increase in BOLD signal, which is referred to as the hemodynamic response (HDR). FMRI is therefore an indirect indicator of neural activity and has inferior temporal resolution and superior spatial resolution compared to EEG. Accordingly, FRMI studies are often combined with simultaneous EEG recording. The most commonly used study design is the "block design" or "subtraction paradigm" where two conditions are alternated in blocks while a certain number of fMRI scans are acquired. Resting state fMRI is a more novel application which allows the detection of relatively independent brain networks and the assessment of circuit integrity. The most frequently assessed circuits include the default mode network, sensory-motor, visual and auditory networks.

2.9   Multi-center Imaging Studies

Standardisation and optimisation of magnetic resonance protocols across multiple sites and MRI platforms is challenging. However, multicentre neuroimaging is routinely used in clinical trials of multiple sclerosis drugs with established cross-platform harmonisation and calibration protocols. Validation of multicentre imaging data normally involves the scanning of the same MR phantoms or controls at all of the participating scanners. Multicentre MR studies have been successfully conducted in Alzheimer's disease, Huntington disease, FTD and ALS. International data repositories have been established by various disease-specific consortia, such as the Alzheimer's disease neuroimaging initiative (ADNI), TRACK-HD or the Neuroimaging society in ALS (NISALS). The cross platform calibration of ADNI utilising travelling MRI phantoms has been comprehensively described and published. The obvious advantage of such collaborations is generating large patient numbers of relatively rare disease phenotypes. The challenges of such initiatives on the other hand include the difficulties around cross-platform harmonisation across different scanner field-strengths and manufacturers, funding and authorship issues, time contribution of participating individuals, data management, storage and protection, ethics approvals etc.

2.10   Neuroimaging Features of Amyotrophic Lateral Sclerosis

Amyotrophic Lateral Sclerosis (ALS) is a relentlessly progressive neurodegenerative disorder. The diagnostic, genetic and clinical aspects of ALS are discussed in detail in Chap. 8. Until relatively recently, ALS has been regarded as pure motor system disorder, however there is now compelling clinical, post mortem and imaging evidence that the disease spreads well beyond the motor cortex affecting frontotemporal, basal ganglia, and cerebellar regions. Standard clinical imaging with T1 and T2-wieghted and Flair imaging is usually performed in the diagnostic phase of the disease to rule out alternative diagnoses. Hyperintensities along the corticospinal tracts are frequently observed on FLAIR and T2-weighted MRI, but these imaging cues are poorly specific to ALS. Hyperintensities along the pyramidal tracts on coronal imaging is sometimes referred to as the "wine glass sign" Fig. 2.4. Motor disability, the degree of cognitive impairment, and the rate of disease progression vary significantly among ALS patients leading the significant clinical heterogeneity which makes the identification of core ALS-specific imaging signatures challenging.

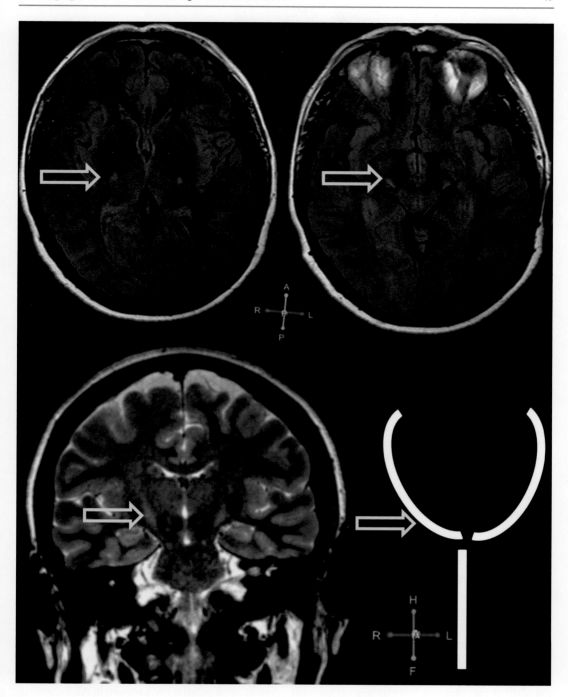

Fig. 2.4 Corticospinal tract hyperintensity in a 57 year old, left handed female patient with ALS, ALSFRS-r: 37, disease duration from symptom onset to scan: 10 months. Axial MRI imaging (*top*) and coronal imaging (*bottom*) is presented. Coronal imaging in ALS occasionally reveals high signal along the bilateral corticospinal tracts, which is sometimes referred to as the "Wine glass sign" or "Wine glass appearance". *Arrows* indicate hyperintensities along the corticospinal tracts

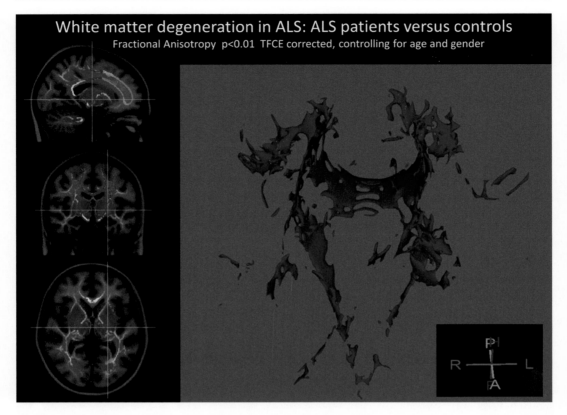

Fig. 2.5 White matter degeneration in ALS demonstrated by diffusion tensor imaging and tract-based spatial statistics based on fractional anisotropy (FA) measurements. The identified white matter regions include the body of the corpus callosum, the descending pyramidal tracts and white matter regions subjacent to the primary motor cortices

Nonetheless, neuroimaging in ALS has contributed significantly to the characterization of ALS-related pathology in vivo, highlighting disease-specific features such as corpus callosum degeneration, corticospinal tract degeneration and motor cortex atrophy Fig. 2.5. Furthermore, multiparametric imaging methods have been successfully utilized to describe the distinctive imaging signatures of key ALS phenotypes, such as patients with bulbar or spinal onset disease. Quantitative MRI techniques and PET has also been extensively utilized in ALS to characterize the distinct pathological patterns associated with the *C9orf72* or SOD1 genotype (Bede et al. 2013).

VBM and SBM studies of ALS consistently highlight grey matter atrophy in precentral gyrus, pre-motor regions, frontal and superior temporal regions Fig. 2.1. VBM studies confirmed that patterns of grey matter atrophy within the motor cortex define the clinical phenotype. Patients with bulbar onset disease have focal atrophy in the bulbar segment of the motor homunculus compared to spinal onset patients and vice versa. Furthermore, the degree of focal cortical pathology measured by VBM or SBM correlates with clinical disability. VBM and SBM studies of ALS also confirmed extra-motor cortical involvement affecting frontal and temporal brain regions especially in patient cohorts carrying the *c9orf72* hexanucleotide repeats. More recently, high resolution structural MRI data has been utilized to assess basal ganglia involvement in ALS confirming significant subcortical grey matter involvement, particularly in the thalamus, accumbens nuclei, caudate nuclei and hippocampi. These findings are consistent with the clinical observations of frontostriatal and corticobasal dysfunction and support the notion that motor disability is complicated by extrapyramidal deficits in ALS. Finally, grey matter studies of ALS confirmed significant cerebellar involvement. White matter studies of ALS invariably highlight corticospinal, corticobulbar and corpus callosum degeneration Fig. 2.4. Similarly to grey matter studies, DTI has also confirmed frontotemporal white matter pathology supporting clinical observations of cognitive and behavioral deficits. The posterior limb of the internal capsule and midbody of corpus callosum are key sites of white matter degeneration in ALS which can be easily detected by DTI studies. Early magnetic resonance spectroscopy studies of ALS reported NAA:Cr ratio reductions in the motor cortex and later studies conformed extra-motor metabolic abnormalities in the frontal cortex and thalamus. Similarly to VBM studies, metabolic changes have been correlated to motor disability and to certain ALS genotypes. Longitudinal MRS studies have shown progressive NAA reductions, and MRS studies have identified metabolic changes in the cervical spinal cord asymptomatic *SOD1* mutation carriers. MRS studies of ALS have shown reductions in cortical levels of GABA suggesting GABA mediated inhibitory dysfunction. Finally MRS was used to demonstrate Riluzole effect in treated patient populations.

FDG PET studies in ALS have shown hypometabolism in the motor cortex, motor association areas and parietal lobes. Patients with predominantly upper motor neuron signs exhibited reduced cortical glucose metabolism compared to lower motor neuron predominant patients. PET studies have identified sensitive correlations between metabolic changes and functional disability measured by rating scales (ALSFRS-r). ALS patients with cognitive impairment have shown additional metabolic changes in the dorsolateral prefrontal cortex, anterior insula, and anterior thalamic nuclei. Finally, FDG PET has been utilized to characterize ALS patients with the *C9orf72* mutation, confirming focal hypometabolism in the cingulate gyrus, insula, caudate, thalamus, superior temporal cortex, globus pallidus and midbrain complementing the structural MRI findings of this patient population. Unsurprisingly, connectivity studies of ALS demonstrated decreased motor network connectivity. However, beyond the motor network, an increased overall functional connectivity has been identified in ALS which is likely to be secondary to inhibitory dysfunction and GABAergic changes. The neuroimaging features of ALS are summarized in Table 2.1.

2.11 Neuroimaging in Frontotemporal Dementia (FTD/FTLD)

Frontotemporal dementia (FTD) or frontotemporal lobar degeneration (FTLD) is an umbrella term that encompasses behavioral variant FTD (Bv FTD), Primary non-fluent aphasia (PNFA), Semantic dementia (SD) and mixed phenotypes. A well-established clinical and pathological overlap exist between FTD and ALS, but FTD may also overlap with Parkinson's disease, progressive supranuclear palsy (PSP), and corticobasal syndromes (CBD). Up to 40 % of FTD cases may be familial and approximately 10 % show autosomal dominant inheritance. A number of genes have been linked to FTD such as microtubule associated protein tau (*MAPT*), pathological GGGGCC hexanucleotide expansions in *C9orf72*, and progranulin mutations (*GRN*). Pathologically, FTD is often classified into FTD with MAPT positive inclusions, TAR DNA-binding protein 43 (TDP-43) positive, and fused in sarcoma (FuS) inclusion positive cases. The clinical, pathological and genetic characteristics of FTD are discussed in detail in Chap. 7. Similarly to ALS, the various FTD genotypes have distinctive imaging signatures; *C9Orf72* positive samples can be distinguished from samples with tau and progranulin based on imaging (Whitwell et al. 2012). The majority of structural studies in FTD described cortical changes associated with BvFTD. These cases exhibit striking orbitofrontal and temporal lobe atrophy. A meta-analysis of 417 BvFTD patients demonstrated additional basal ganglia, insular cortex and thalamus pathology (Schroeter et al. 2014). Studies of non-fluent PPA have confirmed left inferior frontal lobe atrophy, especially in the pars opercularis region, which is consistent with Broca's area.

Table 2.1 Neuroimaging features of ALS

Imaging modality	Main findings
Standard clinical imaging (signs with poor specificity and sensitivity)	Hyperintensities along the corticospinal tracts (the "wine glass" sign of the pyramidal tracts on coronal imaging) (T2-w, FLAIR) Pyramidal tract hyperintensities in the lateral corticospinal tracts in the spinal cord (T2-w axial) Motor cortex atrophy on T1-W Thinning of the corpus callosum on sagittal imaging
Structural imaging	Grey matter atrophy of the motor cortex Extra-motor changes in the frontal lobes, superior temporal regions, and parietal lobes Cerebellar degeneration Basal ganglia changes affecting the thalamus, hippocampus, caudate nucleus and nucleus accumbens Spinal cord atrophy Genotype-specific changes in association with the *C9orf72* hexanucleotide repeat: extensive fusiform gyrus, supra marginal cortex, orbitofrontal, opercular and temporal lobe changes.
DTI	Corticospinal tract degeneration, most frequently captured in the posterior limb of the internal capsule Lateral corticospinal tract degeneration in the spinal cord Corpus callosum changes especially in the body of corpus callosum Corticobulbar tract degeneration Extra-motor frontotemporal white matter degeneration Cerebellar white matter changes *C9orf72*-associated white matter changes in the genu of corpus callosum, anterior commissure, and frontotemporal brain regions.
MR Spectroscopy	Reduction in NAA:Cho and NAA:Cr ratios in the motor cortex Longitudinal studies: progressive reduction in NAA High Myo-inisitol levels reflect glial activation GABAergic dysfunction
PET	FDG PET: hypometabolism in the motor cortex, motor association areas and parietal lobes. C9orf72 associated hypometabolism in the anterior and posterior cingulate gyrus, insula, caudate nucleus, thalamus, left frontal and superior temporal cortex, globus pallidus and midbrain [11C](R) PK11195 suggest microglial activation in the dorsolateral prefrontal cortex, pons, medulla and thalamus Flumazenil PET (GABA marker): reduced uptake in motor and extra motor regions
fMRI	Decreased cortical connectivity: motor network degeneration

PNFA is also associated with middle frontal gyrus, superior temporal pole, and lentiform nuclei changes. Structural studies of semantic dementia have revealed preferential, asymmetric, left-sided temporal lobe pathology as well as fusiform gyrus, hippocampus and amygdala involvement (Hodges et al. 1992). While MAPT mutations have been primarily linked to antero-medial temporal atrophy, orbitofrontal atrophy and fornix changes, GRN mutations are associated with inferior frontal and temporoparietal changes (Rohrer et al. 2010). Relatively symmetric atrophy patterns have been reported in MAPT and asymmetric changes in GRN mutation carriers. These genotype-specific imaging cues may also be relevant in the assessment of presymptomatic mutation carriers.

DTI studies of BvFTD have shown white matter changes in the inferior longitudinal fasciculus, inferior fronto–occipital fasciculus, anterior cingulate and corpus callosum (Diehl-Schmid et al. 2014). Moreover, white matter indices of the genu of corpus callosum have been correlated with measures of emotional blunting and behavioral changes in BvFTD (Lu et al. 2014). White matter studies of semantic dementia have shown changes in the uncinate fasciculus and bilateral inferior longitudinal fasciculus. PNFA is associated with white matter changes in the superior arcuate fasciculus and superior longitudinal fasciculus (Riedl et al. 2014). Resting state fMRI studies of FTD have also revealed phenotype-specific network degeneration (Seeley et al. 2009) Salience network dysfunction has been consistently demonstrated in BvFTD. This network mediates attention and recruits other cognitive networks for the interpretation of complex sensory information. Semantic dementia on the other hand, affects primarily networks connecting the temporal pole, subgenual cingulate, ventral striatum, and the amygdala. In PNFA, network vulnerability involves the frontal operculum, primary and supplementary motor cortices, and the bilateral inferior parietal lobules. The primary function of this network is the integration of motor and language systems. Paradigm-based fMRI studies have shown decreased frontal activity in early-stage FTD during working memory task (Rombouts et al. 2003). PNFA patients exhibit impaired activation of the inferior frontal cortex in language tasks (Wilson et al. 2010). Patients with semantic dementia fail to activate the superior temporal gyrus during reading tasks in comparison to healthy controls.

FDG PET reveals bifrontal and anterior temporal lobe hypometabolism in BvFTD, bilateral temporal lobe hypometabolism in semantic dementia (Diehl-Schmid et al. 2014). and left frontal lobe hypometabolism in PNFA. FDG PET does not only help to classify FTD phenotypes with a predictive value of 78 %, it is also an invaluable tool to differentiate FTD from AD (Matias-Guiu et al. 2014). AD and FTD can be occasionally challenging to distinguish clinically and amyloid PET may sometimes be necessary. The most commonly used amyloid tracer used is 11-C Pittsburg Compound B (PiB), but radiotracers with longer half-life; florbetapir and flutemetamol are now also available. All three are comparable in their affinity for amyloid binding and they are highly specific as they do not bind to tau or alpha synuclein. Most FTD phenotypes do not show amyloid binding. Tau PET tracers are also available, such as the 18F-THK5117 and

18F-T807, but relatively little is known of the Tau-binding profile of FTD phenotypes (Murray et al. 2014).

Single photon emission spectroscopy (SPECT) uses lipophilic compounds that cross the blood brain barrier to measure regional cerebral perfusion. SPECT images may be either interpreted by visual inspection, or quantitative ROI analyses. [99m]Tc Hexamethylpropeleneamine (^{99m}Tc-HMPAO) and ^{99m}Tc-ethyl cystine dimer (^{99m}Tc-ECD) are particularly useful to differentiate FTD from AD. A large meta-analysis of 13 studies including a total of 479 patients found that the sensitivity of SPECT is 65 % and the specificity in differentiating FTD from AD is 72 %. The neuroimaging features of FTD are summarized in Table 2.2.

2.12 Neuroimaging Features of Alzheimer's Disease (AD)

Mesial temporal lobe atrophy and temporoparietal cortical atrophy are the hallmark imaging features of AD on clinical imaging. Mesial temporal lobe volume loss can be observed directly on coronal imaging or indirectly by noting the enlargement of the parahippocampal fissures. Similarly, posterior cortical atrophy is often suspected based on the atrophy of the precuneus and the medial surface of the parietal lobe or the enlargement of the posterior cingulate and parieto-occipital sulci. Changes in the amygdala, hippocampus, entorhinal cortex and temporal horns have been extensively characterized by visual assessment, manual and automated volumetry, surface and voxel-based morphometry. While the visual assessment of the amygdala offers 88 % specificity and 69 % sensitivity, the appraisal of hippocampal changes is associated with 79 % specificity and 70 % sensitivity in the diagnosis of AD. Manual segmentation techniques offer 81 % specificity and 85 % sensitivity in AD. Measurements with automated techniques offer similar diagnostic sensitivity and specificity results. Entorhinal cortex (EC) imaging confirms the diagnosis with 86 % specificity at dementia stage, and 78 % specificity at a mild cognitive

Table 2.2 Imaging features of FTD

Imaging modality	Main findings
Standard clinical imaging	Asymmetric frontal lobe atrophy in bvFTD Volume loss of the caudate heads in bvFTD Thinning of the genu of the corpus callosum on sagittal imaging in bvFTD Marked, asymmetric temporal lobe atrophy in semantic dementia
Structural imaging	BvFTD: Atrophy of the fronto-median cortex, insular cortex, thalamus, left sub callosal area, inferior temporal pole and amygdalae. *C9orf72* mutation: symmetric inferior frontal lobe atrophy and cerebellar atrophy. MAPT mutation – symmetric bilateral changes: antromedial temporal and orbitofrontal atrophy and fornix changes GRN mutation – asymmetrical changes inferior frontal and temporo-parietal atrophy
DTI	BvFTD: white matter degeneration in the anterior superior and inferior longitudinal fasciculus, and genu of corpus corpus callosum. Semantic dementia: uncinate fasciculus and inferior longitudinal fasciculus changes PNFA: superior arcuate fasciculus and superior longitudinal fasciculus pathology Logopenic phenotypes: inferior longitudinal fasciculus, uncinate fasciculus, splenium of corpus callosum, cingulum bundle, and anterior thalamic radiation changes
fMRI- Resting state	BvFTD: Salience Network degeneration Semantic dementia: frontostriatal circuit dysfunction, ventral striatum and amygdala connectivity alterations PNFA: connectivity changes affecting the frontal operculum, supplementary motor cortices, and bilateral inferior parietal lobules.
FDG PET	BvFTD: Frontomedial, thalamic, anterior insular and anterior temporal hypometabolism. Semantic dementia: bilateral temporal hypometabolism PNFA: hypometabolism of the dominant frontal lobe including Broca's area.
Beta Amyloid PET	Usually negative in FTD, may be useful for discriminating logopenic variants of AD from FTD
Tau PET	The sensitivity and specificity profiles of 18F-THK5117 and 18F-T807 are currently studied and are not yet established in FTD.
SPECT	Sensitivity of 65 % and specificity of 72 % in differentiating FTD from AD.

impairment (MCI) stage. More recently, imaging studies demonstrated presymptomatic cingulate gyrus, hippocampus, thalamus and caudate nucleus changes in Presenelin-1 gene carriers (Ryan et al. 2013).

Diffusion tensor imaging (DTI) studies of AD have revealed widespread white matter changes in parietal, temporal, and prefrontal brain regions. More posterior white matter alterations are also commonly reported in AD particularly in the posterior corpus callosum, posterior cingulate gyrus, superior and inferior longitudinal fasciculi, fronto-occipital fasciculus, and in the posterior thalamic radiation. These changes are evidenced by increased radial and mean diffusivity and reduced fractional anisotropy (FA) (Acosta-Cabronero et al. 2010). DTI studies

using tract-based spatial statistics (TBSS) have shown early fornix involvement suggestive of limbic diencephalic network dysfunction in the early stages of the disease.

FDG PET is an important diagnostic tool for both MCI and AD as it sensitively highlights regional temporo-parietal hypometabolism. FGD PET has a diagnostic specificity of 84 % in AD and 74 % in MCI, while sensitivities are 86 and 76 % respectively. Amyloid PET uses radiolabelled markers such as 11-C Pittsburg Compound B (PiB), or radiotracers with longer half-life such as florbetapir and flutemetamol. Both visual inspection and fully automated techniques can be utilized to evaluate ligand binding. Standardized uptake volume ratio (SUVR) and Distribution volume ratio (DVR) measurements are automated approaches which compare regional uptake to reference normative values. ^{11}C- PiB PET has a diagnostic specificity of 83–88 % across various analysis techniques in AD and 53–56 % in MCI. It has a sensitivity profile of 91–100 % in AD and 82–100 % in MCI. ^{18}F Ligands have a specificity of 86 % in AD, and 80 % in MCI while their sensitivity is 87 % in AD and 78 % in MCI (Frisoni et al. 2013).

The core SPECT feature of AD is marked temporo-parietal hypo metabolism. Using ^{99}m Tc- ECD or ^{123}l-IMP this pattern is very specific to AD and can reach a sensitivity of 70 % even with visual interpretation. Metabolic patterns identified on ^{99}Tc-HMPAO SPECT are less specific; 83 % in AD and 64 % in MCI. Functional MRI studies of AD report reductions in default mode network (DMN) integrity and an overall decreased activity at rest. The DMN comprises of the Medial Prefrontal cortex, Posterior Cingulate Cortex, inferior Parietal cortex. This network is active at rest and is physiologically involved in introspective and autobiographic memory processes. Graph-theory based resting-state fMRI connectivity studies have demonstrated DMN dysfunction in pre-symptomatic patient cohorts. The posterior cingulate cortex and precuneus show early and disease-specific vulnerability. The degradation of functional and structural connectivity of the DMN has been demonstrated by combined functional and structural imaging modalities. fMRI studies have confirmed early connectivity alterations in *APOE4* mutation carriers and longitudinal fMRI studies of AD have shown progressive decline in DMN network integrity.

2.13 Imaging Features of Parkinson's Disease Dementia (PDD)

The clinical and pathologic distinction between Parkinson's Disease associated dementia (PDD) and dementia with Lewy Bodies (DLB) can be challenging and imaging may aid the diagnosis. Structural studies of PD, PD with mild cognitive impairment (PD-MCI) and PDD show

incremental cortical atrophy along the cognitive phenotypes of Parkinson's disease. VBM studies show diffuse grey matter loss in frontal, temporal, and occipital lobes, with the relative sparing of parietal regions. Hippocampal volume loss has also been demonstrated in PDD, though less severe than the hippocampal pathology observed in AD. PDD is associated imaging changes in the entorhinal cortex, amygdala and anterior cingulate gyrus. Additional atrophy has been reported in the thalamus, putamen and caudate nucleus. In PD-MCI, prefrontal atrophy has been linked to increased reaction times, and hippocampal atrophy has been correlated with verbal memory impairments. Enlargement of lateral ventricles has been repeatedly reported in PDD, with preferential enlargement of inferior horn of left lateral ventricle.

SPARE-AD (Spatial Pattern for recognition of abnormality for Recognition of Early Alzheimer's disease) has been developed as a quantitative algorithm to identify atrophy patterns consistent with AD. It has also been applied to PD cohorts and has been shown to reliably discriminate between PD and PDD based on hippocampal, and parieto-occipital imaging measures.

The cognitive phenotypes of PD, PD-MCI and PDD are also associated with incremental white matter degeneration, making diffusion tensor imaging a valuable research tool. In PD patients with executive dysfunction, parietal lobe white matter tract degeneration has been reported. PD-MCI patients show fractional anisotropy (FA) reductions in the superior longitudinal fasciculus and corpus callosum. In PDD, there is additional evidence of FA reductions in the inferior longitudinal fasciculus and anterior limb of internal capsule compared to controls. In comparison to PD patients without cognitive impairment, PDD patients exhibit uncinate fasciculus and posterior cingulate degeneration. Resting state fMRI studies of PDD highlighted frontostriatal connectivity alterations in networks relayed through the caudate and the putamen. The identified network dysfunction is distinct from DLB which preferentially involves the Default Mode Network (DMN). Connectivity studies of PDD have successfully correlated cognitive performance with network integrity, and longitudinal studies captured progressive network dysfunction.

Amyloid PET has a limited role in PDD as amyloid burden is generally low and often comparable to the values observed in healthy controls. Only a small minority of PDD patients suffers from amyloid accumulation and their initial cognitive profile is not significantly different from the "low amyloid" PDD cohorts. Longitudinal studies however suggest that those with high amyloid burden, progress into dementia faster than the amyloid negative PD population.

FDG PET is particularly useful to differentiate PDD form PD cases without cognitive abnormalities. PET studies of PDD revealed hypometabolism in the medial frontal and parietal association regions with relatively increased metabolism in the cerebellar vermis and dentate nuclei. The extent of hypometabolism correlates well with cognitive performance especially with measures of executive dysfunction. Longitudinal FDG PET studies reveal progressive metabolic changes, and capture extra-motor changes in PD patients who will later progress into PD-MCI or PDD, well before the clinical development of cognitive changes. The FDG PET signature of PDD and PD-MCI are relatively distinct, so it is possible to differentiate them from other neuro degenerative conditions which may also present with extra-pyramidal symptoms (Poston and Eidelberg 2010).

Dopamine imaging can be undertaken in PD either using PET or SPECT techniques. The agents used for dopaminergic imaging in Parkinson-related conditions can broadly be classified as "Pre-synaptic agents" and "Post-synaptic agents". Pre-synaptic agents include Dopa-decarboxylase ligands which measure dopamine synthesis (^{18}F Dopa, ^{11}C L-Dopa), DAT which identifies functioning dopaminergic terminals, and VMAT-2 which binds to dopaminergic terminals. Post synaptic radioligands measure D2 receptor density in synapses.

In patients with PDD, striatal DOPA decarboxylase activity is reduced by up to 26 % in the caudate nuclei, and by 44 % in the putamen. Additionally, decreased uptake is observed in the anterior cingulate, ventral midbrain and occipital cortex, which is similar to PD cohorts without dementia. Studies using presynaptic ligands such as VMAT-2 show 34 % binding reduction compared to controls in the substantia nigra. Striatal DAT binding is significantly reduced in PDD patients compared to non-demented PD patients especially in caudate and putamen. Imaging studies suggest that the pathophysiological changes in PDD are driven by decreased striatal dopamine synthesis, impaired dopamine storage, reduced dopamine transportation, with increased or normal post synaptic D2 receptor density compared to healthy individuals. The finding of preserved synaptic receptor density distinguishes PDD from DLB, where there is reduced D1 and D2 receptor density.

2.14 Imaging Features of Diffuse Lewy Body Disease (DLB)

In comparison to PDD, DLB shows more widespread grey matter atrophy on structural imaging as demonstrated by voxel-based morphometry (VBM) studies. While imaging studies of DLB are limited by relatively small patient cohorts, there is a consensus that the medial temporal lobes are relatively preserved. DLB is characterized by considerable volume loss in the midbrain, affecting the substantia innominate and the nucleus basalis of Maynert, which is primarily involved in cholinergic pathways projecting to the neocortex. Volume loss in the dorsal meso-pontine grey matter is thought to be disease specific, and is used as an imaging cue for the diagnosis of DLB. In early-stage DLB, there is often already evidence of midbrain, putamen, pons, and basal forebrain atrophy involving both dopaminergic and cholinergic systems. Cortical thickness studies in DLB reveal thinning of mid and posterior cingulate, superior tempor- occipital and lateral orbitofrontal regions. This anatomical pattern of atrophy is distinct from AD which primarily exhibit temporal lobe involvement.

Diffusion tensor imaging studies of DLB show fractional anisotropy reductions in parieto-occipital brain regions, particularly in the precuneal and cingulate gyri. White matter degeneration is also frequently observed in the thalamic and optic radiation. Region of interest (ROI) analyses have shown reduced FA in the inferior longitudinal fasciculus which is associated with the ventral visual pathways. The dysfunction of this tract may explain the abnormal visual phenomena associated with DLB. Several white matter studies have successfully correlated imaging measures with anatomically-associated clinical scales in DLB. Reductions in FA values in cortico-basal fibres for example, correlate sensitively with the third section of the unified Parkinson's disease rating scale (UPDRS) which evaluates motor function.

Resting state fMRI studies of DLB reveal decreased integrity of fronto-parietal, and sensory-motor networks compared to control populations. While the primary visual networks seem to be preserved in DLB, fMRI studies suggest the functional disconnection of the calcarine cortex and lingual gyri may contribute to the visual hallucinations observed in DLB.

Amyloid PET is an extensively evaluated biomarker of DLB, as amyloid burden in DLB is higher than in PDD. Longitudinal studies have shown that those with high amyloid burden are more likely to develop cognitive or behavioral symptoms. FDG PET studies of DLB show predominantly occipital hypometabolism.

Dopaminergic imaging in DLB reveals reduced DOPA uptake by nearly 50 % in the caudate and putamen compared to healthy controls. Patients with DLB also show reduction in VMAT-2 binding in caudate and putamen. DAT binding is reduced by 35 % in DLB in the caudate and putamen compared to controls and reductions are at least 14–22 % more significant than those seen in PD patients.

References

Whitwell JL, Weigand SD, Boeve BF, et al. Neuroimaging signatures of frontotemporal dementia genetics: C9ORF72, tau, progranulin and sporadics. Brain. 2012;135(Pt 3):794–806.

Schroeter ML, Laird AR, Chwiesko C, et al. Conceptualizing neuropsychiatric diseases with multimodal data-driven meta-analyses–The case of behavioral variant frontotemporal dementia. Cortex. 2014;57:22–37.

Bede P, Bokde AL, Byrne S, et al. Multiparametric MRI study of ALS stratified for the C9orf72 genotype. Neurology. 2013;81:361–9.

Hodges JR, Patterson K, Oxbury S, Funnell E. Semantic dementia. Brain. 1992;115:1783–806.

Rohrer JD, Ridgway GR, Modat M, et al. Distinct profiles of brain atrophy in frontotemporal lobar degeneration caused by progranulin and tau mutations. Neuroimage. 2010;53:1070–6.

Diehl-Schmid J, Onur OA, Kuhn J, Gruppe T, Drzezga A. Imaging frontotemporal lobar degeneration. Curr Neurol Neurosci Rep. 2014;14:489.

Lu PH, Lee GJ, Shapira J, et al. Regional differences in white matter breakdown between frontotemporal dementia and early-onset alzheimer's disease. J Alzheimers Dis. 2014;39:261–9.

Riedl L, Mackenzie IR, Förstl H, Kurz A, Diehl-Schmid J. Frontotemporal lobar degeneration: current perspectives. Neuropsychiatr Dis Treat. 2014;10:297.

Seeley WW, Crawford RK, Zhou J, Miller BL, Greicius MD. Neurodegenerative diseases target large-scale human brain networks. Neuron. 2009;62:42–52.

Rombouts SA, van Swieten JC, Pijnenburg YA, Goekoop R, Barkhof F, Scheltens P. Loss of frontal fMRI activation in early frontotemporal dementia compared to early AD. Neurology. 2003;60:1904–8.

Wilson SM, Dronkers NF, Ogar JM, et al. Neural correlates of syntactic processing in the nonfluent variant of primary progressive aphasia. J Neurosci. 2010;30: 16845–54.

Matias-Guiu JA, Cabrera-Martin MN, Garcia-Ramos R, et al. Evaluation of the new consensus criteria for the diagnosis of primary progressive aphasia using fluorodeoxyglucose positron emission tomography. Dement Geriatr Cogn Disord. 2014;38:147–52.

Murray ME, Kouri N, Lin WL, Jack Jr CR, Dickson DW, Vemuri P. Clinicopathologic assessment and imaging of tauopathies in neurodegenerative dementias. Alzheimers Res Ther. 2014;6:1.

Ryan NS, Keihaninejad S, Shakespeare TJ, et al. Magnetic resonance imaging evidence for presymptomatic change in thalamus and caudate in familial Alzheimer's disease. Brain. 2013;136:1399–414.

Acosta-Cabronero J, Williams GB, Pengas G, Nestor PJ. Absolute diffusivities define the landscape of white matter degeneration in Alzheimer's disease. Brain. 2010;133:529–39.

Frisoni GB, Bocchetta M, Chetelat G, et al. Imaging markers for Alzheimer disease: which vs how. Neurology. 2013;81:487–500.

Poston KL, Eidelberg D. FDG PET in the evaluation of Parkinson's disease. PET Clin. 2010;5:55–64.

Role of Neuropsychology in Neurodegeneration

3

Marwa Elamin, Thomas H. Bak, Colin P. Doherty,
Niall Pender, and Sharon Abrahams

3.1   Introduction

A neuropsychological assessment (NPA) can serve as a valuable tool in the investigation of patients with known or suspected neurodegenerative disorders. Common reasons for referral include memory complaints, expressive language difficulties, poor visuospatial awareness, poor decision making, disorganisation, reduced attention, concentration difficulties, changes in personality or behaviour, and deterioration in functioning such as difficulties coping at work or managing one's finances.

The goals of the NPA are often twofold. The first is to confirm or refute the presence of cognitive impairment. This can be a challenging feat for clinicians particularly in cases where cognitive changes are subtle, where premorbid functioning is suspected to be particularly low or high, and where anxiety or depression may be contributing to the patient's symptoms. The NPA can account for these factors in determining the presence of a cognitive deficit and can often detect cognitive and behavioural changes before structural or functional abnormalities emerge on neuroimaging, and as such may be vital for the diagnostic process.

The second goal of the NPA is to delineate the profile of cognitive impairment. This can help to determine whether there is a functional or organic cause to the symptoms, localize organic abnormalities, narrow the differential diagnoses between neurodegenerative disorders, define a patient's functional limitations and his/her residual strengths, and identify targets for rehabilitation, thus facilitating appropriate care pathways. Repeated assessments can also monitor progression or recovery associated with treatment response.

M. Elamin (✉)
Academic Unit of Neurology, Trinity Biomedical
Sciences Institute, Dublin, Ireland
e-mail: marwaelamin08@gmail.com

T.H. Bak
Centre for Cognitive Ageing and Cognitive
Epidemiology , University of Edinburgh,
Edinburgh, UK

The Anne Rowling Regenerative Neurology Clinic,
Centre for Clinical Brain Sciences (CCBS),
University of Edinburgh, Edinburgh, UK

C.P. Doherty
Academic Unit of Neurology,
Trinity Biomedical Sciences Institute,
Dublin, Ireland

Department of Neurology, St. James's Hospital,
Dublin, Ireland
e-mail: colinpdoherty@gmail.com

N. Pender
Department of Neuropsychology, Beaumont Hospital,
Dublin, Ireland

Academic Unit of Neurology, Trinity College Dublin,
Dublin, Ireland
e-mail: niallpender@gmail.com

S. Abrahams
Human Cognitive Neuroscience-Psychology,
Euan MacDonald Centre for Motor Neurone
Disease Research, Centre for Cognitive Aging
and Epidemiology, University of Edinburgh,
Edinburgh, UK

© Springer International Publishing Switzerland 2016
O. Hardiman, C.P. Doherty (eds.), *Neurodegenerative Disorders: A Clinical Guide*,
DOI 10.1007/978-3-319-23309-3_3

3.2 Referring a Patient for Neuropsychological Assessment

Prior to referring a patient for a NPA, a clinician should have a clear idea of the question(s) that he/she hopes to answer following the assessment. This could be a diagnostic question for example, whether a patient is suffering from Alzheimer's disease (AD) or depression, or whether the profile of cognitive impairment may resemble a less common form of dementia such as posterior cortical atrophy or corticobasal degeneration. The referral may simply wish to document whether cognitive impairment is present, for example in diseases where cognitive dysfunction is relatively common such as Parkinson's disease. A repeat assessment may be useful in a patient with known a known cognitive deficit to document progression or treatment response.

It is important to provide the clinical psychologist with the relevant background clinical information for the patient. This helps the psychologist to tailor the assessment to the patient's needs. This includes the medical, neurological, and psychiatric history. Furthermore, any information on premorbid function, ethnicity, and culture may be useful.

It is also essential to consider whether the patient is motivated to undertake the assessment. Conditions that can affect a patient's ability to co-operate include severe illness, active psychiatric difficulties, physical disability and, in rarer circumstances, secondary gain. Milder forms of physical disability can be accommodated by careful tailoring of the neuropsychological tasks. Hearing and visual difficulties should be considered.

It is also worth noting that referring the patient in the early stages of a neurodegenerative condition is more likely to yield a disease specific profile of cognitive abnormalities. In the advanced stages of most neurodegenerative conditions, multiple (if not all) cognitive domains may be affected and thus the original salient features can be difficult to identify. In addition, patients with severe cognitive or behavioural deficits, such as those observed at end stages of a dementing process, are often unable to co-operate with the NPA and require highly specialised assessments.

Finally, if the patient has a poor grasp of the language in which the assessment will be provided, then it would be worth considering the value of the referral or utilising the services of an interpreter to facilitate the assessment.

3.3 The Neuropsychological Assessment

The NPA is usually composed of a clinical interview and a series of neuropsychological tests. The initial interview serves to ascertain background information (such as the patient's age, educational attainment, job history etc.) and to provide insight into the cognitive problems for which he/she was referred.

Observing the patient during the interview can yield valuable information including the ability to communicate effectively, self-care and hygiene, and the presence anxiety and mood disorders. Qualitative assessment can also provide information on the presence of executive dysfunction (e.g. attentional difficulties or perseveration) or behavioural abnormalities (e.g. disinhibition or impulsivity). It is highly desirable to interview an informant after obtaining the patient's consent. Close family members or friends are likely to provide additional and valuable information such as a different perspective with regard to the duration, scope, or severity of any cognitive problems, and the patient's insight into these problems. A separate interview is essential for the assessment of personality or behavioural changes.

The second part of the evaluation involves a comprehensive assessment of multiple cognitive domains that often include memory, language, executive functions, visuo-spatial/perceptual skills, intellectual abilities, processing speed, and behaviour. This takes place in a quiet environment where chances of interruption and distraction are minimized.

In the following section we briefly discuss the major cognitive domains commonly evaluated during a typical NPA. For each cognitive domain, this will include a brief description of its main components and neuroanatomical underpinnings, commonly used tests, and examples illustrating the clinical relevance of testing that domain.

3.4 Memory

Decline in memory is the hallmark of Alzheimer's disease (AD). In addition, memory deficits may also be observed in several other neurodegenerative conditions including frontotemporal dementia (FTD), Parkinson's disease (PD) as well as Huntington's disease (HD), although the cognitive underpinnings of the memory difficulties may differ.

Memory is not a unitary function. We use multiple memory systems to carry out daily activities. A number of models exist which classify these systems. One of the major divisions being short term (or working memory) and long term memory.

The term *working memory* has superseded short term memory and refers to a system which is responsible for temporary storage of information while that information is being manipulated. The temporary nature of this storage is important. Information from working memory will degrade within a matter of seconds. As this memory subsystem is more closely linked to attention and executive functions than to the other memory subsystems, it is discussed in more detail along with other executive functions.

Long term memory can be divided into declarative or non-declarative memory. Declarative memory systems involves the conscious recollection of events (such as remembering that you ate porridge for breakfast this morning), and facts (such as knowing that porridge is a popular oat and milk breakfast cereal). It is assessed through the use of explicit instructions such as 'do you remember the story I read to you?', and as such has been called explicit memory. Most standard neuropsychological tests of memory will assess this type of memory process.

Declarative memory can be further subdivided into episodic and semantic memory. The *episodic memory* system is the system that allows individuals to retain information regarding distinct personally experienced events or "episodes" in their life within the context of a specific time and place. This memory system allows us to determine when and where an event happened. Examples of such experiences would include a

meeting attended this morning, a telephone conversation that took place a week ago, or a friend's wedding which took place a few years ago. Information can be retained for variable periods of time ranging from a few minutes to many years. This involves multiple processes which include registration of the information, encoding the information to memory, consolidating that information within memory, and when required, retrieval of that information.

From a neuroanatomical perspective, the medial temporal lobe, particularly the hippocampus and the extra hippocampal regions (perirhinal, entorhinal, parahippocampal cortices) play a key role in episodic memory. This is evidenced by patients with amnesia and the famous case of HM who underwent bilateral temporal lobe resection for the treatment of focal epilepsy and subsequently developed an inability to retain new memories. Other brain regions implicated in episodic memory involve the fronto-striatal regions, including the basal ganglia and frontal lobes, and the subcomponents of the *Papez circuit*.

The Papez circuit is a neural pathway, first described by James Papez in 1937, which starts and ends in the hippocampus and includes the fornix, mammillary bodies, mammillo-thalamic tract, anterior thalamic nucleus, cingulum, and enterorhinal cortex. The important role this circuit plays in episodic memory is exemplified by the profound memory problem observed following injury to its constituting structures (e.g. mammillary body damage in Korsakoff's encephalopathy or thalamic damage following a stroke).

Within episodic memory there appears to be distinctions between the types of information to be remembered, the mode of recollection, and when the information was acquired. The literature suggests that the left hemisphere, and in particular temporal lobe damage, is associated with verbal memory impairment, while right hemisphere/temporal lobe damage is associated with non-verbal/visuospatial memory impairment. Furthermore, the details of the information is remembered may also provide clues on locality of lesions. Recollection of specific contextual information is dependent on retrieval processes and strategic search. However, recognition memory can also rely on familiarity judgement, here the information may be recognized without retrieval of specific contextual details e.g. "I know that I have seen that man before but I do not know where". In terms of the neuroanatomical underpinnings of these distinctions within the episodic memory, the perirhinal cortex is thought to receive specific item information important for familiarity judgements, while the parahippocampal cortex is concerned with the contextual place information needed for recollection. Both types of information are bound within the hippocampus to form associations which are fundamental to episodic learning.

Associative memory is often evaluated by having patients recall lists of semantically unrelated word pairs (e.g. caterpillar and rocket). Focal hippocampal pathology tends to produce impairment on tasks of associative memory with relative sparing of item memory and familiarity. This type of impairment may be found early in AD.

A final distinction is based on the time of acquisition of information. Retrograde amnesia refers to the loss of information acquired prior to the onset of amnesia. In the early stages of AD, there is typically a temporal gradient with older memories showing less degradation than more recent memories. On the other hand, conditions such as PD and HD are often considered to present with a flat temporal gradient.

Patients with frontal lobe lesions also have significant episodic memory difficulties, particularly in retrieval. However these patients (unlike AD patients) often improve with clues such as category cues (e.g. a type of flower) or context clues, or when asked to identify the correct option from multiple options (recognition tasks). This distinction is often helpful when differentiating behavioural variant frontotemporal lobar degeneration (bvFTD) and AD. Free recall and associative memory will be poor in both cases, but bvFTD patients perform better in cued memory and recognition memory tasks. It is worth noting this distinction in performance is by no means universal as the performance of FTD patients on recognition tasks can be adversely influenced by

response biases (i.e. the patient 's acquiescence and compliance which results in a tendency towards 'yes' responses).

Semantic memory is the memory system involved in retaining facts about the world for example, that polar bears are white, live in the arctic, and are mammals, or that London is the capital of United Kingdom and is a large city with a population of more than 8 million people. Unlike episodic memory, semantic memory is not dependent on a personal time line or on subjective experience. As semantic memory is closely interlinked with language processing and deficits in semantic memory usually present as language difficulties, it is discussed in further detail in the Language section below.

Non-declarative memory systems are involved in situations where there is unconscious retrieval of information and in which learning and recall occur implicitly. The most important example of is *procedural memory* which is an implicit memory system that enables us to learn new skills. It involves unconscious retrieval of a skill acquired through training such as riding a bicycle or playing the piano. Procedural memory is closely linked to supplementary motor cortex, the cerebellum, and the basal ganglia. Patients with damage to these structures, such as patients with PD or HD, have been shown to have impairment in procedural memory. By contrast, patients with AD and bvFTD often have preserved procedural memory including acquisition of new procedural memory skills in the context of impairment of other memory systems such as episodic memory.

Table 3.1 provides a summary of commonly used test of memory. Note that most assessments would include tests of verbal and non-verbal (or visual) memory as patients may display selective deficits (see Fig. 3.1)

3.5 Language Functions

Language difficulties are by definition the presenting and most salient symptoms in patients with primary progressive aphasia. Language abnormalities can also occur in other neurodegenerative

Table 3.1 This table provides examples of commonly used tests of memory

Name of test	Remarks
Wechsler Memory Scale (WMS-III and IV)	Most widely used scale, includes tasks of story recall (Logical memory), recall of word pairs (Verbal paired Associates) and visual memory tasks. (e.g. Visual Reproduction and Design memory)
Doors and People test	The test includes the immediate and delayed recall and recognition of pictures of doors, people, shapes (visual memory) and names (verbal memory)
Rey Osterrieth Complex Figure	The test assesses one's ability to recall and recognise a complex figure after copying it. Limitations include reliance of construction which involves motor function and organisational skills
Rey Auditory Verbal Learning	List Learning Test
California Verbal Learning Test (CVLT)	List Learning Test
BIRT Memory and Information Processing Battery (BMIBP)	This battery includes story recall, figure recall, list and design learning and also includes a test of processing speed
Rivermead Behavioral Memory Test (RBMT-III)	The tasks attempts to mirror everyday life and includes face recognition, story recall and the ability to learn new skills (the Novel task)
Autobiographical Memory Interview	Semi-structured interview that assess the ability to recall facts and incidents from one's past life

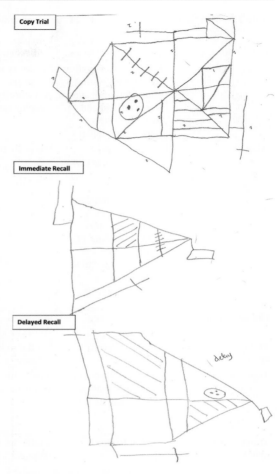

Fig. 3.1 This figure includes copy trial of the Rey Osterrieth Complex Figure as well as the immediate and delayed recall memory. It demonstrates relatively preserved visuo-spatial skills (copy trial) in the context of poor visual memory (recall trials). The patient had a large lesion in the right temporal and parietal cortex

as naming difficulties, and deficits in reading and writing.

3.5.1 Aphasia

Aphasia is a term used to denote impairment in the ability to express one's self and/or to comprehend language. Our understanding of aphasia has been traditionally based on the study of stroke patients. These observations have identified several regions as building blocks of the language network including Broca's area, Wernicke's area,

diseases including AD (in particular younger onset disease), cortico-basal degeneration (CBD), and progressive supranuclear palsy (PSP).

Language is a complex domain with several inter-linked functions. We discuss here some of the most commonly observed language problems including aphasia and associated symptoms such

Table 3.2 This table provides a summary of current classification of aphasia

Type of aphasia	Language expression	Language comprehension	Repetition	Typical site of lesion
Broca' s aphasia	Reduced fluency of speech with halting, effortful speech and word retrieval and paraphasic errors Impaired grammar	Relatively intact except for syntactically complex sentences	Impaired	Dominant Inferior frontal gyrus (Broca's area)
Wernicke's aphasia	Intact sentence structure, fluency of speech, and articulation Empty Meaningless speech content Paraphasic errors with neologisms e.g. call a spoon a "jargle" (May fail to realize they are saying the wrong word)	Markedly impaired	Impaired	Posterior part of superior temporal gyrus (dominant hemisphere)
Global aphasia	Similar to Broca's aphasia	Similar to Wernicke's aphasia	Impaired	Widespread damage to the dominant hemisphere
Transcortical motor aphasia	Similar to Broca's aphasia	Similar to Broca's aphasia	Intact	ACA-MCA watershed region
Transcortical sensory aphasia	Speech is fluent but tends to be empty, vague meaningless	Similar to Wernicke's aphasia	Intact May repeat questions instead of answering them	MCA-PCA watershed region (Brodmann's areas: 37, 22, and 39)
Transcortical mixed aphasia	Similar to Broca's aphasia	Similar to Wernicke's aphasia	Intact	ACA-MCA and MCA-PCA watershed regions
Conduction aphasia	Normal except for mild word finding difficulties	Normal	Impaired	Arcuate fasciculus
Anomic aphasia	Specific deficit in word retrieval and naming object in the context of normal fluency of speech and often normal object knowledge	Intact	Intact	Temporoparietal cortex often including the angular gyrus

the supramarginal and angular gyri. Similarly, the most commonly used classification of aphasia is also based on observation of stroke patients (summarised in Table 3.2). However, Mesulam argues that this classification is not helpful in understanding the impairment in the language network associated with neurodegenerative disease. This is mainly because damage in stroke is due to abrupt, complete destruction of neurons, and the regional distribution is dependent on blood vessel territory. In contrast, the pathological process in neurodegenerative disorders involves gradual, progressive, and selective loss of cortical neurons, and the preferential spread of pathology is believed to be governed by neuronal connectivity within brain networks. This leads to more complex and subtle dissociations and involves brain plasticity. In addition, the model based on stroke patients does not include the anterior temporal lobe (especially on the left hemisphere) which studies from neurodegenerative disorders have shown to be an important part of the language network.

Primary progressive aphasia (PPA) is the prototype of neurodegenerative conditions where the language network is involved. PPA is a heterogeneous group of clinical syndromes often classified under the umbrella of FTD. Although the classification of PPA is still in evolution, it is currently accepted that there are three clinical variants, Agrammatic/non-fluent variant (nfvPPA), the logopenic variant (lvPPA) and the semantic variant (svPPA).

Impaired speech fluency and grammar are the hallmarks of nfvPPA. Fluency of speech is the ability to express oneself in an effortless and articulate manner. This term must not be confused with *verbal fluency* which refers to the ability to generate words based on specific orthographic or semantic criteria (e.g. words starting with the letter "F" or names of animals). The latter is a complex task that has close links to executive functions and is discussed in the section pertaining to that cognitive domain.

The deficits in fluency of speech and grammar observed in nfvPPA are similar to those described in patients with stroke affecting Broca's area. However, nfvPPA patients present in a slowly progressive (as opposed to a sudden) manner. Patients with nfvPPA usually have effortful, halting speech. The breakdown in grammar can include simplification, distorted word order, omissions of function words (such articles and propositions), and poor use of pronouns. These changes extend to writing abilities. Indeed tasks of written language production (such as picture description) are among the most sensitive tasks in early nfvPPA. Other important features of this condition include impaired comprehension of syntactically complex sentences, impaired motor speech production in the form of speech apraxia (described in more detail below), and loss of normal prosody.

Structural and functional imaging in these patients usually shows changes in left posterior fronto-insular region (i.e. inferior frontal gyrus, insula, premotor & supplementary motor areas).

Patients with lvPPA also often have poor fluency of speech associated with the hallmark features of hesitancy due to impaired word retrieval and anomia (difficulty in naming objects while knowing what they are). The fact that grammar is usually intact in these patents is highlighted by Mesulam as an example of the neuropsychological and anatomical dissociation of grammar and fluency observed in neurodegenerative disease but not stroke. In addition, lvPPA patients often have poor comprehension of long unfamiliar sentences lending support to the hypothesis that phonological short-term/working memory impairment is a contributory factor to the deficits observed in this variant. In lvPPA, neuroimaging usually shows structural and functional changes in the left posterior perisylvian tempero-parietal regions (posterior temporal, supramarginal, and angular gyri).

Impaired repetition is a key feature of lvPPA and repetition of long unfamiliar sentences is sensitive in accordance with a phonological working memory impairment. Some impairment in repetition may also be seen in nfvPPA particularly of grammatically complex sentences.

The clinical characteristics of svPPA are described below in the discussion of naming difficulties which form a crucial element of this syndrome.

3.5.2 Naming Difficulties

Difficulties in naming and word retrieval are found across many neurodegenerative diseases and naming abilities are among the most commonly assessed components of language within NPA.

The process of naming objects starts with the initial perception of the object. Impairment at this level is modality specific. For example in visual apperceptive agnosia (discussed in Visuo-spatial skills section) the patient is unable to recognise visual stimuli such as a picture of a key, but can recognise a key via tactile exploration or via auditory modality (e.g. sound of keys jiggling). To exclude modality specific impairment, it is important to test naming using several modalities

Fig. 3.2 This figure provides a simplified schema of the steps involved in the process of naming an object

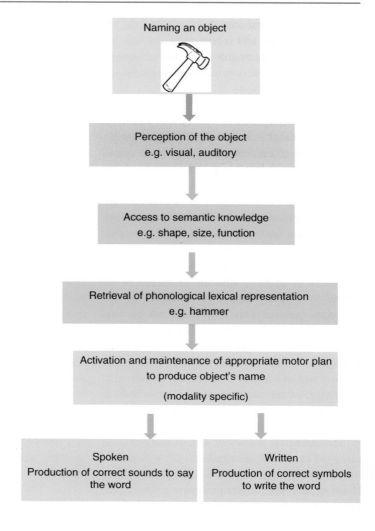

such as picture naming, or naming by description. After the initial perception, naming an item/object requires three main steps: (1) accessing the semantic knowledge relevant to the object; (2) accessing the lexical representation of that object; and (3) activation of the modality specific processes involved in producing the name of that object (e.g. motor speech production in case of spoken language, see Fig. 3.2). Problems can occur at each of these three levels.

The initial step of accessing the semantic knowledge relevant to an object involves access to both the essential and specific attributes of that object (e.g. the characteristics that identify a polar bear from other animals including other types of bears such as its shape, colour, size, etc.)

and to the *conceptual knowledge* about the object (e.g. polar bears live in the arctic, eat fish, are wild animals, can be dangerous, and are considered at brink of extinction). Impaired access to either levels of semantic knowledge can lead to naming difficulties often associated with semantic errors (e.g. saying "cow" instead "bear"). However, impaired access to conceptual knowledge about an object would also cause errors in understanding the function of everyday items. The patient may for example use a spoon to cut food.

Typical examples of naming difficulties due to impaired access to semantic knowledge can be observed in patients with the semantic variant of PPA (svPPA). Imaging svPPA shows abnormalities in both anterio-lateral temporal lobes (usually left greater than right), and it is now recognized that this region plays a key role in semantic memory. Clinical presentation is often with naming problems which may include semantic errors including replacement of low frequency nouns with high frequency nouns (e.g. "dog" for "boar) and the use of supra-ordinate categories as opposed to their specific exemplars (e.g. "animal" for "cow"). Patients also often suffer from surface alexia (discussed below). Sometimes, these patients may understand complex abstract concepts (e.g. is justice more important than mercy?) but not simpler questions dependent on semantic knowledge of common objects (e.g. do people ride pineapples to get to work?). (Please also refer to Chap. 7.)

The second process involved in naming is the modality-independent retrieval of an item's *lexical phonological representation* or *lemma*. This is associated with activation of the occipto-temporal region, the left frontal operculum and insula. Impairments at this level of processing are manifest as an inability to name objects in the context of intact knowledge of what it is. This deficit is termed *anomia* and usually extends to both speech and writing. Clinically this presents as hesitancy, circumlocutions (e.g. that thing … that you put in food). The individual may describe knowing what they want to say, often feeling that the word is at the "on the tip" of their tongue but being unable "to get the words out". Paraphasic errors can occur, most frequently phonemic in nature due partial lemma retrieval e.g. "octoput" for "octopus".

Anomia is often the presenting feature of PPA. Indeed, it is often the most salient and disabling feature of the logopenic variant (lvPPA). However, anomia can be observed in other neurodegenerative disorders affecting the posterior temporal region including AD.

The final process involved in naming takes place once the *lemma* is retrieved and involves activation of a *modality-specific* process depending on whether the output is spoken or written language. Either process can be selectively impaired. In case of spoken language, the *phonologic representation* of the lemma (which includes the correct sounds for producing a specific word and their sequence) is activated and is maintained while motor articulation takes place. This involves complex planning and co-ordination of the muscles that move the tongue, vocal cords, lips and respiratory muscles. Impairment at this level results in errors in sound production which can include erroneous speech sound substitution, insertion, and transpositions. This is termed apraxia of speech and results in the production of spoken words that may have a different meaning (e.g. "horn" for "horse") or have no meaning at all (e.g. "hammot" for "hammock"). This can be difficult to differentiate from phonemic errors observed in patents with anomia. However, patients with apraxia of speech are often aware of their mistake displaying repeated attempt to correct themselves, while patients with paraphasic errors due to anomia are often unaware of their errors. Apraxia of speech is often associated with nfvPPA.

3.5.3 Reading and Writing

Impairment in the ability to read (alexia) or write (agraphia) can have a peripheral or central cause.

Peripheral causes are those external to the central language centres. Peripheral causes of alexia are due to breakdown in the transmission of the visual image of the word to the language centres. Causes of peripheral alexia include reduced visual acuity, visual field defects, ocular motor apraxia, saccadic intrusions and hemi-spatial neglect alexia (due to difficulty perceiving one side of the page/word). Disconnection alexia (also called alexia without agraphia) occurs in lesions affecting the left occipital lobe and splenium of the corpus callosum. It is due to disconnection between the remaining intact primary visual cortex (on the right) and the intact language centres (which are in the left hemisphere). It is usually associated with right hemianopia and preserved writing (because of the intact connections between visual cortex and primary motor cortex). Peripheral causes of agraphia are due to problems in the planning or execution of the motor elements of writing, such as those observed in writing apraxia (often associated with dominant parietal lobe lesions), hemi-spatial neglect, and pyramidal, extrapyramidal, or cerebellar motor deficits.

Central alexia and agraphia are caused by damage to the central language regions, and their classification is based on the dual-route theory of reading and writing. This suggests that two separate mechanisms are involved in these processes. Through the *lexical route*, a skilled reader can visually recognize a "whole word" by sight alone using a mental database (*the internal lexicon*) without the need to resort to letter-by letter reading. Similarly, when attempting to write the word, pre-stored knowledge is used rather than attempting to spell it letter-by letter. The mental lexicon includes all the words an individual knows including words with irregular pronunciation such "yacht" or "cough". The second route is the *phonological one* which is reliant on sounding the word letter by letter using a letter-sound system. This system is used to read/write newly encountered or made up words.

Surface alexia is caused by lack of access to the internal lexicon which forms part of one's semantic knowledge. Patients can read letter by letter (using the phonological route) but struggle when confronted with irregular words. In these cases, patients tend to regularise words (e.g. reading "pint" as "peent").

Similarly, surface agraphia is associated with an inability to spell orthographically irregular words due to lack of access to the internal lexicon. These deficits are caused by damage to the antero-lateral temporal lobes (especially on the left) such as that observed in svPPA.

Conversely, patients with phonological alexia or agraphia have a breakdown in phonological system resulting in complete reliance on the internal lexicon. A patient with phonological alexia can read previously encountered regular and irregular familiar words with similar ease but has significant difficulties reading non-words/pseudo-words (e.g. kjud). These deficits are usually associated with lesions affecting the perisylvian region including superior temporal lobe, angular gyrus, and supramarginal gyrus.

Deficits in patients with deep alexia or agraphia are similar to that observed in the phonological subtypes but there is usually co-existing errors (e.g. reading "horse" as "cow"). This type of language abnormality is usually seen in patients with more widespread left hemispheric damage.

3.5.4 Discourse

Discourse is the term used to describe the complex process of conveying meaning in a concise and accurate manner. These include speech content and non-verbal cues such as prosody (changes in vocal pitch, loudness, and duration to convey emotion or meaning), facial expressions, and gestures. Dysfunctional discourse can cause vague, circumferential speech and poor expression and comprehension of non-verbal clues. The right hemisphere plays a dominant role in the production and comprehension of the different elements involved in effective discourse. Although discourse has rarely been assessed as part of the routine NPA, it can give important clues to the diagnoses and localisation of the cognitive impairment. For instance, poor discourse is commonly reported in patients with bvFTD, who usually have widespread right hemispheric involvement. Table 3.3 includes a summary of commonly used tests of language function.

3.6   Visuo-Spatial Skills

The clinical presentation in posterior cortical atrophy (PCA, also referred to as the posterior variant of AD) is usually dominated by pronounced deficits in visuo-spatial perception. Other neurodegenerative disorders characterized by decline in visuo-spatial skills include classical AD and atypical Parkinsonian syndromes in particular Dementia with Lewy Bodies (DLB) and CBD.

The initial part of processing visual stimuli involves transmission of signals from the retinal cells, via the lateral geniculate body, to the primary visual cortex (V1). Throughout this part of the pathway, and including the primary visual cortex itself, there is prominent retinotopic

Table 3.3 This table provides a summary of commonly used tests of Language function

Name of test	Brief description
Boston Naming Test (BNT)	A test of confrontational naming where the subject is presented with line drawings of objects and animals and asked to name them
Graded Naming Test (GNT)	A test of confrontational naming where the subject is presented with line drawings of objects and animals and asked to name them
Peabody Vocabulary Test (PVT)	The test involves word-picture matching
Pyramids and Palm Trees Test (PPT)	A test of semantic knowledge in which subject is asked to match pictures of objects/animals/plants based on semantic associations
Test for Reception of Grammar (TROG)	A test of comprehension where a subject is presented with a series of sentences of variable syntactic complexity and asked to select (from four options) the picture which matches each sentence best
Token Test	A test of comprehension where the subject is asked to manipulate tokens of varying size, shape and colour according to spoken commands of variable levels of difficulty
Boston Diagnostic Aphasia Examination	A battery of multiple sub-tasks testing both expressive and receptive language skills

localisation. Lesions to this part of visual pathway, including V1 region, leads to visual field defects.

The second part of processing visual stimuli involves appreciation of more complex phenomena such as shape, form, etc. Thus regions within visual pathway distal to striate cortex are organized by function. Lesions affect the whole visual field and lead to impairment of the specific process for which that region is responsible.

The two stream hypotheses is a widely, though not universally, accepted theory of visual processing distal to V1 in human beings. This postulates that visual information flows from the striate cortex to the extra-striate cortex where simple processing of form, shape etc. takes place and from here it flows down two streams.

The ventral stream (or "what pathway") ends in the temporal lobe and its major function is object recognition. The ventral stream has close association with the medial temporal lobe where information can be combined with semantic knowledge, the limbic system (emotional attachment to objects) and dorsal stream (see below). Lesions to the ventral stream are usually caused by bilateral temporal or fusiform lesions and lead to an in ability to visually recognise object (agnosia) colours (acromatosia) and faces (prosopagnosia). Agnosia caused by lesions to the ventral stream is more accurately referred to as *apperceptive* agnosia as there is an inability to recognise objects due to deficits in visual processing. This contrasts with *associative* agnosia where object perception is intact but there is an inability to connect the perceived image with stored semantic knowledge. The latter disorder can be distinguished by the intact ability to copy, draw, or match an object correctly despite the lack of knowledge about its function or meaning.

The dorsal stream (or "where pathway") projects to the parietal lobe and is involved in processing where an object is in space relevant to the viewer and in guiding and perceiving actions . Lesions to the dorsal stream can cause difficulty in perceiving moving objects (akinetopsia), lack of awareness of things/body parts in one hemifield (hemi-spatial neglect), and Balint's syndrome. Balint in his first report of this syndrome described an Engineer who was functionally blind despite having good visual acuity. This was due to a triad of simultanagnosia (inability to perceive more than one component of a scene or object simultaneously), visual optic ataxia: (inability to guide movement visually), and ocular apraxia (inability to direct one' gaze to a visual stimulus/target). Symptoms include searching for a target by moving one's head and in severe cases, functional blindness. Dorsal stream lesions are often caused by bilateral superior parieto-occipital region.

Posterior cortical atrophy (PCA), a variant of AD, often present with deficits in visual perception. Common symptoms include reading difficulties; problems with driving or parking a car; and walking difficulties in the presence of uneven

Table 3.4 This table provides a summary of commonly used tests of visuo-spatial function

Name of test	Brief description
Rey Osterrieth Complex Figure (ROCF, copy trial)	The initial *copy* trial of this test involves the subject copying a complex figure. Performance can be confounded by motor disabilities and/or executive dysfunction leading to poor organisational skills
Clock Drawing Test	The subject is asked to draw clock face including the numbers and the position of the clock hands for a predefined time of day. Several scoring methods are available. Performance can be confounded by motor disabilities and/or executive dysfunction leading to poor organisational skills
Visual and Object Space Perception Battery (VOSP)	The battery includes four tests of object perception (Incomplete Letters, Silhouettes, Object Decision, and Progressive Silhouettes) and four tests of space perception (Dot Counting, Position Discrimination, Number Location, and Cube Analysis).
Benton's Judgment of Line Orientation Test (JLO)	The subject is asked to match the angle between a series of two partial line segments and the angles presented on the response card (11 full lines, all 18° apart from one another, arranged in a semi-circle)
Birmingham Object Recognition Battery (BORP)	Multiple sub-tasks assess variable levels of visual perception e.g. matching of basic perceptual features such as orientation and object size and matching objects different in viewpoint

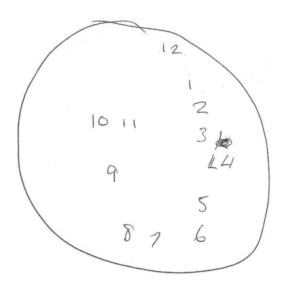

Fig. 3.3 This is a copy of a clock drawing made by a patient with cortico-basal syndrome (CBS) who had significant visuo-spatial deficits

or patterned ground, stairs, sidewalk borders, or escalators due to impaired perception of depth or form. Deficits may affect predominately the dorsal stream (posterior variant of PCA), the ventral stream (ventral variant of PCA), or a combination of both.

Common tasks to test visuo-spatial skills often include replication of complex drawing, judgment of angles, reading disintegrating letters (see Table 3.4). Clock drawing is a common bedside task that can yield useful information (see Fig. 3.3). Both clock drawing and tests involving replication of complex figures (e.g. Rey Osterrieth Figure) can be confounded motor disability (e.g. patients with amyotrophic lateral scleroses or ALS), and by poor organisational skills in patients with poor executive functions in the context of intact visuo-spatial skills (see Fig. 3.4).

3.7 Executive Functions

Impairment in executive function is an early and often the most salient cognitive deficit in bvFTD. Executive dysfunction is also a prominent feature of cognitive change observed in amyotrophic lateral sclerosis (ALS), conditions previously termed "sub-cortical dementias" such as PD, HD, PSP, and DLB and in multiple sclerosis (MS).

Executive functions are a heterogeneous group of skills required for effective planning and execution of goal oriented behaviour. These skills include problem solving, goal recognition, planning goal directed behaviour, error monitoring, the ability to sustain selective attention, inhibition of unwanted responses/impulses, sequencing, mental flexibility as well as the ability to shift strategies in order to adapt to changes in the environment or to unwanted outcomes. Executive

Fig. 3.4 This is the copy trial of the Rey Osterrieth Complex Figure in a patient with bulbar onset amyotrophic lateral scleroses and co-morbid behavioural variant frontotemporal dementia. The figure demonstrates poor planning and organisational skills due to executive dysfunction

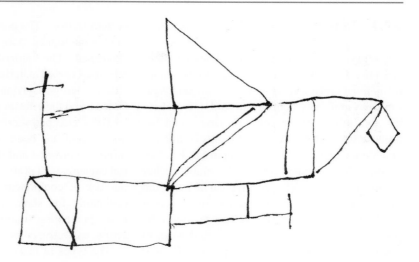

functions are also involved in comprehension of abstract concepts, judgement, and reasoning. Patients with impaired executive functions can display significant difficulties in everyday functioning which can extend to their ability to function independently or maintain their performance at school or work.

The neuropsychological construct of executive functions emerged from observations of patients with frontal lobe lesions. The key role played by the frontal lobes in executive functions was later confirmed using neuroimaging studies. This has led many researchers and clinicians to consider the term "executive dysfunction" to be synonymous with "frontal lobe deficit". This is erroneous not only because it confuses an anatomical construct with a psychological one, but it is also inaccurate. The frontal lobes have functions that extend beyond executive control including motor and sensory functions. Similarly, non-frontal lobe brain regions contribute to executive functions. Of particular importance are brain structures contributing to frontal-subcortical circuitry. For example, the dorsolateral frontal-sub-cortical circuit which projects to and from the dorsolateral prefrontal cortex (DLPC) includes the dorsolateral head of caudate nucleus, the globus pallidus, and the ventro-anterior and medio-dorsal thalamic nuclei. This circuit plays a critical role in multiple executive functions including working memory, problem solving, organizational skills, set shifting, planning,

abstract thinking, and fluency (other fronto-striatal circuits are discussed below).

A comprehensive assessment of executive functions is a challenging endeavour given the heterogeneity of these functions. Performance on one task of executive function is a poor predictor of performance on other executive tasks or indeed of functioning in real world situations. The complexity of executive functions has also resulted in the lack of a universally accepted model or classification. Miyake et al. propose that the fundamental components to executive functions are mental set shifting, information updating and monitoring, and inhibition. On the other hand, Stuss et al. emphasize task setting, monitoring and energization as the building blocks of executive functions. Norman and Shallice proposed a model that involves alternative attentional control systems for thought and behaviour with the predominant system at any one time dependent on whether environmental stimuli are routine/well learned or non-routine. Baddley proposed the concept of the "central executive" which controls attention and supervises several other "slave" sub-systems, a concept that forms the core of a widely accepted model of working memory and is described in more detail below. In the following section we describe some of the major processes which come under the umbrella of executive functions and which are particularly relevant for NPA (for detailed review of executive control function see Diamond A 2013).

3.7.1 Inhibitory Control

Inhibitory control arguably underlines all other executive functions. The term refers to the ability to inhibit unwanted responses and impulses. Impaired inhibitory control can lead to impulsivity and failure to respond to new situations because of overreliance on old habits of thought or action. Cognitive inhibitory control tasks often evaluate the individual's ability to inhibit his/her prepotent response. The most typical tasks are the Stroop colour word test and the more recent Hayling Sentence Completion Test in which the person has to generate an unconnected word to complete a sentence. The latter is particularly sensitive to cognitive deficits in bvFTD (see Table 3.5 for commonly used tasks of executive functions).

Impaired inhibitory control of behaviour is associated with perseveration (in which a person continues to undertake a behaviour which is no longer appropriate for the situation) and environmental dependency. The latter includes behaviours such as imitating other people's speech (echolalia) or action (echopraxia) and utilization behaviour where individuals compulsively pick up items in their environment and use them. Utilization behaviour has been related to focal lesions of the medial prefrontal cortex but can be found in bvFTD.

3.7.2 Set Shifting, Monitoring and Updating

Set shifting, monitoring, and updating are heavily reliant on processes of attention and working memory. Working memory refers to retention of information for brief periods of time often while that information is being manipulated. Intact working memory is essential for understanding and following information over time, and as such is critical for everyday activities e.g. doing simple mental calculations and recalling the start of a paragraph or conversation on reaching its end.

A widely accepted model of working memory (Baddley 1986) proposes a "central executive" which acts as an attentional control system which supervises two "slave systems whose function is to store and manipulate information for brief periods of time. The postulated slave systems are the phonological loop and the visuospatial sketchpad. The phonological loop stores and rehearses *verbal* material and has been associated with the left perisylvian region (posterior part of Broca's and the inferior parietal lobe). The visuospatial sketch pad serves to store and manipulate *images* and has been associated with the right inferior prefrontal and parietal cortex. The "central executive" in prefrontal lobes is involved in a number of component processes including coordinating the slave-systems, sustaining attention, preventing interference, monitoring for errors, and retrieval of the information.

The types of tasks used to assess these functions include reverse digit span, the Trail Making Test and the Wisconsin Card Sort Test. The latter two tasks involve attention switching between concepts in addition to monitoring performance (see Table 3.5 for descriptions of these tasks).

3.7.3 Planning, Problem Solving and Cognitive Flexibility

Planning and cognitive flexibility develop at a later age compared to inhibitory control and working memory, and probably build on these skills. Planning involves the identification of the steps required to achieve a goal and organising these steps in an effective manner to maximize the chances of achieving that goal.

An essential part of planning is strategy formation. To solve a problem a change in strategy is often required. Cognitive flexibility is the ability to change one's strategy to accommodate new demands or changing environment, or because the initial strategy led to an unwanted outcome. Thus, cognitive flexibility is a critical requirement for problem solving. Cognitive flexibility is also closely linked to the ability to shift sets or tasks and to creativity. Impaired cognitive flexibility leads to mental rigidity. Tasks which tap these types of functions include the Wisconsin Card Sorting Test or the Tower of London/Hanoi.

There is considerable evidence linking the ability to plan and organize complex task and to shift strategies to the dorsolateral prefrontal cortex region (DLPC).

Table 3.5 This table provides a summary of commonly used tests of executive functions and processing speed

Name of test	Brief description	Main functions tested
Executive functions		
Wisconsin Card Sorting Test (WCST)	The subject is asked to match a series of stimulus card with four key cards. The subject is not provided with rules used for matching (e.g. by colour or number) but is informed on each occasion if his/her matching is correct. The rules are changed periodically without informing the subject	Cognitive flexibility, problem-solving
Trail Making Test (TMT)	The subject asked to 'connect-the-dots' in a sequential order. The targets in part A are numbers (1, 2, 3, etc.). Part B includes numbers and letters and the subjects is asked to alternate between the two (i.e. A-1-B-2 etc.)	Cognitive flexibility, processing speed
Brixton Spatial Anticipation Test (BSAT)	The task assesses the ability to detect and follow rules and rule changes using a sequence of visuo-spatial stimuli. The subject is asked to predict the position of a black dot on consecutive pages of booklet. The subject is not provided with rules. The rules change periodically every few pages	Cognitive flexibility, problem-solving
Stroop Interference Colour Word Test	In the priming sub-task, subjects are asked to read list of a names of colours as quickly as they can. In the interference sub-task, the subjects are presented with multi-coloured list of names of colours where the names of colours are printed in ink colours not denoted by the name e.g. the word "blue" was printed in red ink. The subjects are asked to name as quickly as possible the *colour* of ink in which each word is printed (e.g. red in this case) while inhibiting the impulse to read the word (e.g. "blue")	Inhibition of unwanted responses
Verbal Fluency (semantic or phonemic)	Semantic fluency (also called category fluency) verbal fluency test, requires the subject to retrieve words that belong to a particular semantic category such as "fruits", "furniture" or "animals". In orthographic fluency (or letter fluency) the subject is asked to generate as many words as possible using a specific letter of the alphabet	Cognitive flexibility, problem-solving, inhibition of unwanted responses, processing speed
Design Fluency	Subjects are asked to generate as many designs as possible using predefined rules e.g. joining a dots using four straight lines	Cognitive flexibility, problem-solving, inhibition of unwanted responses, processing speed
Backward Digit Span	The subjects are asked to recite a series of numbers of increasing length in reverse order	Working memory and attention

(continued)

Table 3.5 (continued)

Name of test	Brief description	Main functions tested
Behavioural Assessment of Dysexecutive Syndrome	The battery includes a self-reporting 20 item questionnaire focused on everyday problems common to individuals with executive dysfunction and a multiple tasks designed to mirror every day activities e.g. Rule shift card test, Key search test, Temporal Judgment Test, Zoo Map Test, Action program Test and Modified Six Element	Multiple
Delis-Kaplan Executive Function System (D-KEFS)	A battery of tasks of executive function which includes verbal and design fluency, sorting test, Colour Word interference test, Trail Making test, Tower test, and Proverb comprehension	Multiple
Test of Everyday Attention	A battery of tasks testing the ability to maintain and switch attention using multiple tasks e.g. searching for symbols on a coloured map, imagining being in an elevator and trying to guess the floor number by counting a series of tape-presented tones etc	Working memory and attention
Processing speed		
Paced Auditory Serial Addition Test (PASAT)	Single digits are presented at regular intervals (e.g. every 3 s) and the subject must add each new digit to the one immediately prior to it	Auditory information processing speed, cognitive flexibility
Symbol Digit Modalities Test (SDMT)	The subject is presented with a sequence of abstract symbols and corresponding specific numbers (key). The task consists of pairing each symbol with its matching number within a specific time period, consulting the key as necessary	Processing speed, attention

3.7.4 Energisation/Initiation

A key function which is assessed commonly within NPA is the ability to rapidly generate responses. Stuss suggested that this process was fundamental to the concept of energisation. Energisation is tested typically by tasks of verbal fluency. During task of verbal fluency, the patient is asked to generate as many words as he/she can using specific orthographic rules (e.g. words starting with the letter "S") or semantic rules (e.g. names of flowers). Verbal fluency tasks assess a number of processes including behavioural spontaneity, intrinsic generation, and strategy formation, in addition to cognitive flexibility. Patients

with frontal lobe lesions produce fewer correct words and commit more rule breaks. Imaging data has shown a strong association between letter fluency tasks (generation of words starting with a specific letter) and the left DLPC and anterior cingulate. Semantic fluency tasks are more dependent on temporal lobe functions (associated with semantic memory).

3.7.5 Reasoning and Abstract Thought

Tests of deductive reasoning assess the person's ability to reason logically and often involve a transitive inference task (If A = B and B = C, then A = C?). Tasks of abstract conceptualisation evaluate the person's ability to work out new concepts and abstract ideas and usually involve the recognition of patterns and similarities between shapes and figures. Metaphorical thinking is often tested using proverb comprehension (e.g. what does the saying "people with glasses houses should not throw stones" mean?). Proverb comprehension tasks are limited by cultural dependency. Poor deductive reasoning and abstract conceptualisation and literal interpretation of metaphors are typically observed in bvFTD patients.

Goel and others have proposed the presence of two types of reasoning. Reasoning about meaningful, familiar, situations (e.g. all parrots are birds; parrots can talk; so all birds can talk?) is thought to rely on background knowledge and beliefs and is linked to the frontal-temporal lobes, particularly left temporal lobe which is associated with semantic knowledge. On the other hand, reasoning about non-specific, unfamiliar situations (where semantic knowledge is not useful) has been shown to activate a parietal system and is postulated to engage visuo-spatial imagery. Both types of reasoning share links to the basal ganglia nuclei cerebellum, fusiform gyri, and prefrontal cortex. In line with this premise, Tireney et al. demonstrated that deficits in deductive reasoning in bvFTD are not a universal phenomenon, with preferential impairment in tasks involving familiar situations (e.g., Spain is west of Italy, Italy is west of Greece, Spain is west of Greece?) compared to similar tasks involving unfamiliar environments (e.g., the AI lab is east of the Roth Centre; Cedar Hall is west of the Roth Centre; Cedar Hall is west of the AI lab).

3.8 Processing Speed

Processing speed is a measure of cognitive efficiency in processing information. It is closely linked to attention and working memory. Impairment in processing speed is one of the most commonly reported cognitive deficits in the so called sub-cortical dementias, such as PD,

HD, and also MS. These reports are limited by the fact that many tasks of processing speed tap into some elements of executive functions and into fluid reasoning (see Table 3.5). In addition, as tests usually measure the time required to complete a specific task, it is difficult to document unbiased estimates of processing speed in disorders where the delay in reaction time can be confounded by motor disability e.g. PD and ALS.

3.9 Social Cognition

Social cognition refers to an emergent, interdisciplinary field devoted to the study of the neurobiological processes underlying social interactions. There is accumulating evidence that bvFTD patients have abnormalities in social cognitive skills, and this impairment has been implicated in the disintegration of social behaviour that is observed in this condition. Indeed, there are reports suggesting that tasks of social cognition maybe more sensitive than those of classical executive functions in detecting changes in early stages of bvFTD. Social cognitive deficits have also been reported in AD, PD, ALS and HD.

Successful social interaction is made possible by at least two overlapping processes. The first is accurate perception and processing of social signals displayed by other individuals. This includes non-verbal cues such as facial expression and tone of voice. The second process is the generation of socially appropriate responses.

Both lesion and imaging studies suggest that multiple brain regions are involved in the processing of non-verbal social signals including the inferio-lateral temporo-occipital cortex, ventromedial prefrontal cortex, the inferior occipital gyrus, the middle/superior temporal sulcus, anterior temporal lobe, basal ganglia, and the amygdala. The right hemisphere is believed to have a dominant role in social cognitive processing.

An essential component of processing of social signal is a skill termed theory of mind (ToM or mentalizing). ToM skills include the ability to attribute independent mental states to other individuals. These mental states may include the individual's knowledge, beliefs, and

Table 3.6 This table provides a summary of commonly used tests of social cognitive skills

Name of test	Brief description
Ekman 60 Test of Facial Affect	A test of the ability to recognise basic facial expressions of emotion using black and white photographs of ten actors depicting six basic emotions (happiness, sadness, anger, fear, disgust and surprise)
Penn Emotion Recognition Test	A computerized test of the ability to recognise basic facial expressions of emotion involving 96 colour photographs of multi-ethnic actors depicting varying intensities of four basic emotions (happy, sad, angry, fearful) as well as neutral expressions
Florida Affect Battery	A test of the ability to recognise and match facial and prosodic expressions of emotions, with and without semantic distraction Battery includes photographs and auditory recordings depicting happiness, sadness, anger, fear and neutral state
The Awareness of Social Inference Test, TASIT	A test uses videoed vignettes in which character depict basic emotions and verbalise sincere, sarcastic or false statement to test the ability to recognise spontaneous emotional expression and to distinguish sarcastic statement from sincere ones or lies with or without contextual clues
Reading the Mind in the Eyes	A test of the affective theory of mind which assesses the ability to recognise the mental state of individuals (e.g. despondent, reflective) from cues in their eye region
Second Order False Belief Order Tasks	A test of the cognitive theory of mind in which subjects are asked to recognise that others may hold false beliefs about other individuals' beliefs or knowledge
Social Faux Pas Recognition Tasks	Vignette or cartoon-based tasks depicting an individual saying/doing something without considering its negative consequences to others and subjects are asked to (1) recognise that speaker lacked the knowledge of the consequences of what he said/did (cognitive theory of mind) and (2) that the listener's mental state would be negatively affected by what they heard/saw (affective theory of mind)

motives which, importantly, may be different from one's own. This skill is critical to our ability as humans to understand, and predict the behaviour of others. It has been proposed that there are two major types ToM. The first type, termed cognitive ToM, is the ability to recognise that another person's knowledge and beliefs may be different from one's own beliefs. Brain regions associated with this skill include the temporo-parietal junctions, and DLPFC. Tasks used to assess these skills include first-order false belief tasks and second-order belief tasks (see Table 3.6).

Affective ToM, on the other hand, denotes the ability to infer another individual's feelings and emotions. Brain regions responsible for affective TOM include the orbitofrontal cortex (OFC) and the ventro-medial prefrontal cortex (VMPC), particularly in the right hemisphere.

The anterior rostral part of the VPMC is part of the ventro-medial frontal-subcortical circuit which includes the anterior cingulate and the nucleus accumbens. This circuit is believed to be critical for motivation. Lesions to this circuit lead to apathy, lack of empathy, and social withdrawal.

The OFC is part of the orbito-frontal cortical-subcortical circuit which includes the venteromedial caudate nucleus. This circuit is associated with the generation of socially appropriate responses based on their potential for reward or punishment. Lesions to this regions lead to socially inappropriate behaviour, disinhibition, and impulsivity.

Impairment in various aspects of social cognition has been reported in a wide range of neurodegenerative conditions (for a detailed review see Elamin et al. 2012). However, there is considerable debate regarding the causal links between the reported deficits on tasks of social cognition and the behavioural changes manifested by patients as well as the contribution of cognitive impairment in other domains to poor performance on these tasks. Examples of tasks used to test social cognition are shown in Table 3.6.

However most of these tests are experimental and are scarcely used within standard neuropsychological assessment.

3.10 Behaviour

Changes in behaviour and personality are the defining feature of bvFTD. However, less prominent change in behaviour is a common complication of many neurodegenerative disorders including language variants of FTD, ALS without co-morbid dementia, HD, and AD.

During a NPA, information regarding behavioural change is usually obtained via a combination of direct observation of the patient (e.g. impulsivity, perseveration, ignoring personal boundaries, inappropriate social behaviour, fixating on certain subjects, utilization behaviour etc.) as well as interviewing an informant. Accurate documentation of behavioural change is a challenging feat because of the subjective nature of this abnormality which is dependent on the patient's premorbid personality and cultural background as well as the informant's characteristics. A discerning informant is likely to give a different report from an overprotective or non-observant one. Multiple behavioural questionnaires have been designed with the aim of standardizing the procedure of evaluating behaviour. Examples include the Frontal Systems Behaviour Scale (FrSBe, Grace and Molloy 2001), the Cambridge Behavioural Inventory (CBI), and the Neuropsychiatric Inventory Questionnaire (NPI-Q).

The most frequently reported behavioural change in neurodegenerative diseases is apathy. Other commonly reported behaviours include irritability, aggressiveness and lack of empathy. Behavioural changes in neurodegenerative disorders have been reported to be linked to right hemispheric involvement and are often similar to those observed in patients with known social cognitive deficits. However, social cognitive deficits are yet to be confirmed to be predictive of the behavioural deficits observed in these patients.

The severity of behavioural change relative to any co-existing cognitive abnormalities and the pattern of behavioural deficits offer clues to the underlying neurodegenerative disorder. In bv-FTD, disintegration of behaviour is the most salient abnormality and can occur in the context of intact cognitive functioning. Research criteria for diagnosing bvFTD include five domains of behavioural disinhibition, apathy, loss of empathy, simple or complex stereotyped/perseverative behaviour and changes in eating behaviour/hyper-orality with an increased consumption of sweet food. It has been suggested that bv-FTD can be subdivided into apathetic variant, disinhibited variant and a stereotyped-compulsive syndrome at onset of symptoms. However, these symptoms frequently co-occur, making the distinction often difficult (see Chap. 7 for a more detailed discussion).

Patients with language variants of FTD often also develop behavioural changes, though these usually follow and are less prominent than the language deficits. A similar spectrum of behavioural change has also been reported in ALS which is known to clinically overlap with bvFTD. Mild behavioural changes have been reported in up to 25 % of ALS patients with another 10–15 % displaying marked changes that fulfil the criteria for co-morbid bvFTD.

Behavioural changes reported in AD include apathy, withdrawal, agitation, irritability and aggression. HD is another disorder where behavioural changes are a prominent feature including apathy, impulsivity, risk-taking behaviour, obsessive-compulsive behaviour, lack of empathy, mental rigidity, irritability, lack of insight, disinhibition, and social misconduct.

The identification of the behavioural complications of neurodegenerative disorders is important as it is often a cause of significant strain on patient's relationship with his family and carer. Indeed, there is evidence suggesting that behavioural changes are a more reliable predictor of carer burden than physical disability or cognitive impairment.

3.11 Apraxia

Apraxia is a term used to describe difficulties in performing motor tasks that cannot be explained by motor or sensory weakness, or inability to comprehend the command. Patients can have limited insight into their deficits which are more frequently noticed by family member and work colleagues. Therefore, it is important to specifically ask both the patient and the informant about activities of daily living such getting dressed, washing one's self and other activities or hobbies that the individual normally engages in such as cooking, gardening or DIY.

In addition to intact motor and sensory system, the ability to carry out complex motor actions (praxis) requires at least two processes. The first process is accessing semantic information regarding how to perform a specific task. This includes knowledge regarding what a tool such as a hammer is, and how to use it. The second process is accessing the stored sensorimotor "action plan" required to successfully perform the action. These stored action plans include multiple elements such as the position the limbs need to be placed in, the speed and tempo of the action required, and the appropriate sequence. Apraxia is most frequently associated with in the left frontal premotor and fronto-parietal cortex where these action plans are believed to be stored. Once activated, the information is transmitted to primary motor cortex to carry out the action with contribution from the cerebellum and BG.

Apraxia is frequently seen in many neurodegenerative conditions particularly corticobasal syndrome (CBS) and mid to late stages of AD and PPA. We discuss here the main types of apraxia.

3.11.1 Ideational Apraxia

Unfortunately, this term is used in the literature to describe two very different types of apraxia. We will describe both types here and provide an alternative term less prone to confusion.

The term ideational apraxia was classically used to describe impairment in the first process described above i.e. accessing the semantic information related to the action. The alternative term used for this type of apraxia is *conceptual apraxia* because the patient has impaired access to the concepts involved. Patients not only have difficulties producing the correct action on demand,

but are also unable to imitate the examiner or recognise the action when presented with several options. Patients may not be able to recognise a situation that needs intervention (problem unawareness) or select the correct tool required to carry out a specific action (e.g. may use a hammer to cut paper). Notably, the ability to name tools is intact. Conceptual apraxia is commonly observed in AD.

The second type of apraxia often referred to as ideational apraxia is a disorder characterized by difficulties in performing an action in the correct sequence. Understandably, an alternative term for this apraxia is *sequencing apraxia*. To test for this type of apraxia the subject is asked to perform a multi-step action such as putting a letter in an envelope or making a sandwich. Lesions causing sequencing apraxia are most often in the left occipito-parietal cortex.

3.11.2 Ideomotor Apraxia

Ideomotor apraxia describes a situation where access to semantic information regarding a specific action is maintained, but activation of the specific action plan is impaired. Patients with this condition can recognise a problem, select the correct tool to use, and can correctly identify the action when performed by the examiner. However, they are unable to perform the action themselves either on verbal command or following a demonstration by the examiner (imitation). Lesions leading to ideomotor apraxia are most commonly in the left frontal premotor and parietal cortex.

Ideo-motor apraxia can lead to multiple types of errors in performing motor tasks including using the wrong part of the body, incorrect spatial alignment of limbs, moving the limbs or tool in the wrong spatial plane (e.g. flexing and extending the wrist when using a pair of scissors), and persistent use of body part as a tool despite verbal correction (e.g. using finger as a pen when asked to write or as toothbrush when asked to demonstrate how to use a toothbrush). In addition the patient may display errors in the timing and tempo of action.

Both ideational apraxia and ideomotor apraxia are commonly observed in CBS, but it is important to note that changes can be confined to one hand as the initial clinical presentation in CBS is usually highly asymmetrical.

3.11.3 Other Types of Apraxia

In *conduction apraxia*, there is difficulty in imitating action performed by the examiner despite having no problems performing the action on verbal command. The opposite phenomenon is called *verbal dissociation apraxia*. The anatomical correlates of these types of apraxia are less well understood.

Limb-kinetic Apraxia is term is used to describe reduced dexterity or difficulty in performing fine motor movements, such as buttoning a shirt or putting on jewellery. It is described mainly following damage to primary sensorimotor cortex and cortico-spinal tract and less frequently the premotor cortex.

Dressing Apraxia is a disorder characterized by difficulty in getting dressed, for instance a patient can try to clothes items inside out or upside down. This can be assessed by asking a patient to put on garment such as sock or a shirt after it has been turned inside out.

Constructional apraxia is the term used to describe difficulties in copying two or three dimensional drawings (e.g. dissecting pentagons or a cube).

It is interesting to note that some experts view dressing and constructional apraxia not as true apraxic syndromes, but rather manifestations of visuo-perceptual abnormalities. This view is supported by the fact that these are the only forms of apraxia associated with right (as opposed to the left) hemispheric (usually parietal lobe) damage.

3.12 Other Domains

The NPA often included tests of premorbid function and intelligence quotient (IQ). The Wechsler Adult Intelligence Scale (WAIS) is a large assessment designed to measure current IQ. It is a comprehensive battery of tests, now in its fourth revision, which includes both verbal and non-verbal/visuo-perceptual tasks as well as tests of processing speed and working memory. Each subtest can also be used individually to assess a component function.

To confirm if an individual's current IQ level represents a decline (due to disease or aging) from a previous level of functioning, it is essential to estimate his/her premorbid level functioning. Many tasks of premorbid IQ involve testing the individual's vocabulary or reading abilities. Examples include the Test of Premorbid Functioning – UK Version (ToPF[UK]) and its predecessors the Wechsler Test of Adult Reading (WTAR) and the National Adult Reading Test (NART). These tasks consist of a list of mostly orthographically irregular words (e.g. cough or xenophobia) which the patient is asked to pronounce correctly. The rationale behind these tasks is that performance relies on person's knowledge base while placing minimal demands on memory and executive function, and therefore would be expected to remain relatively stable in the presence of general cognitive decline. However, an obvious caveat to this assumption is surface dyslexia, often observed in svPPA patients, where patients cannot access their internal lexicon and will display difficulty in reading irregular words resulting in spuriously low estimates of premorbid IQ. A further caveat is that these tests are highly sensitive to level of English (only suitable for those with English as a first language), cultural background and education.

A quantitative estimate of anxiety and depression can be helpful in interpreting a patient's overall performance. Simple questionnaire like the Hospital Anxiety and Depression Scale (HADS, Zigmond and Snaith 1983) can be used.

3.13 Pitfalls in Interpreting a Neuropsychological Report

The results of the NPA should be interpreted in the context of the patient's clinical picture and background including age and educational attainment. It is essential to consider potential confounding factors such as physical disability, severe attentional deficits, anxiety, depression or apathy.

Performance on neuropsychological tasks is usually judged against a large cohort of healthy controls producing norms. These may provide a cut-off for abnormal performance usually less the second or fifth percentile of the normative dataset. Limited conclusions can be drawn about an individual's performance if he/she is significantly different from the population from which the normative data was drawn. This is particularly relevant in case of differences in IQ and/or cultural background. Age and on occasion education appropriate normative data can be found for assessment of memory and executive functions.

In addition, neuropsychological tasks are never domain pure. For example patients with severe language deficits (e.g. PPA patients) are likely perform poorly on all tasks involving verbal communications. Thus a PPA patient is likely to have poor scores on verbal memory tasks. This usually contrasts sharply with normal performance on tests of non-verbal (e.g. visual) memory. Similarly, PCA patients who often have severe visuo-perceptual deficits, often struggle with tasks requiring intact visuoperceptive skills regardless of the domain the tasks was designed to evaluate.

Finally, poor motivation or "effort" on the part of the subject being tested can lead to spuriously poor scores. Most professional neuropsychological organisations now recommend that effort tests, also known as symptom/performance validity tests, are administered as part of a routine neuropsychological assessment. Effort tests can be either stand-alone (for example, the Rey-15 item test) and are administered as specific tests of validity or they can be embedded into the testing process. Most effort tests are based on the principle that patients with significant impairments can successfully complete the test and that excessive variation from the expected performance level indicates invalid performance and, in turn, an invalid neuropsychological assessment. Poor effort can be due to a deliberate attempt to misrepresent ability or it can be a secondary effect of other processes such as organic apathy, psychiatric symptoms or pain. Regardless of the aetiology effort should be measured and recorded as part of the assessment process.

3.14 Summary of the Neuropsychological Profiles of Common Neurodegenerative Disorders

The neuropsychological profiles of common neurodegenerative disorders are summarised in the table below (Table 3.7).

Table 3.7 This table provides a summary of the neuropsychological profiles of common neurodegenerative disorders

	Most salient deficits	Associated features
AD	Early impairment of episodic memory	Deficits in visuospatial functions, language, executive functions Apraxia
PCA	Early and prominent visuo-spatial deficits including those mediated via the dorsal stream (e.g. Balint's syndrome) and ventral stream (e.g. object agnosia, prosopagnosia,, environmental agnosia)	Gerstmann's syndrome (agraphia, acalculia, finger anomia, right-left disorientation) Language problems Working memory and executive dysfunction
bvFTD	Early deterioration in behaviour (which may or may not be accompanied by cognitive change) Executive dysfunction most prominent cognitive change	Recent evidence suggests that Bv-FTD (particularly early onset disease) can be also associated with significant memory impairment

Table 3.7 (continued)

	Most salient deficits	Associated features

nfvPPA	Language impairment is the most salient deficit
	  Reduced fluency and agrammatism
	  Impaired repetition and comprehension of syntactically complex sentences
	  Abnormalities in speech production including apraxia of speech and dysprosody
		Dyscalculia ± other elements of Gerstmann's syndrome
		Behavioural changes can be observed

svPPA	Language impairment is the most salient deficit
	  Marked naming problems and impaired object knowledge
	  Single word comprehension (esp. low frequency items) is impaired
	  Repetition usually intact	

lvPPA	Language impairment is the most salient deficit
	  Main problem is impaired word retrieval
	  Repetition usually impaired
	  Sentence comprehension can be impaired especially for long improbable sentences	

PD	Executive dysfunction and working memory Poor memory recall	Visuo-spatial skills may be impaired Procedural memory may be impaired
LBD	Executive dysfunction Deficits in visuo-spatial skills	
PSP	Executive dysfunction Prominent verbal (particularly letter fluency) fluency deficit Poor memory recall	Behavioural changes can be observed
CBD	Deficits in language and visuospatial functions Executive functions are also affected Apraxia	Numerical calculation problems common Behavioural changes can be observed
MSA	Cognitive impairment uncommon	Behavioural changes can be observed
HD	Executive function (in particular processing speed) and recall memory are predominantly affected Behavioural and psychiatric changes often prominent	Procedural memory may be impaired Subtle language changes reported including impaired comprehension of prosody
MS	Executive function (in particular processing speed) and recall memory are predominantly affected	
ALS	Letter fluency deficits, executive dysfunction, language deficit, and poor social cognition	Memory changes can occur although often secondary to executive dysfunction

AD Alzheimer's type dementia, *PCA* posterior cortical atrophy, *bvFTD* behavioural variant frontotemporal dementia, *nfvPPA* non-fluent of primary progressive aphasia, *svPPA* semantic variant of primary progressive aphasia, *lvPPA* logopenic variant of primary progressive aphasia, *PD* Parkinson's disease, *DLB* dementia with Lewy bodies, *PSP* primary supranuclear palsy, *CBD* corticobasal degeneration, *MSA* multiple system atrophy, *HD* Huntington's disease, *ALS* amyotrophic lateral scleroses, and *MS* multiple sclerosis

3.15 Cognitive Screening Tools

Cognitive screening tools are essential tools that allow clinician to evaluate patients within clinic in a short period of time and to decide whether more detailed neuropsychological investigation is warranted.

The most widely used bed-side cognitive screening tasks include the Mini-Mental State Examination (MMSE), the Montreal Cognitive Assessment (MoCA), Addenbrooke's Cognitive Examination (ACE), and the Frontal assessment Battery (FAB).

The MMSE is a structured test of mental status first introduced in 1975. The test examines orientation and attention, memory, calculation, language, and constructional praxis. The MMSE is widely used and validated test that takes about 10 min. It is considered a sensitive test for identifying AD. However, it is less sensitive to mild cognitive impairment (MCI) and to dementia syndromes where the main cognitive deficits lie in executive functions (e.g. FTD). In addition, the test does not include adjustments for age, education or cultural background.

The MoCA and ACE were both designed to address the weaknesses of the MMSE, in particular the lack of executive tasks, and as such are more useful in differentiating AD from FTD. The MoCA (Nasreddine et al. 2005) is a brief test (10 min). It examines the same domains as the MMSE but includes additional tests of executive functions (a simplified Trail Making Tests, a test of verbal fluency, and a finger tapping test of inhibitory control and task of abstract/conceptual thinking). The authors provide two versions of the MoCA in an effort to reduce learning effects on repeat testing and thus provide a more accurate measure of progression over time. It is available in 36 languages. Performance on the MoCA is affected by educational attainment and the instructions suggest adding an extra point in patients who had less than 12 years of education though it is unclear if this adjustment is sufficient. The MoCA has been reported to have a high sensitivity in distinguishing healthy controls from patients with AD (88–100 %), MCI (77–96 %), PD with dementia (81 %), HD (97.4 %) and FTD (78 %). The reported sensitivity is in many cases (e.g. HD and FTD) superior to that reported with the MMSE. However, the reported specificity in distinguishing dementia patients from controls is very variable (30–98 %).

The ACE assesses five cognitive domains, namely attention/orientation, memory, verbal fluency, language and visuospatial abilities. The ACE was developed in 2000 (Mathuranath et al. 2000), revised in 2006 (ACE-R, Mioshi et al. 2006), and a third version was published in 2013 (ACE-III, Hsieh 2013). The revisions aimed to address weaknesses in previous versions. Administration of the ACE takes 15–20 min, slightly longer than the MMSE or MoCA. The ACE is one of the most widely used tests in both a clinical and research context. The positive predictive value for the presence of dementia at cut-off of 82/100 approached 100 %. The test has also been shown differentiate AD from non-AD with high sensitivity and specificity (74 % and 85 % respectively). It has been translated to multiple languages. The sensitivity and specificity of the more recently published ACE-III for the presence of dementia is similarly high (e.g. 100 and 96 % at cut-off score of 88/100).

The Frontal Assessment Battery (FAB, Dubois et al. 2000) is a brief test designed to identify cognitive changes in patients with executive dysfunction due to frontal lobe pathology. It is comprised of six tasks that tests abstract reasoning, verbal fluency, motor programming and executive control of action including Luria motor sequences, resistance to interference and conflicting instructions, inhibitory control (go–no go test), and environmental dependency. The FAB has been shown to differentiate AD and FTD with high levels of sensitivity (77 %); and specificity (87 %).

There is an increasing interest in disease specific screening tools. These can be designed with the cognitive profile of a specific disease in mind. For example, the Executive and Social Cognitive Battery Screening test for FTD (Torralva et al. 2009) was designed to mirror everyday tasks involving executive function and social cognitive skills (described in more detail in Chap. 7). Other tools take into account not only the cognitive profile of the disease in question but also the disease factors that may confound cognitive testing. For example the Edinburgh Cognitive and Behavioural Assessment Scale or ECAS (Abrahams et al. 2014) was designed to

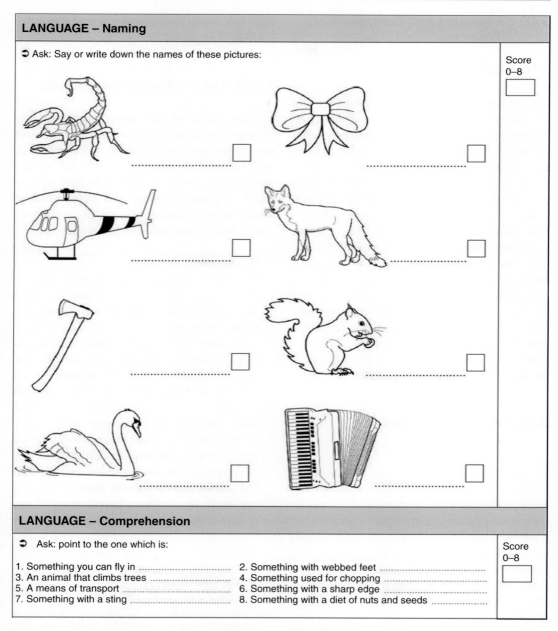

LANGUAGE – Naming

➲ Ask: Say or write down the names of these pictures:

Score
0–8

LANGUAGE – Comprehension

➲ Ask: point to the one which is:

Score
0–8

1. Something you can fly in .... 2. Something with webbed feet ....
3. An animal that climbs trees .... 4. Something used for chopping ....
5. A means of transport .... 6. Something with a sharp edge ....
7. Something with a sting .... 8. Something with a diet of nuts and seeds ....

Fig. 3.5 This is the first page of the Edinburgh Cognitive and Behavioural Assessment Scale (ECAS). All tests in the ECAS were designed to minimize the confounding effect of physical disability

distinguish cognitive deficits typically observed in ALS (executive functions, language, letter fluency, and social cognition) from those often encountered in the aging population and in mild cognitive impairment (e.g. memory). The informant based behavioural questionnaire is focused on behavioural changes frequently reported in ALS. Importantly, the tool sub-tasks were specifically designed to minimize bias due to physical disability, a major confounding factor in the neuropsychological assessment of ALS patients see Fig. 3.5). The value of the ECAS in other motor disorders where disability can confound cognitive performance is under investigation.

3.16 Emerging and Controversial Theories

3.16.1 Cognitive Reserve

The concept of cognitive reserve emerged from the observation that the disease burden on autopsy, such AD type pathology, was a poor predictor of clinical symptoms during life. The hypothesis suggests that individuals with higher initial cognitive abilities, due to engaging in intellectually enriching activities, are able to compensate for the brain insults induced by disease or aging for longer periods of time, thus manifesting cognitive change at later stage. Multiple factors have been postulated to contribute to cognitive reserve including higher premorbid IQ, higher educational attainment, engaging in occupations that place high demands on cognitive function, bilingualism, and having large social networks. Most of the evidence supporting the concept of cognitive reserve comes from AD studies. However, the literature to date is inconsistent and the theory is still subject to considerable debate.

3.16.2 Hebb's Theory and Its Extensions

In its most simplified version Hebb's theory refers to the hypothesis proposed by Donald Hebb in 1949 in which he postulated that persistent or repetitive excitatory activity between two neurons tends to induce permanent lasting changes (structural or biochemical) to the connections between the two neurons, leading to improved efficiency in future communications. The theory is often summarized as "*Cells that fire together, wire together*".

More recently Bak and Chandran extended this theory following the observation that in patients with ALS, a disease characterized by significant motor disability, there is evidence of impairment of verb (as opposed to noun) knowledge in these patients. As brain structures related to words pertaining to motion are likely to be well connected brain structures that initiate the motor aspects of movement, the authors proposed that in neurodegenerative disease spreads along such functional connections ("*neurons that fire together die together*").

3.16.3 The Weakest Link Hypothesis

Mesulam proposes that phenotypic expressions of some neurodegenerative disorders may reflect underlying subtle/subclinical developmental vulnerabilities. This theory is supported by the increased frequency of dyslexia in PPA patients and in their first-degree relatives and proposes to explain how the same genetic defect can manifest with different phenotypes in different kindreds.

Conclusion

Over the last few decades, neuropsychological assessments have been increasingly applied successfully to aid in the clinical diagnosis of neurodegenerative disorders. The unique information provided by these assessments helps to confirm and delineate the cognitive and behavioural changes manifested by patients facilitating accurate diagnoses as well as objectively document progression over time and response to therapy. This chapter provided a review of the process of the NPA, a process which if undertaken correctly, starting with appropriate referrals and ending with valid interpretation of the resultant reports, can result in significant improvement of the quality of care provided to patients.

Further Reading

Abrahams S, Newton J, Niven E, Foley J, Bak TH. Screening for cognition and behaviour changes in ALS. Amyotroph Lateral Scler Frontotemporal Degener. 2014;15(1–2): 9–14. doi:10.3109/21678421.2013.805784. Epub 19 Jun 2013.

Alvarez JA, Eugene Emory E. Executive function and the frontal lobes: a meta-analytic review. Neuropsychol Rev. 2006;16(1):17–42.

Baddeley AD. Working memory. Oxford: Oxford University Press; 1986.

Baddeley A. Working memory: theories, models, and controversies. Annu Rev Psychol. 2012;63:1–29. doi:10.1146/annurev-psych-120710-100422. Epub 27 Sep 2011. Review.

Bak TH, Chandran S. What wires together dies together: verbs, actions and neurodegeneration in motor neuron disease. Cortex. 2012;48(7):936–44.

Chan RC, Shum D, Toulopoulou T, Chen EY. Assessment of executive functions: review of instruments and identification of critical issues. Arch Clin Neuropsychol. 2008;23(2):201–16.

Diamond A. Executive functions. Annu Rev Psychol. 2013;64:135–68. doi:10.1146/annurev-psych-113011-143750. Epub 27 Sep 2012.

Dubois B, Slachevsky A, Litvan I, Pillon B. The FAB: a frontal assessment battery at bedside. Neurology. 2000;55(11):1621–6.

Duke LM, Kaszniak AW. Executive control functions in degenerative dementias: a comparative review. Neuropsychol Rev. 2000;10(2):75–99.

Elamin M, Pender N, Hardiman O, Abrahams S. Social cognition in neurodegenerative disorders: a systematic review. J Neurol Neurosurg Psychiatry. 2012; 83(11):1071–9.

Eustache F, Desgranges B. MNESIS: towards the integration of current multisystem models of memory. Neuropsychol Rev. 2008;18:53–69.

Grace J, Stout JC, Malloy PF. Assessing frontal lobe behavioral syndromes with the frontal lobe personality scale. Assessment. 1999;6:269–84.

Harciarek M, Kertesz A. Primary progressive aphasias and their contribution to the contemporary knowledge about the brain-language relationship. Neuropsychol Rev. 2011;21:271–87.

Harvey PD. Clinical applications of neuropsychological assessment. Dialogues Clin Neurosci. 2012;14(10): 91–9.

Heilman KM. Apraxia. Continuum (Minneap Minn). 2010;16(4 Behavioral Neurology):86–98.

Hillis AE. Naming and language production. Continuum (Minneap Minn). 2010;16(4 Behavioral Neurology): 29–44.

Hsieh S, Schubert S, Hoon C, Mioshi E, Hodges JR. Validation of the Addenbrooke's cognitive examination III in frontotemporal dementia and Alzheimer's disease. Dement Geriatr Cogn Disord. 2013;36(3–4):242–50.

Jurado MB, Rosselli M. The elusive nature of executive functions: a review of our current understanding. Neuropsychol Rev. 2007;17(3):213–33. Epub 5 Sep 2007. Review.

Lowndes G, Savage G. Early detection of memory impairment in Alzheimer's disease: a neurocognitive perspective on assessment. Neuropsychol Rev. 2007;17:193–202.

Martin RC. LANGUAGE PROCESSING: functional organization and neuroanatomical basis. Annu Rev Psychol. 2003;54:55–89.

Mathuranath PS, Nestor PJ, Berrios GE, Rakowicz W, Hodges JR. A brief cognitive test battery to differentiate Alzheimer's disease and frontotemporal dementia. Neurology. 2000;55(11):1613–20.

Mesulam MM, Rogalski EJ, Wieneke C, Hurley RS, Geula C, Bigio EH, Thompson CK, Weintraub S. Primary progressive aphasia and the evolving neurology of the language network. Nat Rev Neurol. 2014;10(10):554–69.

Mioshi E, Dawson K, Mitchell J, Arnold R, Hodges JR. The Addenbrooke's cognitive examination revised (ACE-R): a brief cognitive test battery for dementia screening. Int J Geriatr Psychiatry. 2006;21(11):1078–85.

Nasreddine ZS, Phillips NA, Bédirian V, Charbonneau S, Whitehead V, Collin I, Cummings JL, Chertkow H. The montreal cognitive assessment, MoCA: a brief screening tool for mild cognitive impairment. J Am Geriatr Soc. 2005;53(4):695–9.

Rogalski E, Johnson N, Weintraub S, Mesulam M. Increased frequency of learning disability in patients with primary progressive aphasia and their first-degree relatives. Arch Neurol. 2008;65(2):244–8.

Royal J. Executive functions. Annu Rev Psychol. 2013;64:135–68.

Salmon DP, Bondi MW. Neuropsychological assessment of dementia. Annu Rev Psychol. 2009;60:257–82.

Stuss DT. Functions of the frontal lobes: relation to executive functions. J Int Neuropsychol Soc. 2011;17(5):759–65.

Vakil E. Neuropsychological assessment: principles, rationale, and challenges. J Clin Exp Neuropsychol. 2012;34(2):135–50.

Zigmond AS, Snaith RP. The hospital anxiety and depression scale. Acta Psychiatr Scand. 1983;67:361–70.

Alzheimer's Disease

4

Damien Gallagher, Robert F. Coen,
and Brian A. Lawlor

4.1 Introduction

Alzheimer's disease (AD) is a progressive neuro-degenerative disorder of the brain characterized by an insidious onset of memory impairment, progressive cognitive deterioration, emergence of neuropsychiatric symptoms, and functional decline. Pathologically, it is characterized by the accumulation of amyloid plaques and intraneuronal neurofibrillary tangles, which are associated with neuronal dysfunction and eventual cell death. It is the most common form of dementia accounting for between 50 and 60 % of all cases. The global prevalence of dementia is increasing and it has been projected that the number of people affected will double every 20 years to an estimated 81.1 million by 2040. AD is therefore the most common neurodegenerative disorder affecting between 20 and 30 million individuals worldwide. It is primarily an age-related disorder. The prevalence of dementia is low (approximately 1 %) in individuals aged 60–64 but increases exponentially with age so that in individuals aged 85 years or over, the prevalence in the Western world is between 24 and 33 %. AD has a complex multifactorial etiology and apart from age, genetic and environmental factors play important roles in the onset and progression of disease.

4.2 Risk Factors

4.2.1 Genetic Factors

From a genetic point of view, Alzheimer's disease is a heterogeneous disorder with both familial and sporadic forms. The vast majority of Alzheimer's disease is sporadic and of late onset (≥65 years), while a small proportion of all cases (<2 %) may inherit the disease in autosomal dominant fashion. These variants are generally of early onset (<65 years). Autosomal dominant forms are mostly related to mutations in one of three genes: amyloid precursor protein gene (APP) on chromosome 21, presenilin 1 gene (PS1) on chromosome 14, and presenilin 2 gene (PS2) on chromosome 1 (Table 4.1). PS1 accounts for the majority of mutations while APP and PS2 mutations occur less frequently. All of these

D. Gallagher (✉)
Geriatric Psychiatry, Sunnybrook Health Sciences Centre, University of Toronto, Toronto, ON, Canada
e-mail: damien.gallagher@sunnybrook.ca

R.F. Coen
Memory Clinic, Mercer's Institute on Aging, Dublin, Ireland

St. James's Hospital, Dublin, Ireland
e-mail: rcoen@stjames.ie

B.A. Lawlor
St. James's Hospital, Dublin, Ireland

Department of Psychiatry, Trinity College Dublin, Dublin, Ireland
e-mail: BLAWLOR@stjames.ie

© Springer International Publishing Switzerland 2016
O. Hardiman, C.P. Doherty (eds.), *Neurodegenerative Disorders: A Clinical Guide*,
DOI 10.1007/978-3-319-23309-3_4

Table 4.1 Established Alzheimer's genes and their functional relevance

Gene (protein)	Chromosome	Inheritance	Role in AD pathogenesis
APP (amyloid precursor protein)	21	Autosomal dominant	Mutations in the APP gene promote cleavage at b or g sites leading to overproduction of Aβ
PSEN1 (presenilin 1)	14	Autosomal dominant	Mutations in the PS1 gene promote cleavage at the g site leading to overproduction of Aβ
PSEN2 (presenilin 2)	1	Autosomal dominant	Mutations in the PS2 gene promote cleavage at the g site leading to overproduction of Aβ
APOE (apolipoprotein E)	19	Modifies age of onset	Promotes the deposition of Aβ?

genes impact upon the production of the beta amyloid protein (Aß), which is the principal component of senile plaques hypothesized to play a central role in the evolution of Alzheimer's pathology. The vast majority of AD patients, however, have sporadic late-onset disease, which has a complex etiology attributed to interactions between environmental risk factors and individual genetic susceptibilities. Twin studies have estimated the heritability of late-onset sporadic AD to be approximately 76 %.

The most well-established genetic risk factor for late-onset AD is the apolipoprotein E gene (APOE). Three APOE alleles have been identified: e2, e3, and e4. The APOE e4 allele has been linked to the development of AD, whilst epidemiologic as well as pathologic studies have suggested a possible protective effect for the e2 allele. There is an apparent gene-dosing effect according to the actual genotype. One meta-analysis reported the odds of developing AD in heterozygous carriers of the APOE e4 allele as threefold, while the odds for homozygous carriers was almost 15-fold.

The APOE e4 allele operates mainly by decreasing the age of onset with each allele copy lowering the age of onset by almost 10 years. It is therefore a marker of susceptibility rather than a determinative gene. The mechanism whereby APOEe4 influences the development of AD is complex and may be modified by other genes and environmental factors. APOE acts as a cholesterol transporter in the brain, which mediates neuronal protection and repair and is believed to participate in early Aß deposition. The APOE e4 allele has been associated with increased severity of illness including faster cognitive decline, increased risk of conversion from mild cognitive impairment to AD, more neuropsychiatric symptoms, decreased survival time, and increased amyloid load at autopsy. The use of APOE genotype as a diagnostic tool has been examined in several studies but low sensitivity and specificity limit its usefulness and it is not currently recommended for diagnostic use. Table 4.1 summarizes established Alzheimer's genes and their functional relevance.

Although the APOE e4 allele has been calculated to account for most of the genetic risk in late-onset alzheimer's disease, a number of candidate genes of smaller effect have also been identified. The advent of large Genome Wide Association Studies (GWAS) has allowed identification of several genes of small effect and findings are collated in the online AlzGene database which allows researchers to compare results and search for consistency between international groups. It is hypothesised that genetic mutations of modest effect in concert with other genetic and environmental factors, may precipitate clinical disease in vulnerable individuals. For example, variant of genes for CLU (clusterin/apolipoprotein J), CR1 (complement receptor 1), and PICALM (phosphatidylinositol-binding clathrin assembly protein) have achieved genome-wide significance in independent GWAS studies. These genetic variants may be involved in reduced clearance of Aß. It is hoped that improved understanding of underlying mechanisms of action may lead to new therapeutic targets to delay the onset and progression of disease.

4.2.2 Lifestyle and Vascular Risk Factors

Although several AD risk factors are genetic in nature, others are determined by environmental or lifestyle influences and may be amenable to modification. Recent years have seen an expansion in the number of epidemiological studies in AD and several risk factors that were traditionally considered as "vascular" have been associated with increased risk of AD (Table 4.2). Longitudinal studies such as the Cardiovascular Risk Factors, Aging, and Dementia (CAIDE) study have found midlife hypertension, hypercholesterolemia, and obesity to be associated with increased risk of dementia and AD in later life.

Clustering of risk factors was observed to increase the risk in an additive fashion. A dementia risk score using data gathered during the CAIDE study predicted dementia with a sensitivity of 0.77, specificity of 0.63, and negative predictive value of 0.98 over 20 years of follow up. This score included variables such as age ($\geq$47 years), low education (<10 years), hypertension, hypercholesterolemia, and obesity. There is now a great deal of interest in developing approaches to help reduce the risk of AD in later life through identifying individuals who

Table 4.2 Potentially modifiable risk factors found to be associated with Alzheimer's disease in population studies

Risk factors for Alzheimer's disease	Protective factors for Alzheimer's disease
Hypertension/hypotension	Physical activity
Obesity	Cognitive and social stimulation
Diabetes mellitus	Diet (fish consumption > once/week)
Hypercholesterolemia	Alcohol (light to moderate intake)
Hyperhomocysteinemia	Higher educational status (>15 year vs. <12 year)
Stroke	Purpose in life and conscientiousness
Smoking	Social engagement
Depression, distress, and loneliness	
Sleep disturbances	

might benefit from intensive lifestyle consultations and pharmacological interventions in earlier life. However, not all studies have replicated these findings and one systematic review concluded that the evidence for single clinically defined vascular risk factors was inconsistent at best while the strength of the association was increased by identifying interactions between risk factors such as hypertension and diabetes. In addition, the relationship between cognition and blood pressure is complex with hypertension in midlife and hypotension in later life both associated with increased risk of AD. Although initial case control studies reported a protective effect for smoking, longitudinal studies have now established that smoking is associated with increased risk of AD. Longitudinal studies show that stroke increases the subsequent risk of AD and hyperhomocysteinemia has similarly been reported to increase risk.

Other factors, that have been reported to be protective from population studies, include regular fish consumption, moderate wine intake, and higher educational status. There is also now a significant amount of epidemiological data, which suggests that individuals who are more socially and physically active and engage in more cognitively stimulating activities are at decreased risk of developing dementia and AD. In fact, a recent review concluded that after accounting for non-independence between risk factors, around a third of Alzheimer's diseases cases worldwide might be attributed to potentially modifiable risk factors. Psychological risk factors are also important. In particular, depression has been found to behave as both a risk factor for and prodromal symptom of AD. Late onset depression may occur as part of the prodrome of early AD but depression, which occurs decades in advance of cognitive decline, is also known to increase risk of AD in a dose-dependent fashion. Psychological distress and loneliness have similarly been reported to increase risk. A number of mechanisms for the association between depression and AD have been proposed. Depression has been independently associated with increased risk of cerebrovascular disease and the chronic neurotoxic effects of elevated glucocorticoids upon hippocampal neurogenesis and repair may also diminish cognitive reserve. Finally, depression may have a more direct neuropathological effect as stress and exogenous glucocorticoids have been shown to increase β-amyloid production in animal models of AD. Having a greater sense of purpose in life and conscientiousness appear to be protective and have both been independently associated with reduced risk of AD. Sleep disturbances, particularly reduced sleep duration, sleep fragmentation, and sleep-disordered breathing, have been implicated as potentially remediable causes of cognitive decline. However, further research is needed to better define the nature of these associations and determine mechanisms which might allow further exploration of preventive and therapeutic strategies. There are already many good reasons why maintaining good psychological health and promoting a physically, cognitively, and socially active lifestyle may be advisable and beneficial for patients.

4.2.3   Other Risk Factors

Data from epidemiological studies reported an association between nonsteroidal anti-inflammatory (NSAID) use and decreased risk of AD while interventional studies in this area have been negative to date. Lipid-lowering medications have similarly been reported to be associated with decreased risk while interventional studies of statins have been largely negative to date. Hormone replacement therapy (HRT) was associated with decreased risk of AD while an interventional study reported an increased risk of dementia, again highlighting the caution with which observational findings must be interpreted. Severe head injury and exposure to toxins such as defoliants and fumigants have been associated with increased risk. Static risk factors include a family history of trisomy 21. Female gender has also been associated with increased prevalence AD. There are many possible reasons for this variable observation although a number of investigators have concluded that it is due to the longer life expectancy in females rather than gender-specific risk factors for the disease.

4.2.4   Pathogenesis

The exact cellular mechanisms leading to neuronal cell death in AD remain uncertain but multiple etiological and pathogenetic hypotheses have been put forward. Macroscopically, the brain in established AD shows a variable degree of cortical atrophy with widening of cerebral sulci and compensatory ventricular enlargement. Microscopically, the disease is characterized by amyloid plaques and neurofibrillary tangles (Fig. 4.1). The current criteria for a pathologic diagnosis of AD require the presence of both amyloid plaques and neurofibrillary tangles in excess of that anticipated for age-matched healthy controls. Amyloid plaques consist of a central core of amyloid protein surrounded by astrocytes, microglia, and dystrophic neurites. Neurofibrillary tangles contain paired helical filaments of abnormally phosphorylated tau protein that occupy the cell body and extend into the dendrites. Neuronal loss or atrophy in the nucleus basalis, locus ceruleus, and raphe nuclei of the brainstem leads to deficits in cholinergic, noradrenergic, and serotonergic transmitters, respectively. The deficit in cholinergic neurotransmission and the observation that this correlated strongly with the degree of cognitive impairment led to the "cholinergic hypothesis" of AD and the subsequent development of cholinesterase inhibitors to redress this deficit.

4.2.5   Amyloid Hypothesis

The amyloid hypothesis remains the best-defined and most studied conceptual framework for AD (Fig. 4.2). Over time, this hypothesis has undergone alterations primarily due to the fact that increased beta amyloid protein (Ab) and plaque formation are no longer considered to be sole triggering factors for deleterious events leading to AD. The exact cellular mechanisms leading to neuronal cell death in AD remain uncertain. The amyloid cascade hypothesis holds that an imbalance between Ab production and clearance plays a critical role in progression of AD. Ab is derived from the much larger transmembrane

Fig. 4.1 Low power (**a**) and high power (**b**) views of hippocampus with neuritic amyloid plaques (*P*), which consist of a central core of amyloid protein surrounded by astrocytes, microglia, and dystrophic neurites and neurofibrillary tangles (*T*), which contain paired helical filaments of abnormally phosphorylated tau protein. The current criteria for the histopathological diagnosis of Alzheimer's disease require the presence of both entities

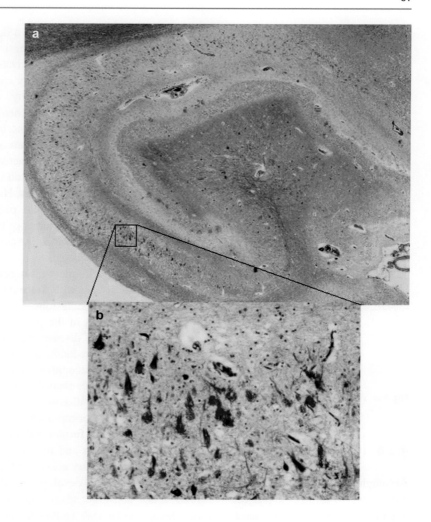

protein, amyloid precursor protein (APP), by the action of two proteases referred to as beta (b) and gamma (g) secretase. The initial cleavage of APP is mediated by b secretase and then, depending on the exact point of cleavage by g secretase, three principle forms of Ab comprising 38, 40, or 42 amino acid residues, respectively are produced. Most mutations in the APP or presenilin genes alter APP processing resulting in increased levels of Ab. At a certain critical concentration, Ab monomers associate to form neurotoxic oligomers, which then further associate into insoluble fibrils and are deposited as amyloid plaques. The relative amount of Ab 42 formed is important as this longer form of Ab is more prone to aggregate and form oligomers. Ab oligomers could directly inhibit hippocampal long-term potentiation and

impair synaptic function in addition to the inflammatory and oxidative stress caused by aggregated and deposited Ab. Much is yet to be learned about the formation and toxicity of these soluble forms of Ab and how they may trigger deleterious changes. The central significance of Ab in the pathogenesis of AD has recently been called into question given negative outcomes from trials of therapeutic agents targeting this pathway. A more current view of the amyloid cascade hypothesis is that other events as well as Ab are important in triggering degenerative processes. The concept of Ab as only one of the factors that causes AD, explains it's less than perfect correlation with disease severity and it seems increasingly likely that Ab, although necessary, is not by itself, sufficient for AD to occur.

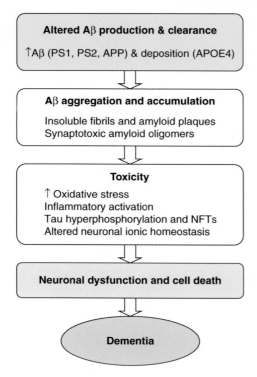

Fig. 4.2 Amyloid cascade hypothesis

4.2.6   Other Proposed Mechanisms

Although amyloid has received much attention with regard to halting the progression of AD, it is not the only target for disease-modifying therapies. Neurofibrillary tangles, which consist of aggregations of hyperphosphorylated tau protein, are another pathologic hallmark of AD. Tau binds to and stabilizes microtubules that are elongated polymers intrinsic to axonal structure and function. When tau is hyperphosphorylated, it aggregates into tangles with resulting destabilization of microtubules and compromised neuronal function. It is unclear whether neurofibrillary tangles are a cause or consequence of AD but their formation may be critical to AD-related cell death. Inflammatory mechanisms have long been known to play an important role in the evolution of AD pathology and many studies have shown a broad variety of inflammatory mediators, including acute phase proteins, cytokines, and chemokines within the vicinity of AD plaques. Neuroinflammation is

still considered to be a downstream consequence in the amyloid hypothesis whereby Ab within the CNS brings about activation of microglia, initiating a proinflammatory cascade that results in the release of potentially neurotoxic substances, including cytokines, chemokines, reactive oxygen and nitrogen species, and various proteolytic enzymes, leading to neurodegeneration. It has also been suggested that activation of microglia may lead to phosphorylation of tau and formation of neurofibrillary tangles. However, the exact role of inflammation in the pathology of AD and its mechanisms in terms of the cells involved, which include microglia, astrocytes, and T lymphocytes are still debated.

The frequent co-occurrence of cerebrovascular disease with AD and the fact that fewer neuropathologic lesions of AD appear to result in dementia in the presence of comorbid cerebrovascular disease has been well documented (as per the landmark Nun cohort study). In fact, it is now recognized that mixed pathology is the rule rather than the exception and that cerebrovascular disease is clinically under-recognized and under-reported. The vascular hypothesis of AD goes further and proposes that cerebral hypoperfusion and microvascular pathology may be the primary etiological factor in AD. It proposes that AD develops when two biological events converge; advancing age and the presence of vascular risk factors to create a critically attained threshold of cerebral hypoperfusion (CATCH). This leads to dysregulation of endothelial nitric oxide (NO) production, capillary degeneration, and mitochondrial oxidative stress. The resulting crisis leads to cellular and subcellular pathology involving protein synthesis, development of plaques, inflammatory response, and synaptic damage leading to the manifestations of AD.

4.2.7   Clinical Features

The typical clinical presentation of AD is that of insidious progressive impairment of episodic memory representing early involvement of medial temporal lobe structures with the emergence of additional deficits such as aphasia, apraxia, agnosia, and executive deficits as the disease progresses. Findings from longitudinal studies indicate that neuropsychological deficits in multiple cognitive domains are evident several years in advance of a diagnosis of AD. One meta-analysis reported that the largest deficits in pre-clinical AD exist in the domains of perceptual speed, executive functioning, and episodic memory with smaller deficits in the domains of verbal ability, visuospatial skills, and attention. This is characterized clinically by initial forgetfulness for daily events with progressive involvement of language skills, decision making, judgment, orientation, recognition, and motor skills. Neuropsychiatric symptoms are frequently observed and occur in 60–98 % of patients with dementia. They are a significant source of distress for patients and families and a major determinant of outcomes such as length of hospital stay and nursing home placement. They ordinarily increase with increasing disease severity but are observed early in the disease process and have been documented in 30–75 % of patients with mild cognitive impairment. Apathy, anxiety, depression, and agitation occur most frequently. Delusions are also common and include themes of theft, intruders, imposters, or other ideas of persecution, reference, or infidelity. Visual and auditory hallucinations are the most common perceptual abnormalities although somatic, olfactory, and tactile hallucinations have also been reported. Functional decline starts with the impairment of higher order (instrumental) functions, such as the management of the house-hold affairs or finances before more gross functions relating to basic self-care are affected. Atypical presentations of AD occur in approximately 6–14 % of cases and are more prevalent in those with younger onset disease. Atypical presentations have been divided into a number of variants including a frontal variant, which may present with executive dysfunction or behavioural symptoms and is difficult to distinguish clinically from frontotemporal dementia. There is also a logopenic variant where there is more prominent impairment of language and a posterior variant where deficits in visuospatial function predominate. These presentations remain relatively uncommon,

particularly in late onset disease, where the typical clinical course is one of insidious episodic memory decline with progressive involvement of other cognitive skills as outlined above.

4.2.8 Mild Cognitive Impairment

Neurodegeneration is estimated to start 20–30 years before clinical onset. During this pre-clinical phase, the burden of plaque and tangle pathology gradually increases until the threshold for clinical expression is reached. Mild Cognitive Impairment (MCI) is a clinical classification of patients who manifest cognitive deficits in excess of that expected for normal aging but who do not have significant functional impairment.

The initial diagnostic criteria specified the presence of subjective and objective deficits in memory, with the purpose of detecting patients with the earliest clinical signs of Alzheimer's pathology for recruitment to clinical trials. Patients in these studies were observed to convert to Alzheimer's disease at a rate of approximately 10–15 % annually. The diagnostic criteria have since been broadened to include patients with deficits in domains other than memory, to reflect the heterogeneity of both progressive and non-progressive pathologies represented within this classification. Patients with amnestic deficits in addition to deficits in other domains have the greatest risk of progression to Alzheimer's disease. Significant variation in rates of conversion to Alzheimer's disease has been observed depending on the diagnostic criteria used and populations investigated. A recent review of longer-term follow-up studies (5 years or more) indicated that the annual conversion rate of 10–15 % only held true in samples monitored over a short observation period and that the conversion rate was highest shortly after presentation with a marked decline in subsequent years. The authors reported an average cumulative conversion rate of 31.4 % over a mean observation period of 6 years in a sample, which included patients derived from both clinic and community populations. Reported variations in conversion to AD likely reflect variations in the underlying aetiology with conversion rates at the higher end of the range anticipated in individuals with MCI due to AD.

4.2.9 Diagnosis and Revised Diagnostic Criteria

Regarding the diagnosis of Alzheimer's disease there have been two conceptually overlapping but differing revisions of the National Institute of Neurologic and Communicative Disorders and Stroke – Alzheimer's Disease and Related Disorders Association (NINCDS-ADRDA) criteria. One developed etc by the International Working Group (IWG) for new Research Criteria for the Diagnosis of Alzheimer's Disease (AD), the other by the National Institute on Aging – Alzheimer's Association (NIA-AA) workgroups on diagnostic guidelines for Alzheimer's disease. Both revisions incorporate biomarkers but differ in how this information is used. Biomarkers are a core requirement in the IWG criteria which are research diagnostic criteria. The NIA-AA revision provides different sets of diagnostic criteria for the different stages of AD, namely the asymptomatic preclinical phase, the symptomatic pre-dementia phase (mild cognitive impairment due to AD), and the dementia phase. The NIA-AA pre-dementia and dementia criteria can be clinically applied even in the absence of biomarkers which are incorporated on a basis of increased or decreased likelihood. Both the NIA-AA criteria and more recently revised IWG criteria (IWG-2) address the issue of atypical presentations of AD which can present as a posterior variant (occipitotemporal or biparietal subtypes), a logopenic (language prominent) variant, or a frontal variant. The IWG-2 criteria outline criteria for diagnosis of typical, atypical and mixed presentations of the disease.

The IWG research criteria differ from previous criteria in that they do not require the presence of significant functional decline to diagnose Alzheimer's disease given the increasing emphasis on identifying patients in the early clinical or preclinical stages of the disease for recruitment to clinical trials. In contrast, the NIA-AA approach retains the NINCDS-ADRDA two-step approach to the diagnosis of dementia due to AD in which there is initial identification of a dementia syndrome and then the application of criteria based on the clinical features of the AD phenotype. It is important that disorders, which may mimic a dementia syndrome such as delirium or depression, are first excluded. A detailed history of the clinical features and longitudinal course as outlined above should be elicited. This is best obtained from a reliable informant, given the patient's judgment and insight is frequently impaired. The symptom profile will help distinguish Alzheimer's disease from other dementia syndromes such as vascular, Lewy body, or frontotemporal dementia. A general neurological and physical examination should be performed to both exclude comorbid medical conditions, which may have an adverse effect on cognitive function and detect other neurological disorders. The neurological examination is ordinarily unremarkable in early AD but focal neurological or atypical features may be an indicator of pathologies such as normal pressure hydrocephalus, neoplasm, Parkinson's plus syndromes, or motor neuron disease, and should prompt appropriate referral. Motor or sensory abnormalities or disturbance of gait and seizures are uncommon until the later stages of the disease. A mental state examination should detect the presence of mood or anxiety symptoms, which can mimic or complicate cognitive decline. This also provides an opportunity to exclude psychotic symptoms such as delusions or perceptual abnormalities. Neuropsychiatric symptoms must be enquired for as they may not be disclosed by patients or caregivers until they become intolerable or precipitate a crisis. A number of instruments have been designed to quantify the frequency and severity of neuropsychiatric symptoms in patients with AD such as the Neuropsychiatric Inventory (NPI) and Behavioral pathology in Alzheimer's disease (BEHAVE-AD) rating scale. Function should equally be assessed through the use of structured questionnaires of basic activities of daily living (ADL) such as feeding and toileting and instrumental activities of daily living (IADL) such as shopping, cooking, managing finances, and

Table 4.3 Summary of NIA-AA and IWG-2 research criteria for probable and typical presentations of AD

NIA-AA criteria	Revised research criteria (IWG-2)

Criteria for probable AD
1. Must meet criteria for dementia
  A. Insidious onset
  B. History of worsening of cognition by report or observation.
  C. The initial & most prominent cognitive deficits are evident on history & examination in one of the following categories
    (a) Amnestic presentation: with evidence of cognitive dysfunction in at least one other cognitive domain
    (b) Non-amnestic presentations: could be language, visuospatial or dysexecutive presentation with dysfunction in other cognitive domains.
  D. The diagnosis of probable AD dementia should not be applied when there is evidence of other contributory pathology (e.g. substantial cerebrovascular disease, core features of dementia with Lewy bodies & others)
	Criteria for typical AD (A plus B at any stage)
	  A. Specific clinical phenotype
	    Presence of an early and significant episodic memory impairment (isolated or associated with other cognitive or behavioural changes that are suggestive of a mild cognitive impairment or of a dementia syndrome) that includes the following features:
	    Gradual and progressive change in memory function reported by patient or informant over more than 6 months
	    Objective evidence of an amnestic syndrome of the hippocampal type, based on significantly impaired performance on an episodic memory test with established specificity for AD, such as cued recall with control of encoding test.
	  B. In-vivo evidence of Alzheimer's pathology (one of the following)
	    Decreased Aβ1–42 together with increased T-tau or P-tau in CSF
	    Increased tracer retention on amyloid PET
	    AD autosomal dominant mutation present (in PSEN1, PSEN2, or APP)
	Exclusion criteria: An atypical history, atypical clinical features or other medical conditions severe enough to account for memory & related symptoms.

medication. More complex instrumental functions are typically impaired in the earlier stages. The extent of cognitive testing will be determined by the clinical context and presentation as outlined below.

Regarding biomarkers these include atrophy of medial temporal lobe structures determined through qualitative or quantitative MRI ratings, abnormal concentrations of amyloid beta 42 and total/phospho-tau in cerebrospinal fluid, hypometabolism (typically temporoparietal in AD) on positron emission tomography (FDG PET) and determination of amyloid load using amyloid binding PET ligands such as Pittsburgh compound B (PIB). IWG-2 draws a distinction between Diagnostic (pathophysiological) markers which reflect in-vivo pathology (amyloid beta 42 and total/phospho-tau in csf; amyloid binding PET) and Progression (topographic or downstream) markers which indicate clinical severity (staging marker) and might not be present in the early stages. Their refined criteria for AD require the presence of Diagnostic markers (Table 4.3).

Amyloid beta 42 is reduced in the CSF of AD patients (possibly as a result of deposition of the protein in senile plaques) and tau is increased (possibly a reflection of the release of tau in CSF with neuronal loss). The determination of optimal thresholds for detecting incipient AD according to CSF concentrations of amyloid beta 42 and total tau/phospho-tau continues to be refined. Three large multicenter studies (ADNI, DESCRIPTA, SBP) have confirmed that the combination of amyloid beta 42 with either tau or phospho-tau has the highest predictive accuracy for AD.

4.3 Investigations

4.3.1 Cognitive Testing

The extent and the type of cognitive testing to be undertaken will be determined by the clinical context and presentation. The Mini Mental State Examination (MMSE) is one of the best known and simplest bedside cognitive tests to administer. It takes 5–10 min to complete and is a useful measure of global cognitive function. A total score of 23 or less out of a possible perfect score of 30 is considered dementia, but it is important to note that thresholds vary according to age and education. In an educated population, an MMSE cut-off of 26 or below should raise suspicion of dementia, as this is the cut-off utilized in more recent research studies. The MMSE may not be sensitive to very subtle cognitive impairment, but can be useful as a general screening tool or to monitor performance over time. The MMSE declines by approximately 2.8 points per year in patients with Alzheimer's disease, with a slower decline in the milder stages and faster decline in the moderate to severe stages of the disease. The Montreal Cognitive Assessment (MOCA) is a more recently developed widely used screening test with a similar 30-point format to the MMSE. It includes additional tests of visuo-spatial and executive function, which make it more sensitive in patients with mild cognitive impairment. Other lengthier tests of global cognitive function include the Addenbrookes Cognitive Examination (ACE-III), Cambridge Cognitive Examination (CAMCOG-R), Alzheimer's Disease Assessment Scale – Cognitive (ADAS-Cog) and Mattis Dementia Rating Scale (DRS-2). Patients with minor impairments, high levels of educational attainment, or atypical clinical features can perform deceptively well on bedside tests and may require more comprehensive assessment in specialist centers. Measures of free recall, particularly verbal recall, have consistently been shown to be impaired in the earliest clinical stages of Alzheimer's disease and predict early conversion from mild cognitive impairment. Predictive accuracy may be increased by combining tests of free recall with tests of executive function, processing speed, and semantic fluency.

4.3.2 Blood Tests

The bloods tests, which are routinely ordered as part of a cognitive screen include full blood count, B12/folate, renal/liver/bone profile, and thyroid function tests. This may be supplemented by screening for vascular risk factors with a fasting lipid profile and fasting glucose. Syphilis serology may be requested but is not routinely screened in many centers depending on the risk profile of the patient. Nonspecific markers of inflammation,

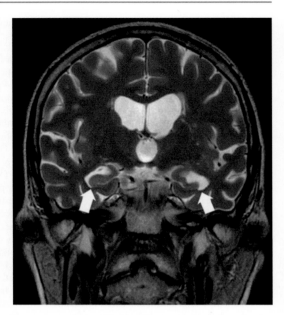

Fig. 4.3 Alzheimer's disease. Coronal T2-weighted fast spin echo (FSE) sequence. Note the pattern of generalized atrophy with preferential involvement of the medial temporal lobes (hippocampi) bilaterally (*arrows*). There is little or no white matter disease indicating a reasonably pure form of plaque and tangle disease

such as ESR or CRP may be helpful where infective or inflammatory diseases are suspected.

4.3.3 Neuroimaging

Structural neuroimaging should be used in the evaluation of every patient suspected of dementia. Non-contrast CT can be used to identify surgically treatable lesions and vascular disease. MRI (with a protocol, including T1, T2, or FLAIR sequences, and susceptibility weighted sequences) can increase sensitivity for subcortical vascular contributions to cognitive decline and exclude other intracranial pathology or identify regional atrophy. Atrophic changes in medial temporal lobe structures such as the entorhinal cortex and hippocampus, as well as in parietal cortices may be seen on neuroimaging, which may become more marked and generalized as the disease advances (Fig. 4.3). However, volumetric changes may be minimal or absent in the very early stages of Alzheimer's disease. Functional neuroimaging with positron emission tomography (PET) or

Table 4.4 Summary characteristics of the cholinesterase inhibitors

	Mechanism of action	Common adverse effects	Starting dose	Usual treatment dose
Donepezil	Acetylcholinesterase inhibitor	Nausea/vomiting/insomnia/diarrhea	5 mg od. (p.o.)	10 mg od. (p.o.)
Galantamine	Acetylcholinesterase inhibitor and modulates presynaptic nicotinic receptors	Nausea/vomiting/insomnia/diarrhea	4 mg bd or 8 mg XL od. (p.o.)	12 mg bd or 24 mg XL od. (p.o.)
Rivastigmine	Acetylcholinesterase and butyrylcholinesterase inhibitor	Nausea/vomiting/insomnia/diarrhea	1.5 mg bd (p.o.) or 4.6 mg od (top)	6 mg bd (p.o.) or 9.5 mg od (top)

single photon emission computed tomography (SPECT) may usefully augment structural imaging where uncertainty exists regarding the clinical features and presentation. A reduction in blood flow or glucose hypometabolism in temporoparietal areas is most commonly described in AD. The use of amyloid PET scans has been largely confined to research settings to date although with increasing availability and standardization of methods this may play a greater role over time.

4.3.4 Other Investigations

Electroencephalography (EEG) may be a useful adjunct and should be included in the diagnostic workup of patients suspected of having Creutzfeldt–Jakob disease or transient epileptic amnesia. CSF analysis is mandatory when inflammatory disease, vasculitis, or demyelination is suspected. The use of CSF biomarkers such as amyloid beta 42, total tau and phospho-tau has been largely confined to clinical research settings to date with considerable variability in results between laboratories. However, with improved standardization of methods and publication of consensus criteria, CSF biomarkers are likely to play a greater role, and are increasingly recommended in young onset and atypical presentations.

4.4 Management

4.4.1 Cognitive Symptoms

Acetylcholinesterase inhibitors are currently the mainstay of pharmacological therapy for Alzheimer's disease. The acetylcholinesterase inhibitors in use are donepezil, galantamine, and rivastigmine, which act to increase cholinergic neurotransmission through inhibition of the enzyme, acetylcholinesterase. The three compounds have certain unique pharmacological properties although no difference in efficacy between the three medications has been consistently demonstrated. Prescriber choice is ordinarily determined by side effect profile and individual familiarity (Table 4.4). Donepezil and galantamine are selective acetylcholinesterase inhibitors while rivastigmine inhibits acetylcholinesterase and butyrylcholinesterase with similar affinity. Galantamine also allosterically modulates presynaptic nicotinic receptors. The efficacy of these medications has been studied in over 30 randomized double-blind clinical trials and they have been shown to have a treatment effect on average of 2.5–3.5 points on the Alzheimer's disease assessment scale, cognitive subscale (ADAS-Cog, range 0–70) over 6 months compared with patients receiving placebo. There is some variability between studies but approximately twice as many patients who receive a cholinesterase inhibitor have a 4-point difference on the ADAS-Cog (25–50 % vs. 15–25 %) and approximately three times as many patients who receive a cholinesterase inhibitor have a 7-point difference (12–20 % vs. 2–6 %) on the ADAS-Cog compared to those taking placebo. A 7-point difference is equivalent to slowing the symptoms by approximately 1 year and more patients have less decline rather than a measurable improvement in symptoms. It is important to discuss this point with patients and their families who may anticipate improvement rather than a reduction in the rate of decline.

A Cochrane review concluded that donepezil, rivastigmine, and galantamine are efficacious in mild-to-moderate Alzheimer's disease and that treatment benefits included small improvements on measures of activities of daily living and behavior in addition to cognitive measures. There is nothing to suggest that the effects are less for patients with severe dementia although there fewer studies in this regard. More recently, a study which randomized patients with moderate to severe AD who had been stable on donepezil to either continue or discontinue the treatment found a functional and cognitive advantage for those who continued donepezil.

Overall, these medications are well tolerated and adverse effects such as nausea, vomiting, or diarrhea are most frequently reported. This can ordinarily be avoided by starting at a low dose, which is then titrated upward. Coadministration with food also delays absorption and can reduce gastrointestinal side effects. Rivastigmine is available as a daily patch, which has a more favorable gastrointestinal side effect profile than oral rivastigmine. Other important possible adverse effects to consider include cholinergically mediated exacerbation of chronic obstructive pulmonary disease, peptic ulcers, or atrioventricular conduction abnormalities. Both donepezil and galantamine are metabolized by the cytochrome P450 enzymes, CYP2D6 and CYP3A4, and can thus interact with drugs that inhibit these enzymes. Rivastigmine has less potential for interaction given that it is metabolized at the site of action and does not have a hepatic metabolism.

A beneficial response to a cholinesterase inhibitor may be determined by the clinician's global assessment of cognitive, functional, and behavioral symptoms taking into account the report of the primary caregiver. Observation for up to 6 months may be necessary to assess for potential benefit. Brief tests of cognitive function may be relatively insensitive to the cognitive effects of acetylcholinesterase inhibitors. Medication should be discontinued if it is poorly tolerated or if deterioration continues at the pretreatment rate. There is some evidence that patients who either do not tolerate or respond to one cholinesterase inhibitor may benefit from another. It is important to note that acetylcholinesterase inhibitors are a symptomatic treatment and do not alter the underlying neurodegenerative process which is progressive.

Acetylcholinesterase inhibitors have been used in a number of interventional studies to see if they can delay transition to Alzheimer's dementia in patients with mild cognitive impairment. There is currently little compelling evidence to recommend their use in such patients given that the majority of studies to date have failed to meet their primary efficacy objectives. One group reported delayed progression to Alzheimer's disease over 12 months but not over 3 years, while another noted a small beneficial effect on cognition, which did not translate into improved function. Various explanations for these largely negative findings have been proposed, including the heterogeneity of patients under study, the possibility that there is simply less cholinergic dysfunction in patients with mild cognitive impairment, or that current outcome measures are insufficiently sensitive to changes in patients with mild disease.

Memantine is a noncompetitive NMDA receptor antagonist, which is believed to protect neurons from glutamate-mediated excitotoxicity, which may occur in Alzheimer's disease. Memantine has been shown to have a small beneficial effect on measures of cognition, function, and behavior in moderate-to-severe Alzheimer's disease with a barely detectable clinical effect in patients with milder disease. Memantine is generally well tolerated with few adverse events. There is conflicting evidence regarding whether the addition of memantine to donepezil in patients with moderate-to-severe disease may yield additional symptomatic benefit. Despite the theoretically neuroprotective properties of memantine, it is felt that current drug trials are too short to assess if the drug has any disease-modifying effects.

4.4.2 Neuropsychiatric Symptoms (See Also Chap. 12)

Neuropsychiatric symptoms (NPS) occur in approximately 80 % of individuals with dementia during the course of the disease. Neuropsychiatric symptoms (NPS) are distressing for the patient, lead to increased caregiver stress and are associated with greater likelihood of institutional care and increased costs. Non-pharmacological interventions are ordinarily first line and should be exhausted before pharmacological approaches are considered. The type of neuropsychiatric symptoms together with their frequency, diurnal pattern, and identifiable triggers or reinforcers should be documented. A number of instruments have been designed to quantify the frequency and severity of NPS including the neuropsychiatric inventory, the behavioural pathology in AD scale and Cohen-Mansfield agitation inventory among others. Accurate documentation of frequency, severity and relevant triggers will help in the formulation of a tailored and targeted treatment approach. A person-centred care approach which aims to understand the reasons for the behavior from the patient's perspective are central to any intervention. First, consider unmet medical needs, such as pain, delirium, or a recent change in medication. Environmental and psychosocial factors, which increase the likelihood of behavioral disturbance, include overcrowding, lack of privacy, noise, or poor communication between carers and patients. Orientation through the use of a memory book, family photographs, and a calendar around the patient's bed can help decrease agitation. Motor disturbances may alternately be an expression of discomfort, fear, paranoia, or simply boredom. Education for carers regarding the behavioral management of such symptoms is helpful and should be considered as part of an initial treatment approach.

Pharmacological treatments are only helpful for specific symptoms and their use should be targeted (discussed in more detail in Chap. 12). There is some evidence to support the use of antidepressant medication for the treatment of depression in Alzheimer's disease although there have also been a number of negative studies and symptoms may sometimes resolve with other supportive measures. When an antidepressant is chosen, SSRIs are generally favored and medications such as older tricyclic agents are generally avoided. Benzodiazepines should generally be avoided except for short term or occasional use for anxiety symptoms and should be limited to shorter acting agents. Cholinesterase inhibitors have not been associated with notable improvement of NPS and there are conflicting findings regarding memantine with a number of negative studies. There is some emerging evidence that certain SSRIs such as citalopram may reduce agitation in AD and further studies in this area are required.

The best-studied pharmacologic agents for NPS are antipsychotic medications and there is evidence to support the use of risperidone, olanzapine and aripiprazole for agitation and aggression in AD. However, antipsychotic medications have been associated with increased risk of cerebrovascular events, mortality and cognitive decline limiting their use to circumstances where alternate approaches have been ineffective and there is severe distress or risk. It is important to obtain informed consent where possible, discuss the risks/benefits with the next of kin and document the relevant considerations before starting such a medication. Medication should be reviewed regularly and discontinued if the risks outweigh the benefits. It is known that a proportion of patients may have antipsychotic medication safely discontinued after 3 months while those with more severe symptoms at baseline may require ongoing treatment.

4.4.3 Supporting Caregivers and Legal Considerations

The physical and emotional health of the primary caregiver is critical to optimal care of the patient with Alzheimer's disease. Caregivers have increased rates of psychological and physical morbidity, which in turn predict early transfer to long-term care and escalation of costs. One of the most widely used tools to assess the demands of caregiving on the care-giver is the Zarit burden inventory, which is a 22-item, self-administered questionnaire. Multimodal and multidisciplinary interventions tailored to the needs of individual caregivers have been shown to achieve improved outcomes for patients and carers and can delay time to institutional care. Legal issues should also be addressed with patients and carers such as advance directives and power of attorney as appropriate. Voluntary organizations such as the Alzheimer's association (www.Alz.org) and the Alzheimer's society (www.alzheimer.org.uk) have an important role to play and can provide patients and their families with useful information regarding Alzheimer's disease and the availability of daycare and respite services locally.

4.4.4   Lifestyle Issues, Cognitive Stimulation, and Alternate Therapies

In recent years, there has been an increasing amount of epidemiological evidence, which links low educational level, vascular risk factors, and decreased social activation with increased risk of Alzheimer's disease. These findings, coupled with an increased under-standing of neural plasticity, have stimulated interest in the area of lifestyle interventions to improve cognitive function.

Several observational studies have documented decreased risk of cognitive decline and dementia in adults who exercise more and are more physically active. However, interventional studies in individuals with AD or individuals at risk of AD are less frequent and further studies are required. One interventional study, which randomized 170 participants with memory complaints (60 % of whom had mild cognitive impairment) to either a 24 week home-based program of physical activity or to education and usual care reported a 1.3 point difference on the ADAS-Cog in favor of the intervention. Exercise has also been shown to benefit the physical functioning of patients with AD and has been associated with fewer falls during the course of a 1-year intervention.

The utility of cognitive training techniques and whether gains on neuropsychological test scores translate into everyday functional improvement continues to be explored. A recent systematic review of cognitive training and rehabilitation in patients with mild to moderate AD concluded that cognitive training was not associated with positive or negative outcomes but that the overall quality of the trials was low to moderate. Further research is warranted in clearly defined at-risk populations to determine whether cognitive training may prevent or delay incident dementia.

Vascular risk factors such as hypertension, hypercholesterolemia, obesity, diabetes, and smoking in midlife and later years have been associated with increased risk of AD (as discussed in more detail above). It is already known that comorbid cerebrovascular disease facilitates the clinical expression of Alzheimer's pathology, but there is now increasing knowledge regarding converging and shared pathogenic mechanisms. There is mixed evidence regarding the treatment of hypertension for prevention of dementia, and interventional studies of statins have had negative results on cognitive outcomes to date. There remain compelling cardiovascular and cerebrovascular indications for the detection and treatment of vascular risk factors, which should ordinarily be addressed in the course of cognitive screening.

Patients sometimes enquire about the benefit of alternative therapies such as Gingko biloba or vitamin E. Recent systematic reviews have concluded that there is no consistent evidence to recommend their use in patients with AD or to prevent progression from MCI to AD. One systematic review of interventional studies using omega-3 fatty acids reported improvement in specific cognitive domains for participants with Cognitive Impairment No Dementia (CIND) but not in healthy subjects or those with AD.

4.5   Recent Advances

4.5.1   Disease-Modifying Therapies

In addition to ongoing research in cognitive and lifestyle interventions to delay or prevent the onset of Alzheimer's dementia (as outlined above), there are currently a large number of clinical trials underway in the area of potentially disease-modifying pharmacological therapies. Given the projected expansion in Alzheimer's disease worldwide, the public health implications of an intervention, which would delay disease onset by even a modest

Table 4.5 Summary of disease-modifying agents and approaches to Alzheimer's disease

Therapy	Mechanism
Amyloid-based therapies	
Secretase inhibitors and modulators	Reduce production of Ab(beta)-42
Anti-aggregation agents	Prevent the oligomerization and fibrillization of Ab(beta)
Statins	Decrease Ab(beta) production
Active and passive amyloid vaccines	Promote clearance of amyloid plaques and oligomeric forms of amyloid
Tau-related therapies	
Kinase inhibitors	Decrease hyperphosphorylation of tau
Neuroprotective therapies	
Antioxidants	Reduce oxidative injury
Anti-inflammatory agents	Reduce inflammation-mediated injury
Neurorestorative therapies	
Nerve growth factor (NGF) and neurotrophins	Promote neuronal survival and repair Neuronal regeneration
Stem cell therapy	Replacement of cells
Cell transplantation	

interval, would be highly significant. Disease-modifying therapies would differ from existing symptomatic therapies in that they should delay disease progression through impacting upon underlying pathophysiological processes with resultant long-lasting changes in disability. Accurate characterization of the underlying pathophysiology of Alzheimer's disease, as outlined above, has suggested a number of targets for potential disease-modifying treatments. Therapeutic agents under investigation may be broadly considered under the headings of anti-amyloid, tau related, neuroprotective, and neurorestorative therapies (Table 4.5).

4.5.2 Anti-amyloid Therapies

Anti-amyloid agents generally act upon the production, aggregation, or clearance of the Ab peptide. These therapies target different parts of the amyloid cascade and include agents that reduce

amyloid production through inhibition or modulation of γ and β secretases, agents, which prevent the oligomerization and fibrillization of Ab and immunotherapeutic agents, which facilitate clearance of Ab. The central significance of amyloid in the pathogenesis of AD has recently been called into question given negative outcomes from trials of a number of agents targeting this pathway. Tarenflurbil, an agent that modulates g secretase activity, failed to achieve significance on its primary endpoints in a phase III trial and another agent, Tramiprosate, which binds soluble Ab(beta), thus preventing amyloid deposition, was also negative. Epidemiological studies which linked cholesterol-lowering statin medication with reduced risk of AD and laboratory data indicating a possible mechanism through which statins might reduce production of Ab(beta) triggered further investigation of statins for AD. However, randomized controlled trials of statins for AD have been negative to date. There has also been interest in antihypertensive agents such as calcium channel blockers and those acting on the angiotensin system. Nilvadipine is a calcium channel blocker which has been shown to enhance Ab clearance and restore cortical perfusion in mouse models of AD. There have been promising findings from early clinical studies in patients with AD and a large phase III study of this agent is currently underway.

Immunotherapy forms another potential strategy in anti-amyloid therapy,. A number of hypotheses have been proposed to explain how immunotherapy may result in Ab(beta) clearance. It has been proposed that microglial activation with endocytosis and phagocytosis of Ab(beta) plaques facilitates clearance while alternately, it has been proposed that circulating antibodies may draw soluble Ab(beta) across the blood-brain barrier, thus preventing detrimental binding within the CNS. Research into this area began in earnest when it was found that it was possible to prevent or reverse Ab(beta) accumulation in the brain of an animal model by active immunization with Ab(beta)42. A phase II trial utilizing this method demonstrated effective removal of Ab(beta) plaques but was stopped prematurely because 6 % of patients developed meningoencephalitis. The specificity of Ab(beta) antibodies has since been investigated and active immunization therapies targeting different regions of Ab(beta)42 are under investigation. It was similarly found that passive immunization by peripheral infusion of Ab(beta) antibodies facilitated Ab(beta) clearance in animal models while other investigators utilizing intravenous immunoglobulin containing naturally derived human antibodies against Ab(beta) also presented promising results.

More recently, the results of two Phase III trials utilizing humanized monoclonal antibodies, bapineuzumab and solanezumab, in patients with mild to moderate AD were published. Both antibodies failed to demonstrate positive results on their primary cognitive and functional outcomes measures. The authors concluded that the initiation of anti-amyloid treatment after dementia develops may be too late to affect the clinical course of the disease. The point at which anti-amyloid therapy should be commenced is a critical consideration and studies in samples with earlier stages of the disease are now underway.

4.5.3 Tau-Related Therapies

The formation of neurofibrillary tangles is dependent upon hyperphosphorylation of tau and tau phosphorylation is regulated by a balance between multiple kinases and phosphatases. Glycogen synthase kinase 3 (GSK-3b(beta)) is a key tau kinase, and medications, which are known to inhibit GSK 3b(beta), such as lithium, have shown positive effects in animal studies. Valproic acid has similarly been reported to inhibit GSK 3b(beta). The need to expand therapies for AD beyond amyloid-based approaches means that kinase inhibitor therapeutics now forms an expanding area of research with ongoing exploration of new and existing compounds, which target GSK 3b(beta) and other kinases implicated in the hyperphosphorylation of tau.

4.5.4 Neuroprotective Therapies

These therapies target the neurotoxic effects of Ab through numerous secondary pathways. These include oxidation, inflammation, and demyelination. Astrocyte activation has been hypothesized to play a role in AD pathogenesis and astrocyte-modulating compounds in patients with AD are under investigation. The receptor for advanced glycation end-products (RAGE) is a ubiquitous cell surface receptor, which has been postulated to mediate many of the toxic and neuroinflammatory effects of Ab(beta) and may have potential as a therapeutic target. AMPA type glutamate receptors are believed to mediate most fast synaptic neurotransmission in the brain and positive modulation of these receptors may potentially enhance cognition. An antihistamine (dimebon) with postulated mitochondrial stabilizing properties was tested in a trial in patients with mild-to-moderate Alzheimer's disease and demonstrated significant efficacy on cognitive, functional, and neuropsychiatric outcome measures, although these findings were not replicated in phase III studies which were subsequently discontinued.

4.5.5 Neurorestorative Therapies

These approaches consist of nerve growth factor (NGF) and neurotrophin therapies, stem cell approaches, and transplantation that may assist in cell survival or replacement and regeneration. NGF, like other neurotrophins, promotes cell survival by signaling through specific tyrosine kinase receptors to effectively block apoptosis from occurring in either a developing or damaged neuron. The impermeability of the blood–brain barrier to exogenous NGF and other neurotrophins is a significant challenge for the development of potential therapeutic agents in AD and strategies to circumvent this difficulty are being researched.

4.5.6 Novel Biomarkers

Diagnosis of Alzheimer's disease in its earliest clinical stages can be difficult and biological markers of underlying Alzheimer's pathology have become an increasingly important component of early diagnostic evaluation. This not only improves diagnostic accuracy but assists with prognosis and evaluation of response to potential disease-modifying therapies, which are likely to be of greatest benefit if used before the onset of significant functional impairment. Novel neurochemical, structural, and functional neuroimaging methodologies increasingly augment standard neuropsychological investigations and clinical evaluations as outlined above. These include cerebrospinal fluid levels (CSF) of amyloid beta 42, total tau, and hyperphosphorylated tau, which have displayed good accuracy in identifying incipient AD among subjects with MCI. Methods of CSF analyses continue to be refined and there have been increased efforts to overcome variability between centers with recent publication of consensus criteria to facilitate standardization of CSF biomarker testing. A variety of potential plasma biomarkers for incipient AD have been identified including plasma amyloid beta 42 or plasma amyloid beta 42/40 ratio and additional proteins identified through the use of proteomic methodologies. To date, no single plasma biomarker of Alzheimer's pathology has displayed sufficient sensitivity or specificity although combining biomarkers from different metabolic pathways may increase diagnostic accuracy and further studies of this approach are underway.

4.5.7 Neuroimaging Biomarkers

Recent advances in neuroimaging techniques have greatly enhanced clinical research in early Alzheimer's disease. In particular, PET tracers, which can bind to amyloid-beta, now allow the detection of amyloid pathology in vivo. The majority of studies published to date have utilized 11C-Pittsburgh Compound B (PiB), but a number of 11-F tracers with a much longer half-life, have also been developed. The vast majority of patients with a clinical diagnosis of AD have evidence of amyloid on PET imaging studies and antemortem amyloid PET imaging correlates well with findings at autopsy. A consistent finding across studies is that approximately 30 % of cognitively normal older individuals have evidence of amyloid pathology, consistent with the hypothesis that the pathophysiological process of AD may begin years, if not decades prior to the diagnosis of clinical dementia. Early detection of amyloid burden in individuals at risk of cognitive decline and AD has facilitated investigation of anti-amyloid therapies in individuals who are presymptomatic or in the very early stages of disease. It is also possible to track the activity and efficacy of novel therapeutic agents upon amyloid burden with serial imaging. However, PET tracers remain largely a research tool as there are still methodological variations between centres and not all individuals with amyloid pathology necessarily progress to AD. Novel tracers have also emerged to allow in vivo assessment of tau pathology in patients with AD opening new possibilities for the measurement and assessment of novel therapeutic agents targeting this other key pathologic hallmark of AD.

Novel methods for structural MRI continue to evolve, including measures of cortical thickness and tensor morphometry. These techniques have demonstrated evidence of subtle atrophy in MCI and very mild AD. Other neuroimaging techniques which are also under active investigation, include functional magnetic resonance imaging (fMRI) and fluorodeoxyglucose (FDG) PET. FDG PET measures glucose metabolism and decreased FDG uptake is an indicator of impaired synaptic function. In patients with AD there is typically decreased uptake in the lateral temporoparietal or posterior cingulate-precuneus areas with similar changes in patients with early disease. fMRI has consistently shown abnormal hippocampal function during memory encoding in patients with mild AD. fMRI studies have also examined functional connectivity, and have demonstrated disruptions in the default network in patients with AD. Similar disruptions in functional connectivity have been reported in MCI and even in amyloid-positive normal older individuals, suggesting that alterations in this network may be an early sensitive marker of brain dysfunction.

4.5.8 Future Directions

The AD field continues to evolve toward earlier diagnosis, in the hope that earlier intervention with potential disease-modifying therapies will be more efficacious. There have been recent changes to refine diagnostic criteria and incorporate greater use of biomarkers so that older individuals with memory impairment and evidence of amyloid pathology or atrophy should be considered to have very mild AD. Clinical trials of amyloid-lowering agents in these individuals with very early disease and even in the preclinical stages of disease are currently ongoing.

New research criteria have described the category of "preclinical" AD, which encompasses individuals with evidence of amyloid pathology on PET imaging or CSF markers, but who have no clinical symptoms or only very subtle cognitive decline. Several recent studies have demonstrated that clinically normal older individuals with high amyloid burden demonstrate functional and structural brain alterations similar to those observed in MCI and AD. Furthermore, these studies suggest that amyloid-positive older individuals may already have subtle memory impairment, particularly evident when level of cognitive reserve or baseline intellectual capacity is taken into account. However, further longitudinal study is required to determine if the presence of amyloid in cognitively normal individuals is both necessary and sufficient to reliably predict progression to the clinical dementia of AD. An international effort to acquire longitudinal biomarkers in presymptomatic carriers of autosomal dominant mutations (the Dominantly Inherited Alzheimer Network—DIAN study) is also developing methods to track disease progression in the preclinical stages of AD. These studies are critical to moving the field toward a different treatment paradigm. Similar to cardiovascular disease and cancer, the optimal treatment for AD may be at these very early stages, perhaps prior to the emergence of any clinical impairment.

Further Reading

Albert MS, DeKosky ST, Dickson D, Dubois B, Feldman HH, Fox NC, et al. The diagnosis of mild cognitive impairment due to Alzheimer's disease: recommendations from the National Institute on Aging-Alzheimer's Association workgroups on diagnostic guidelines for Alzheimer's disease. Alzheimers Dement. 2011;7(3): 270–9.

Ballard C, Gauthier S, Corbett A, Brayne C, Aarsland D, Jones E. Alzheimer's disease. Lancet. 2011;377(9770): 1019–31.

Dubois B, Feldman HH, Jacova C, Hampel H, Molinuevo JL, Blennow K, et al. Advancing research diagnostic criteria for Alzheimer's disease: the IWG-2 criteria. Lancet Neurol. 2014;13(6):614–29. doi:10.1016/S1474-4422(14)70090-0.

Gallagher D, Mhaolain AN, Coen R, Walsh C, Kilroy D, Belinski K, et al. Detecting prodromal Alzheimer's disease in mild cognitive impairment: utility of the CAMCOG and other neuropsychological predictors. Int J Geriatr Psychiatry. 2010;25(12):1280–7.

Hampel H, Wilcock G, Andrieu S, Aisen P, Blennow K, Broich K, et al. Biomarkers for Alzheimer's disease therapeutic trials. Prog Neurobiol. 2011;95(4):579–93.

Herrmann N, Lanctot KL, Hogan DB. Pharmacological recommendations for the symptomatic treatment of dementia: the Canadian Consensus Conference on the Diagnosis and Treatment of Dementia 2012. Alzheimers Res Ther. 2013;5 Suppl 1:S5.

Lawlor B, Kennelly S, O'Dwyer S, Cregg F, Walsh C, Coen R, et al. NILVAD protocol: a European multicentre double-blind placebo-controlled trial of nilvadipine in mild-to-moderate Alzheimer's disease. BMJ Open. 2014;4(10):e006364.

McKhann GM, Knopman DS, Chertkow H, Hyman BT, Jack Jr CR, Kawas CH, et al. The diagnosis of dementia due to Alzheimer's disease: recommendations from the National Institute on Aging-Alzheimer's Association workgroups on diagnostic guidelines for Alzheimer's disease. Alzheimers Dement. 2011;7(3):263–9.

Dementia and Cerebrovascular Disease

5

Joseph Harbison, Sean P. Kennelly, and Rose Anne Kenny

5.1   Introduction

The nature of the association between cerebrovascular disease (CVD) and dementia has been debated for many years. At one point, CVD was considered the dominant cause of dementia, then, it was conversely thought in fact to be an uncommon cause. Vascular dementia (VaD) is a heterogeneous term and comprises dementias resulting from all types of vascular pathologies: cortical vascular dementia; subcortical ischemic dementia; strategic-infarct dementia; hypoperfusion dementia; haemorrhagic dementia; and dementias resulting from specific arteriopathies.

Under the most widely accepted diagnostic criteria the diagnosis of VaD requires the presence of cognitive decline (loss of memory and deficits in at least two other domains) resulting in impaired functional abilities. Evidence of CVD must be confirmed by neuro-imaging for a diagnosis of probable VaD, and the onset of dementia and CVD must be reasonably related temporally. Several specific diagnostic criteria are used to assist the diagnosis of VaD including the *Diagnostic Manual on Mental Disorders*, 5th edition (DSM-V) criteria, the *International Classification of Diseases*, 10th edition (ICD-10), the National Institute of Neurological Disorders and Stroke Association International pour le Recherché at L'Enseignement en Neurosciences (NINCDS-ARIEN) criteria, and the Hachinski Ischemic score. Unfortunately however, as with many neurocognitive disorders, consistency of diagnosis between these tools and with neuroimaging is poor. For example, a population based clinic-pathologic study in the United Kingdom, found that the NINCDS-ARIEN diagnostic criteria had a sensitivity of 43 % and a specificity of 95 %. Similarly, in a US based cohort study of patients diagnosed with dementia, application of the NINCDS-ARIEN criteria gave a proportionate risk for VaD of 4 %, whereas application of the DSM-IV criteria in the same patient population gave a rate of VaD of 29 %. Neither estimate correlated closely with the ultimate neuropathologic diagnosis. Overall the NINCDS-ARIEN criteria appear to be the most specific (see Table 5.1), and are used most commonly in research. The Hachinski Score (Table 5.2) is a

J. Harbison • R.A. Kenny (✉)
Department of Medical Gerontology, Trinity College, Dublin, Dublin, Ireland

Department of Medical Gerontology, Mercer's Institute for Successful Ageing, St James's Hospital, Dublin, Ireland

S.P. Kennelly
Medical Gerontology, Trinity College, Dublin, Dublin, Ireland

Acute Medical Unit, Tallaght Hospital, Dublin, Ireland

© Springer International Publishing Switzerland 2016
O. Hardiman, C.P. Doherty (eds.), *Neurodegenerative Disorders: A Clinical Guide*,
DOI 10.1007/978-3-319-23309-3_5

Table 5.1 NINDS-ARIEN criteria for diagnosing vascular dementia

Cerebrovascular disease
Focal central nervous system signs
Evidence of cerebrovascular disease by neuroimaging
A relationship between the two manifest by one or more of the following
Dementia onset within 3 months after having a stroke
Abrupt deterioration in cognition or fluctuating stepwise course

Table 5.2 Hachinski ischaemic score

Item no.	Description	Value
1	Abrupt onset	2
2	Stepwise deterioration	1
3	Fluctuating course	2
4	Nocturnal confusion	1
5	Preservation of personality	1
6	Depression	1
7	Somatic complaints	1
8	Emotional incontinence	1
9	History of hypertension	1
10	History of stroke	2
11	Associated atherosclerosis	1
12	Focal neurological symptoms	2
13	Focal neurological signs	2

Items distinguishing vascular dementia from Alzheimer's Dementia: fluctuating course (odds ratio (OR): 7.6), stepwise deterioration (OR: 6.1), focal neurological symptoms (OR: 4.4), hypertension (OR: 4.3) and history of stroke (OR, 4.30)

useful tool for distinguishing between Alzheimer's Type Dementia and Vascular Dementia with about a 90 % sensitivity and specificity for this determination with a score ≥ 7 being suggestive of Vascular dementia. It is understandably less useful in distinguishing from mixed types . Unlike the NINDS ARIEN criteria it does not require the availability of brain imaging to apply.

As not all patients fulfil the strict criteria for dementia, and many may be significantly cognitively impaired without memory loss, the term vascular cognitive impairment (VCI) has been suggested and reinforced in the recent DSM V criteria. VCI includes VaD, but also encompasses

mixed Alzheimer's disease (AD) and VaD as well as vascular cognitive impairment without dementia and hereditary disorders.

5.2   Prevalence

VaD is historically considered the second most common cause of dementia in the elderly after AD. Between 1 and 4 % of people over 65 years suffer from VaD and the prevalence appears to double every 5–10 years after the age of 65 years. Although the prevalence increases more with age than Alzheimer's dementia, no large population cohort has been studied to date in any ethnic or racial group where prevalence of VaD exceeds that of Alzheimers. Cognitive decline of any severity may be present in over 80 % of stroke patients ranging in age from 55 to 85 year. Prevalence of post stroke dementia depends on criteria used but probably exceeds 30 %. While it is clear that AD and VaD often co-exist in the elderly population, it has been much harder to estimate the prevalence of this "mixed dementia". Autopsy series report that co-existing vascular pathology occurs in 24–28 % of AD cases and conversely half of patients with vascular disease who become demented also have AD pathology. Patients often have clinical features of both AD and VaD, and both conditions share similar risk factors and pathogenic mechanisms.

5.3   Clinical Features

Due to the variety of pathogenic mechanisms, the clinical manifestations of VaD can be varied and are determined by the size, location, and type of cerebral damage. There are several conditions that can mimic the appearance of dementia which should always be excluded at the outset of investigation (see Table 5.3). Classically the clinical features include an abrupt onset, stepwise deterioration, fluctuating course, and are often accompanied by focal motor and sensory abnormalities including early onset of urinary incontinence and gait disorders (see Table 5.4). However

Table 5.3 Conditions which can mimic dementia

Worried well – not demented
Mild cognitive impairment – reduction from baseline in one or several cognitive domains but no functional impairment
Affective disorders: Depression, manic-depressive disease
Other psychiatric conditions: obsessive compulsive disorders, old age psychosis, and paranoid (delusional) disorder
Acute or prolonged confusion (Up to 6 months) – delirium
Adverse effects of medications
Unrecognized complex partial seizures
Unrecognized drug or alcohol abuse
Single-domain cognitive deficits such as Korsakoff's disease

Table 5.4 Key differential diagnostic features of vascular dementia (VaD)

Features typical of a classic presentation of VaD
Focal neurological symptoms and signs (e.g., visual disturbances, sensory or motor symptoms, hemiparesis, visual field defects, extrapyramidal signs, etc.)
Presence of cerebrovascular lesions on brain imaging
Preservation of emotional responsiveness and personality
Depression
Impairment of executive function (ability to plan, strategize, and execute commands)
Stepwise deterioration in cognition
Incontinence
Somatic symptoms
Visuospatial dysfunction
Dysphasia
Emotional lability
Nocturnal confusion and wandering
Features that make a diagnosis of pure VaD unlikely
Early onset of memory deficit
Progressive decline of memory deficit and other cognitive functions (e.g., Language, perception, and motor skills)
Absence of cerebrovascular lesions on brain imaging

subcortical VaD can present with a gradual onset and deterioration similar to the pattern seen in AD. Even within VaD, the clinical features can be further subdivided:

5.3.1 Cortical VaD

This is predominantly characterised by the abrupt onset of unilateral sensorimotor changes along with aphasia, apraxia, or agnosia (cortical cognitive impairments). Most patients have an element of executive dysfunction, as expressed by difficulties in areas such as initiation, planning, and organisation of activities. There may be day-to-day fluctuations in severity with long plateaus between events.

5.3.2 Strategic Infarct

Single strategic infarcts have the potential to cause cognitive and other deficits that are dependant on the area of the brain affected. Particular cerebral regions, known to produce symptoms of acute onset VaD when affected include the thalamus, basal forebrain, and caudate. From a cognitive perspective, memory impairment, dysexecutive syndrome, confusion, and fluctuating levels of consciousness can occur. Behavioural changes include apathy, lack of spontaneity, and perseveration.

5.3.3 Subcortical VaD

Cerebrovascular lesions in the subcortical area tend to cause slow but episodic deterioration in executive functioning and abstract thought, as well as mood changes including depression, personality changes, and emotional lability. Although in many instances memory deficits are less severe, the difficulties with complex tasks lead to decreased performance in activities of daily living. Binswanger disease (also known as subcortical leukoencephalopathy) is due to diffuse white matter disease. In Binswanger disease (see Fig. 5.1), vascular changes observed are fibrohyalinosis of the small arteries and fibrinoid necrosis of the larger vessels within the brain.

With regard to the clinical course of the disease as a whole, the median survival from dementia onset to death is 3.9 years for patients with VaD, as compared with 7.1 years for patients

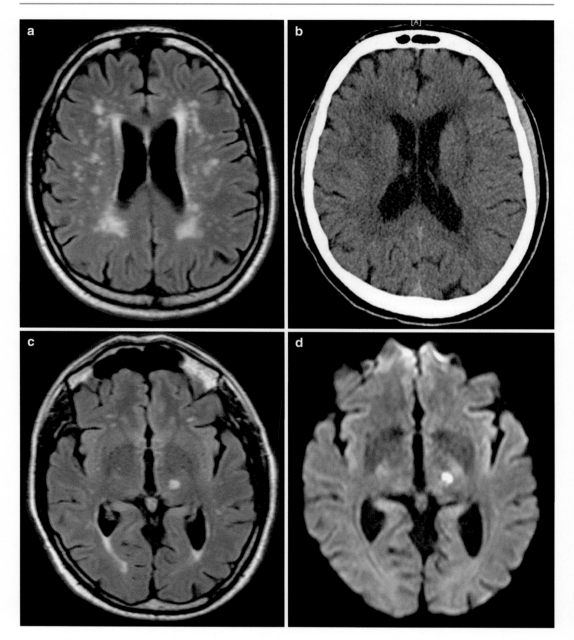

Fig. 5.1 Brain Imaging from a 68 year old man with a history of sub-cortical (Binswanger's) Vascular Dementia who presented with an episode of right arm and face paraesthesia. (**a**) MR FLAIR sequence at level of lateral ventricles showing multiple small ischaemic areas in white matter. (**b**) Non-Contrast CT image at same level showing hypodensity within white matter. (**c**) FLAIR image showing acute infarct in left medial thalamus. (**d**) Diffusion Weighted Image at same level

with AD, and 5.4 years for patients with mixed dementia.

Subjects suffering primary intracerebral haemorrhage are also reported as having an increased risk of cognitive impairment and dementia. Assessment of this is more complicated due to the coexistence of amyloid angiopathy, a common cause for primary intracerebral haemorrhage, and Alzheimer's disease, both being associated with the pathological deposition of beta amyloid protein.

5.4 Neurodegeneration and VaD

VaD arises as a consequence of hypoxia and ischemic insults including haemorrhage and hypoperfusion, that trigger neurodegeneration by depriving neurons of oxygen and glucose. Hypoxia and ischaemia initiate a neurodegenerative signaling cascade, involving the release of glutamate, activation of the NMDA receptor, accumulation of free calcium intracellularly, free radical formation, and subsequent necrosis and apoptosis. Acute hypoxia also leads to microglial activation and the synthesis of inflammatory mediators, which are also injurious to neurons in the ischaemic penumbra.

5.5 Biomarkers and Vascular Dementia

Unlike AD, there are currently no established biochemical markers for VaD. Commonly AD and VaD pathology coexist in what is termed "mixed" dementia (MD). As a result of this coexistence, in many cases an exact diagnosis of either AD or VaD can be difficult on clinical grounds alone, and therefore biological markers may be of use in assisting this distinction. Recent studies have suggested that levels of neurofilament light protein (NFL) in the cerebrospinal fluid (CSF) may correlate with the degree of white matter lesions on magnetic resonance imaging. Studies investigating CSF levels of Amyloid-β40 (Aβ-40), Amyloid-β42 (Aβ-42), total Tau (Tt), and phosphorylated tau (Tp), have shown inconsistent results, but overall patients with VaD have lower CSF levels of Tt and Tp, and higher levels of Aβ-40 and Aβ-42, than either MD or AD. Many studies have failed to find a difference in the levels of these biomarkers in patients with VaD, when compared to non-demented populations. No serum or plasma biomarkers have shown consistent results to date.

Neuroimaging findings, in particular presence of probable ischaemic lesions on Magnetic Resonance Imaging of the brain, are the most widely used biomarker for Vascular Dementia. However, even this has not been shown to correlate with neuropathological findings on necropsy. White matter disease is associated with neuronal loss but also with demyelination and inflammatory cell infiltrate. It is also associated with a disproportionate increase in vascular permability and loss of the blood brain barrier and it is thought that an increase in interstitial fluid, particularly in periventricular areas, may contribute to extent of apparent white matter hyperintensities where neuronal tissue is still functional.

5.6 Cardiovascular Risk Factors and Dementia

Many links exist between vascular disease and AD. Cerebral atherosclerosis is associated with a higher risk of AD. Cardiovascular risk factors are associated with clinically diagnosed AD and VaD. The commonalities in associations between cardiovascular risk factors and dementia labelled as AD or VaD underline the relevance of vascular disease to dementia in general, and the flaws in simplistic diagnostic categories.

When discussing the cardiovascular risk factors for VaD, it is best to categorise them into modifiable and non-modifiable risk factors.

The most important non-modifiable risk factors are gender and age, followed by genetic predisposition, ethnicity, and a previous history of stroke. Both incidence and prevalence of VaD increase with age and tend to be higher in men. Dementia affects about 7 % of the general population older than 65 years and 30 % older than 80. Genetic defects for several monogenic disorders have been identified. These include cerebral autosomal dominant arteriopathy with subcortical infarcts and leucoencephalopathy (CADASIL), which is a cause of small vessel disease, migraine and stroke leading to cognitive impairment within 20 years of the onset of symptoms. Other genetic disorders include hereditary cerebral haemorrhage with amyloidosis- Dutch type (HCHWA-D), a syndrome of primarily haemorrhagic strokes resulting in cognitive impairment and dementia in the majority of cases. Ethnicity appears to be of importance given that previous studies suggest that VaD represents over 50 % of all dementias in Japan, however there may have been an over-diagnosis of VaD in some of these studies. Recent regional Chinese studies have demonstrated comparable prevalence rates for all dementia subtypes in Chinese and Western countries. There is a history of prior stroke in 76 % of patients with VaD and in 57 % of those with VCI, as compared with only 5–7 % of people with AD.

Modifiable risk factors for VaD are those that reduce ones risk for cardiovascular disease i.e., hypertension, atrial fibrillation, diabetes mellitus (DM), hyperlipidaemia, and smoking. Epidemiological data shows that hypertension (especially in midlife) is one of the most potent risk factors for VaD, and it has been shown that control of hypertension can reduce ones risk of VaD. Patients with diabetes are three times more likely to develop stroke-related dementia than the general population. Dyslipidaemia, although a well established risk factor for ischemic heart disease, has been convincingly demonstrated as a risk factor for AD or VaD. Elevated levels of non-high-density lipoprotein cholesterol (non-HDL-C), and low density lipoprotein cholesterol (LDL-C), and decreased levels of high-density lipoprotein cholesterols, have been shown to be weak risk factors for the development of VaD. The evidence for smoking and dementia is also somewhat ambivalent, although recent studies have suggested that smokers have twice the risk of developing VaD, compared to ex-smokers and non-smokers.

There is also an overlap between cardiac disease and the development of dementia. Cognitive impairment is seen in 26 % of patients discharged from hospital following treatment for heart failure. The degree of cognitive impairment correlates with the degree of left ventricular impairment, and systolic blood pressure levels less than 130 mmHg. This highlights the potential for hypotension and diminished cardiac reserve to exacerbate cerebral hypoperfusion,

contributing to subsequent dementia. Similarly, following coronary artery bypass graft (CABG) surgery the reported incidence of "early" cognitive impairment ranges from 33 to 83 %. In this group of patients, widespread atherosclerotic disease can predispose to vascular sequele leading to neurologic dysfunction. Long-term cognitive outcomes are more favourable for off-pump CABG, but late postoperative dementia is predicted by early cognitive deterioration. Aggressive postoperative risk factor control appears to impact favourably on cognitive outcomes.

5.7   Primary Prevention of VaD

Primary prevention aims to reduce the incidence of VaD by early detection and optimum treatment of known vascular risk factors for cardiovascular disease and stroke, prior to the onset of such diseases. With the exception of treating hypertension, the evidence for this policy is primarily based on that for prevention of other vascular diseases and biological plausibility. Targeting high risk groups, particularly those patients with hypertension, possibly affords the best opportunity for reducing the incidence of dementia in the general population. Initial results from trials examining the effects of antihypertensive therapy on dementia were conflicting. Longitudinal data from the Rotterdam study of 7046 elderly participants showed that the relative risk of VaD was reduced by over one third, over a mean 2.2 years follow up in those who were receiving antihypertensives at baseline. Two subsequent prospective randomised studies, the Medical Research Council [MRC] (diuretic/β blocker based therapy), and the Systolic Hypertension in the Elderly Programme [SHEP] (Diuretics ± β blocker therapy) studies, showed no benefit in preventing dementia. However further evaluation of the latter trial revealed that cognitive and functional evaluations may have been biased towards the null effect by differential dropout. Another randomised trial, the Systolic Hypertension in Europe [Syst-Eur] trial, demonstrated that treatment with the dihydropyridine calcium channel blocker nitrendipine reduced the incidence of dementia (both AD and VaD) by 55 % over 2 years, although only small numbers of new cases were identified in either group. Further studies are underway examining the possible neuroprotective properties of certain antihypertensive agents, and how these may be responsible for the reduced incidence of dementia following treatment. Given the strength of mid-life hypertension as a risk factor for the development of dementia, perhaps one of the strongest indications for aggressive management of high blood pressure at this stage of life is the reduction in the incidence of dementia seen in later life.

5.8 Secondary Prevention of VaD

Secondary prevention of VaD mainly focuses on stroke management and the prevention of recurrent stroke. Treatment with anti-platelet agents should be initiated as indicated by the nature of the patient's underlying vascular pathology. The Perindopril Protection Against Recurrent Stroke Study (PROGRESS) trial confirmed the benefits of blood pressure lowering in secondary prevention. Although the primary outcome of PROGRESS was stroke incidence, dementia and cognitive function were secondary outcomes. Treatment with the long-acting angiotensin- converting enzyme (ACE) inhibitor perindopril, combined with the diuretic indapamide significantly reduced the incidence of dementia by 34 % in patients with recurrent stokes. Similarly, less cognitive decline was noted in patients who received active treatment. It was also observed in this study that treatment with combination therapy led to greater reductions in BP, and was more effective at reducing the risk of dementia than monotherapy. A PROGRESS magnetic resonance imaging (MRI) substudy investigated the effect of antihypertensive therapy on the progression of white matter intensities (WMH). We know that WMH are associated with vascular cognitive impairment and VaD, and are often observed on brain MRI in elderly patients. There was a significant reduction in the total volume of new WMH's in patients who received perindopril ± indapamide. Therefore

active management of high BP stopped or delayed the progression of WMH's in patients with known cardiovascular disease.

Two randomised studies, the Heart protection Study (Simvastatin) and the Prospective Study of Pravastatin In the Elderly at Risk study (PROSPER), failed to identify a treatment benefit of statin therapy on cognition or dementia. However it has been suggested that the follow up period in these studies may have been too short to clearly demonstrate a treatment benefit, if one was present.

5.9 Treatment of VaD

The mainstay of management of VaD is the prevention of new stokes, as discussed above. There are currently no pharmacological agents licensed for the treatment of VaD. Studies of vasodilators, nootropics, ergot alkaloids, antioxidants, and hyperbaric oxygen have largely failed to demonstrate any symptomatic benefit to treatment. However, low numbers of participants, short follow up periods, and the absence of clear endpoints has limited the power of several of these trials. Therefore further studies are necessary to investigate the role these agents may play in the treatment of VaD.

Propentofylline is a xanthine derivative with purported neuroprotective effects, by acting as a glial cell modulator. Several double-blinded randomised placebo controlled trials have demonstrated significant symptom improvement and long term efficacy, when used for the treatment of VaD. The use of certain dihydropyridine calcium channel blockers (DHP-CCB), such as nimodipine and nicardipine have been associated with favourable outcomes in clinical trials, however the beneficial effects were greater in subcortical dementia, and were short lived. While the exact mechanism of action is unclear, certain DHP-CCB's have been associated with increased cerebral perfusion and reduced cellular apoptosis, as well as generally lowering blood pressure.

Autopsy reports of patients with VaD have shown significantly reduced choline acetyl-transferase activity in several brain regions including the caudate and putamen, hippocampus, and temporal cortex, supporting evidence for a role for cholinergic depletion in the pathogenesis of VaD. While the magnitude of the loss of cholinergic neurons is less in VaD compared to AD (40 % versus 70 %), it is reasonable to hypothesize that in a similar way to AD, enhancing cholinergic transmission may be a rational treatment approach for VaD. Several trials have examined the use of the three acetycholinesterase inhibitors (AChI) used for the treatment of AD (donepezil, rivastigmine and galantamine) in patients with VaD. Rivastigmine is a second generation AChI with the capacity to inhibit both acetylcholinesterase and butyrylcholinesterase. In a randomised open-label 1 year study, 208 patients with VaD were treated with rivastigmine. There was a slight improvement in executive function (clock drawing tests) and in behaviour, however the results of further blinded, placebo-controlled trials are awaited. Galantamine is an AChI that also modulates central nicotinic receptors. The analysis of two large studies involving VaD patients failed to demonstrate a significant improvement in overall cognition and memory scores with treatment, however there did appear to be a slight improvement in executive function. The most positive results have been seen with donepezil. Donepezil is a piperidine-based agent, and is a non-competitive, reversible antagonist of cholinesterase, and is highly selective for acetylcholinesterase. Efficacy and safety has been shown in two large randomised placebo-controlled trials, and confirmed in a Cochrane review. Altogether 1219 patients with VaD, according to NINDS-ARIEN criteria, were recruited for 24-week trials. The patients were randomised to placebo, donepezil 5 mg, or donepezil 10 mg per day. There was a statistically significant improvement in cognition, global functioning and activities of daily living in both treatment groups compared to placebo. Overall there is evidence to suggest that the use of certain AChI's in VaD may offer some symptomatic relief. The degree of improvement on cognitive measures although statistically significant, does appear to be small and may be short lived. The presence of side effects associated with these medications may limit their use in patients with pure VaD. There are still no guidelines recommending the use of Cholinesterase inhibitors in subjects with VaD but consideration may be given to the treatment on an individual basis.

There is limited evidence for the use of N-methyl-D-asparate receptor antagonist Memantine in VaD. It has evaluated in two trials of patients with mild/moderate VaD. There was significant but minor improvement in cognitive function, and a slight improvement in behaviour from baseline over placebo but no improvement in activities of daily living. Although it appeared to be well tolerated it probably has no use currently in the management of VaD.

5.10   Future Directions in VaD

Given that AD, VaD, and a mixture of both account for the vast majority of cases of dementia, a discussion on future directions for VaD must also look at the future directions for all dementias. There are several aspects of neuroimaging that are likely to make a significant contribution to our diagnostic capabilities over the coming years. Functional imaging techniques such as MR spectroscopy, Diffusion Tensor Imaging or functional MRI can highlight levels of impaired cerebral perfusion, neuronal dysfunction and damage to tracts and pathways, even in the absence of any structural abnormalities on conventional MR. New positron emission tomography (PET) techniques using ligands such as Pittsburgh Compound-B, have enabled visualisation and quantification of amyloid within the brain and may help improved discrimination of dementia subtypes. These techniques will assist with an earlier diagnosis of dementia, perhaps before the clinical onset of symptoms enabling earlier treatment, however further research is required to establish appropriate cut-off values that are specific and sensitive enough to differentiate patient from normals.

As discussed earlier there are currently no established biomarkers to assist the diagnosis of VaD or other cerebrovascular diseases.

The identification and understanding of bio-markers for AD, has led to their introduction in many of the new criteria for diagnosis of AD. There have been numerous studies looking for blood biomarkers for those at high risk of stroke. In the future one would hope that our understanding of these AD biomarkers and their correlation with neuropathology, as well as the identification of new vascular biomarkers, would lead to a greater understanding in the crossover between vascular disease and VaD, and an ability to distinguish between the two and an ability to better characterise subtypes of VaD that may differ in risk factor and likely treatment.

Despite these predicted advances in biotechnol-ogy, it is likely that the mainstay of treatment for VaD will depend on aggressive management of vascular risk factors prior to stroke, and careful monitoring and follow-up post stroke. Future stud-ies are required to develop a predictive risk score for post-stroke dementia, and to evaluate sort cog-nitive screening instruments identifying high risk patients with vascular cognitive impairment.

It will become increasingly important as newer treatments for AD and VaD become avail-able, that we have an understanding of the inter-play between the two pathological mechanisms for both conditions.

Conclusions

Despite being the second most common form of dementia after AD, with which it shares important pathologic features and symptoms, VaD frequently goes undiagnosed. There is likely to be an exponential increase in the inci-dence of VaD over the coming years, given the aging demographic profile of countries world-wide, especially in developing countries. Although no treatments are currently licensed for the symptomatic treatment of VaD, there does appear to be mild symptomatic benefit to treatment with certain cholinesterase inhibi-tors and memantine. Without doubt, the pri-mary treatment goal currently is to reduce ones risk of suffering a primary cerebrovascu-lar event, and where one has occurred, to limit the risk of recurrent events. This requires aggressive vascular risk factor management.

Suggested Reading

Craig D, Birks J. Rivastigmine for vascular cognitive impair-ment. Cochrane Database Syst Rev. 2005;(2):CD004744.

Forette F, Seux ML, Staessen JA, Thijs L, Babarskiene MR, Babeanu S, Bossini A, Fagard R, Gil-Extremera B, Laks T, Kobalava Z, Sarti C, Tuomilehto J, Vanhanen H, Webster J, Yodfat Y, Birkenhäger WH, Systolic Hypertension in Europe Investigators. The prevention of dementia with antihypertensive therapy: new evi-dence from the systolic hypertension in Europe (syst-eur) study. Arch Intern Med. 2002;162(18):2046–52.

Kalaria RN, Ballard C. Overlap between pathology of Alzheimer disease and vascular dementia. Alzheimer Dis Assoc Disord. 1999;13 Suppl 3:S115–23.

Mok V, Lam W, Chan Y, Wong K, editors. Post stroke dementia and imaging. New York: Nova Science pub-lishers incorporated; 2009.

Malouf R, Birks J. Donepezil for vascular cognitive impairment. Cochrane Database Syst Rev. 2004;(1): CD004395.

Moroney BE, Desmond DW, Hachinski VC, Mölsä PK, Gustafson L, Brun A, Fischer P, Erkinjuntti T, Rosen W, Paik MC, Tatemichi TK. Meta-analysis of the Hachinski Ischaemic score in pathologically verified dementias. Neurology. 1997;49:1096–105.

O'Brien J, Ames D, Gustafson L, et al., editors. Cerebrovascular disease, cognitive impairment and dementia. 2nd ed. New York: Taylor 2005.

Paul RH, Cohen R, Ott BR, Salloway S, editors. Vascular dementia: cerebrovascular mechanisms and clinical management. Totowa: Humana Press Inc; 2005.

Snowden D. Aging with grace: the nun study and the science of old age. How we can live longer, healthier, and more vital lives. London: Harper Collins Publishers; 2002.

Parkinson's Disease

6

Diana A. Olszewska, Stanley Fahn,
Richard A. Walsh, and Tim Lynch

Parkinson's disease (PD) is the second most common neurodegenerative disorder after Alzheimer's disease affecting 6.3 million people worldwide. Due to the population aging, it is thought that the prevalence will double by the year 2030. Annual European cost of Parkinson's disease is estimated at 13.9 billion euro. The majority of cases are sporadic, commonly referred to as idiopathic Parkinson's disease (IPD). The cardinal clinical features are bradykinesia, rigidity, rest tremor and postural instability. A flexed posture and the freezing phenomenon are also commonly seen. There has been increasing awareness of the non-motor symptoms of IPD including depression, dementia, sleep disruption and autonomic disturbance. These can equal the motor symptoms in terms of their functional impact, particularly in advanced stages of the disease.

6.1 Pathology

IPD arises as a result of degeneration of neurons in the substantia nigra pars compacta. The pathological hallmark is the α(alpha)-synuclein containing Lewy body, an eosinophilic, proteinaceous cytoplasmic inclusion seen in surviving neurons (Fig. 6.1).

Staining for Lewy pathology with antibodies to α(alpha)-synuclein indicates that the first location of pathologic change is in the olfactory apparatus and caudal brainstem, especially the dorsal motor nucleus of the vagus in the medulla. Neural involvement is thought to spread progressively rostrally up the brainstem in a fashion hypothesised by Braak and colleagues, who studied the pattern of α(alpha)-synuclein involvement in autopsied brains. The cerebral cortex is involved late in this schema, in keeping with the evolution of cognitive impairment, (if not frank dementia) in patients with long-standing IPD. When the motor symptoms of IPD are evident, the substantia nigra already has lost about 60 % of dopaminergic neurons, and the dopamine content in the striatum is about 80 % less than normal. Involvement of non-dopaminergic neurons including cholinergic

D.A. Olszewska • T. Lynch (✉)
Department of Neurology,
Dublin Neurological Institute,
Mater Misericordiae University Hospital,
Dublin, Ireland
e-mail: diana.angelika.olszewska@gmail.com;
tlynch@dni.ie

S. Fahn
Department of Neurology,
Columbia University Medical Center,
New York, NY, USA

R.A. Walsh
Department of Neurology, Tallaght Hospital,
Dublin, Ireland
e-mail: Richard.Walsh@amnch.ie

© Springer International Publishing Switzerland 2016
O. Hardiman, C.P. Doherty (eds.), *Neurodegenerative Disorders: A Clinical Guide*,
DOI 10.1007/978-3-319-23309-3_6

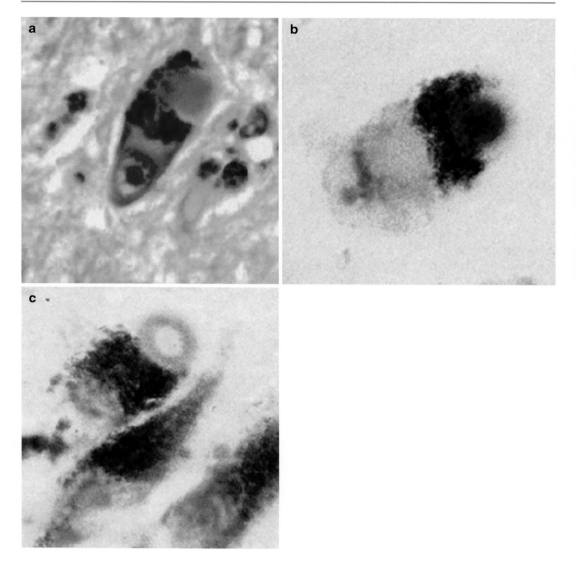

Fig. 6.1 (**a**) H&E staining of a substantia nigra neuron containing a Lewy body; (**b**) The core of each Lewy body stains more strongly for α(alpha)-synuclein than the characteristic halo (**c**) which is strongly immunoreactive for ubiquitin

neurons in the nucleus basalis of Meynert, noradrenergic neurons in the locus coeruleus and serotonergic neurons in the midline raphe may be significant in the non-motor symptoms.

6.2   Diagnosis

The diagnosis of IPD remains essentially a clinical one. If made by a neurologist, the diagnosis based on clinical impression has been shown to have a positive predictive value of 76 % up to 98.6 % for

those working in a specialist movement disorders service. The United Kingdom Parkinson's Disease Society Brain Bank criteria are typically used in Research studies of PD; bradykinesia with one of tremor, rigidity and postural instability are required in the absence of exclusion criteria (Table 6.1). Retrospective application of these criteria to patients diagnosed with PD in life demonstrates positive predictive values of between 82 and 92 %. This diagnostic accuracy may be improved if a levodopa response and asymmetry are also sought but sensitivity may be lost.

Table 6.1 Exclusion criteria for Parkinson's disease

History of repeated strokes with stepwise progression
History of repeated head injury
History of definite encephalitis
Oculogyric crisis (unless drug induced)
Neuroleptic exposure at time of diagnosis
Sustained remission
Supranuclear gaze palsy
Cerebellar signs
Early severe autonomic involvement
Early severe dementia
Babinski sign
Presence of cerebral tumour or communicating hydrocephalus on imaging
Failure to respond to an adequate dose of levodopa (up to 2000 mg)
Scans without evidence of dopaminergic deficit (SWEDDs)

Some physicians will use the 'levodopa challenge' where a response to a single dose of up to 300 mg of levodopa supports the diagnosis of PD. Tremor predominant forms of IPD may not however demonstrate any response to levodopa and some atypical forms of parkinsonism will, thus causing diagnostic confusion. Others avoid this challenge, particularly in younger patients, given concerns that even a single dose of levodopa may 'prime' the basal ganglia for dyskinesia.

An important aspect of the initial and subsequent clinical assessments is to look for atypical features suggesting an alternative diagnosis, having important implications for predicting survival and treatment response. Some conditions mimicking IPD will require alternative treatment strategies (Table 6.2). Also, it is not uncommon for IPD to present with symptoms not readily attributed to the disease. Some of these patients will carry alternative diagnoses before the more obvious parkinsonian features appear (Table 6.3).

6.3 Subtypes of Parkinson's Disease

Parkinson's disease can be classified into subtypes. The most common classification is based on the time of onset of PD: young versus late onset and secondly on the dominant feature:

Table 6.2 Clinical features of the Parkinson-plus (atypical) disorders

Progressive supranuclear palsy
Early falls
Prominent axial rigidity
Pure freezing of gait and early freezing
Arm abduction when walking
Frontalis overactivity (startled appearance)
Deep naso-labial folds
Vertical gaze palsy or 'round the houses' vertical saccades
Blepharospasm
Prominent Square-wave jerks
Slowing of horizontal saccades
Apraxia of eye opening
Characteristic voice is a hoarse, throaty growl, with some hesitation between words
Multiple systems atrophy
Prominent cerebellar or autonomic features
Flexed posture
Anterocollis
Myoclonus or polyminimyoclonus
Laryngeal stridor (may only be nocturnal)
Early orofacial dyskinesia with levodopa
Pyramidal tract signs (e.g. extensor plantar responses, spastic 'catch' in addition to rigidity)
Purple discolouration of the feet due to abnormal vascular autonomics
Corticobasal degeneration
Unilateral dystonia
Alien-limb phenomenon
Unilateral stimulus sensitive myoclonus
Cortical sensory loss
Dyspraxia

Table 6.3 Parkinsonian symptoms and signs commonly attributed to other disorders

Fatigue
Dyspnea
Bradyphrenia
Depression
Joint pain (particularly shoulder pain)
'Radicular' pain (true radicular pain may worsen in 'off' states)
Foot cramps/dystonia
Dysphonia
Anxiety/panic attacks
'Weakness' affecting ability to rise from chairs or apparently unilateral weakness

tremor-predominant versus akinetic-rigid pheno-type with the mixed category falling in between those two. Below are discussed the main features of the different subtypes.

1. Young onset Parkinson's disease: age of onset between 20 and 40, with associated rigidity and dystonia, good response to L-dopa, but with an early development of dyskinesias, slower progression of the disease than in the late-onset PD. Associated with Parkin muta-tion (discussed in a genetics section) in 1/3 of the cases.
2. Late-onset Parkinson's disease: age of onset over 60, with a rapid disease progression.
3. Tremor-predominant PD: often misdiagnosed as an essential tremor, good prognosis, with a slow progression.
4. Postural instability and gait difficulty (PIGD) also called akinetic-rigid subtype: with an early cognitive decline and higher frequency of dementia, depression and apathy.
5. Mixed PD: features of tremor predominant and PIGD.

6.4 Differential Diagnosis of Parkinsonism

6.4.1 Atypical Parkinsonism

Approximately three quarters of patients present-ing with parkinsonism have typical motor fea-tures, and are most likely to have pathologically confirmed IPD. The remaining 25 % of patients will have so-called atypical parkinsonism, also called Parkinson-plus syndromes. This group of primary degenerative parkinsonian disorders includes progressive supranuclear palsy (PSP), multiple system atrophy (MSA) and corticobasal degeneration (CBD) and are covered in Chap. 9. All may start with an asymmetrical clinical syn-drome indistinguishable from IPD. These forms of parkinsonism all share a tendency to be poorly responsive to levodopa, be largely symmetrical (with the exception of corticobasal degeneration) and have little or no rest tremor (although myoc-lonus mimicking tremor may be evident).

Table 6.2 highlights clinical features that should raise suspicion of an atypical parkinsonism.

6.4.2 Dementia with Lewy Bodies

Patients presenting with dementia before, or within 1 year of manifesting parkinsonism, are by convention given a diagnosis of dementia with Lewy bodies (DLB). Visual hallucinations are common and the course of cognitive impairment is typically fluctuating, often with dramatic vari-ability from 1 day to the next. Some patients will have prominent autonomic dysfunction. Patients with dementia beginning after 1 year are diag-nosed with PD with dementia (PDD). Both these conditions may represent different points on the spectrum of 'Lewy body disease' with a larger cortical burden of Lewy bodies than in patients with IPD.

6.4.3 Secondary Parkinsonism

6.4.3.1 Drug-Induced Parkinsonism
Parkinsonism can follow exposure to drugs with an antagonistic effect at D_2 receptors. This is the most common cause of secondary parkinsonism and is typically seen in patients requiring anti-psychotic (neuroleptics, major tranquillizers) treatment. Newer, 'atypical' neuroleptics with less affinity to the D_2 receptor are less likely to result in extrapyramidal side-effects and are pre-ferred when treating psychosis in IPD. The com-monly used anti-emetic drugs metaclopramide and prochlorperazine also have a D_2 antagonist effect. Other drugs known to induce parkinson-ism include lithium, tetrabenazine, reserpine, val-proate, and the calcium channel blockers, cinnarizine and flunarizine.

Drug withdrawal typically results in a slow improvement although latent parkinsonism may have been unmasked and full recovery may not occur.

6.4.3.2 Vascular Parkinsonism
This is also known as 'lower body parkinsonism' due to prominent gait disturbance and relatively

less arm involvement. Often, these patients will have early freezing which is not typically seen in IPD. This is an important cause of parkinsonism in older patients and those with a history of vascular risk factors (particularly hypertension). The pathophysiology is related to small vessel disease with prominent periventricular ischemia. Patients with basal ganglia infarcts are more likely to respond to levodopa. Magnetic resonance imaging (MRI) of brain is useful to identify those patients who may have a vascular cause of parkinsonism. Other clinical features that can help differentiate vascular from idiopathic parkinsonism are a postural more than resting tremor and preserved olfaction.

6.4.3.3 Fragile X Pre-mutation

The pre-mutation state of Fragile X can present with tremor, parkinsonism and autonomic features and may therefore be misdiagnosed as essential tremor, IPD or MSA. An accurate family history is vital, looking for a history of a related child with learning disability or autism. The presence of ataxia is another important clue. In one series of 26 patients with premutations of the FMR1 gene, 57 % of cases had mild bradykinesia, resting tremor was present in 40 % and 71 % had upper limb rigidity.

6.4.3.4 Others

Secondary parkinsonism can also occur following toxin exposure, including manganese (miners, intravenous drug abuse), carbon disulphide and 1-Methyl-4-phenyl-1,2,3,6-tetrahydropyridine (MPTP) (described by Langston JW and Palfreman J in "The Case of the Frozen Addicts").

Rarely parkinsonism can arise as a consequence of strategically-placed structural lesions such as large Virchow-Robin (perivascular) spaces or central nervous system (CNS) tumors, more commonly supratentorial meningiomas causing basal ganglia compression than by direct tumor infiltration.

Functional parkinsonism is well recognized but rare. Clues to the diagnosis are a history of previous psychogenic illness, an abrupt onset, entrainment of tremor, selective disability and distractibility.

6.4.4 Disorders That Can Mimic Parkinsonism

6.4.4.1 Essential Tremor

Essential tremor (ET) is one of the most common disorders mistaken for IPD, characterized by a postural and kinetic tremor without rest tremor. Patients with ET can have cog-wheeling but without rigidity. Where there is a combination of a resting hand tremor with essential tremor, the physician should consider rest tremor appearing late in ET, or the combined resting-postural tremor syndrome.

Parkinsonism and essential tremor could also represent the co-occurrence of two common movement disorders.

6.4.4.2 Dystonic Tremor

Dystonic tremor usually occurs in a dystonic body part. Some distinguish this from 'dystonia with tremor', tremor observed in an unaffected body part with dystonia elsewhere. Dystonic upper limb tremor will sometimes have a 'null-point' where rotation of the affected limb will reach a point where the tremor is abolished. Like ET, dystonic tremor of the upper limbs will not have the latent period before re-emerging on changing position as seen in IPD (re-emergent tremor). Dystonic tremor tends to be more irregular and jerky in character and may have a torsional component.

6.4.4.3 Normal Pressure Hydrocephalus

Normal pressure hydrocephalus (NPH) presents with one or all features of a triad of gait apraxia, urinary incontinence and cognitive impairment. Gait can be similar to that of vascular parkinsonism because of involvement of periventricular descending corticospinal tracts. Imaging is essential in demonstrating dilatation of all ventricles out of proportion to the degree of cortical atrophy. Diagnosis is made most reliably by removal of a large volume (at least 40 ml) of cerebral spinal fluid (CSF) via lumbar puncture, which can also predict the potential for improvement with shunt placement although this remains controversial. Video of gait and cognitive assessment performed pre and post lumbar puncture is useful for later assessment.

6.4.5 The Role of Imaging in Diagnosing Parkinson's Disease

With a classical clinical picture, there is little or no role for neuroimaging in making a diagnosis of PD. Positron emission tomography (PET) with the fluordopa ligand and single photon emission computed tomography (SPECT) are the principal options.

In SPECT studies, radioligands of the dopamine transporter (DAT) are used to determine the pre-synaptic integrity of nigrostriatal neurons. The DAT is exclusively localised to dopamine-producing neurons. Advantages of the technique are the wide availability of SPECT scanners and the ability to continue dopaminergic medication at the time of imaging. Patients with IPD will demonstrate reduced radiotracer uptake in the striatum bilaterally which tends to be asymmetrical, particularly affecting the posterior (dorsal) putamen (Fig. 6.2). Scans without evidence of dopaminergic dysfunction (SWEDDs) is the term

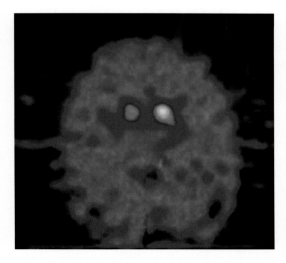

Fig. 6.2 Transaxial sections of a I-123 Ioflupane SPECT (DaTSCAN) from a patient with idiopathic Parkinson's disease demonstrating bilateral loss of uptake in the posterolateral aspect of the putamen bilaterally in a pattern typically seen soon in early disease

applied to normal scans of patients with a clinical diagnosis of IPD. The diagnosis in these patients likely represents a false positive as no long-term data or post-mortem studies have subsequently proven a diagnosis of IPD. Many of these patients will have a true diagnosis of essential or dystonic tremor, and some may have dopa-responsive dystonia, in which parkinsonism is often a feature, but the clue is the DAT scan is normal.

SPECT imaging has no role in differentiating atypical parkinsonism from IPD, because both have reduced DAT imaging. Its main use is in differentiating IPD from ET, drug-induced tremor/parkinsonism or psychogenic tremor, all of which should have normal imaging. Transcranial sonography has emerged as an alternative imaging modality, with nigral hyperechogenicity having a sensitivity of up to 90 % for IPD. Correlation with disease stage or severity has not been proven, and the significance of abnormalities in approximately 10 % of clinically unaffected individuals has yet to be established.

While the DAT scan remains the only approved PD diagnostic tool, recent research shows the possibility of a 3 T-susceptibility-weighted (SWI) MRI being a new accurate test for PD. The healthy nigrosome-1 (largest of the five described) is easily visualized on 3 T SWI as a presence of a 'swallow tail' of the dorsolateral substantia nigra, which is absent in PD. Resting state fMRI also holds a promise to aid the early diagnosis of PD with the latest research showing reduced resting functional connectivity in the basal ganglia in PD patients with an intact cognition.

6.5 Genetics

Case–control studies have confirmed a higher prevalence of IPD amongst first-degree relatives of affected patients supporting a genetic component to the disease. However the relative contribution of environmental and genetic factors to the pathophysiology of idiopathic PD is unclear. A number of Mendelian single gene mutations are associated with familial clustering of Parkinson's disease, although this accounts for less than 10 % of all PD.

Familial PD has both clinical and pathological overlap with IPD but commonly has a younger age at onset. The first single gene mutation identified 17 years ago as a cause of familial PD was in the gene coding for α(alpha)-synuclein. There has been more recent interest in the study of common variants or single nucleotide polymorphisms (SNPs) in the genes associated with familial PD. Common variants may be associated with an increased risk of sporadic PD although effect sizes are small and larger study populations are required to adequately power case–control studies. Some of the genes and their products associated with familial PD are discussed below.

6.5.1 α(alpha)-synuclein (PARK 1)

The *SNCA* gene encoding the α(alpha)-synuclein protein is located on chromosome 4q21.3. *α(alpha)*-Synuclein is an abundant presynaptic protein of unclear function. The resulting parkinsonism transmits in an autosomal dominant pattern. It is rare, being reported only in a handful of families from Greece, Italy, Germany, and Spain. The protein, *α(alpha)*-synuclein, is present in Lewy bodies. Duplication and triplication of the *α(alpha)*-synuclein gene also causes familial parkinsonism (PARK4), indicating that overexpression of the normal (wild-type) synuclein protein is sufficient to provoke dopaminergic neurodegeneration. This supports a pathogenic role for *α(alpha)*-synuclein in IPD. There is debate as to whether Lewy bodies are contributing to the pathogenesis of PD or if the aggregation of *α(alpha)*-synuclein fibrils to form Lewy bodies is an effort of the cell trying to protect itself from toxic *α(alpha)*-synuclein oligomers.

6.5.2 Parkin (PARK 2)

The Parkin gene is found on chromosome 6q25.2–27 and is the most common genetic cause for early-onset PD (before age 50), accounting for 50 % of familial and 20 % of sporadic early onset disease. *Parkin* mutations give rise to autosomal recessive PD that can have typical features

of IPD, but may also demonstrate hyperreflexia, dystonia at presentation and sleep benefit. Rest tremor is not prominent. Post-mortem studies have shown nigral degeneration in patients with *Parkin* mutations without Lewy bodies. There is an ongoing debate whether the heterozygote carrier state predispose to later onset PD in families.

6.5.3 PINK1 (PARK 6)

After *parkin* mutations, *PINK1* mutations are the second most common cause of early onset PD, sharing autosomal recessive inheritance. Disease progression is usually slow with early levodopa-induced dyskinesias. The parkinsonism is often preceded by anxiety and depression. The *PINK1* gene codes for a mitochondrial protein that is a recognized component of Lewy bodies seen in late onset IPD, and the few available autopsy studies have identified typical neuropathological findings.

6.5.4 DJ-1 (PARK 7)

Mutations in the *DJ-1* account for 1–2 % cases of early-onset familial PD. The presentation is with a typical early onset parkinsonism, often with dystonic and neuropsychiatric features. Unlike the unaffected heterozygous state with Parkin and PINK1 mutations, carriers do not demonstrate functional neuroimaging evidence of nigrostriatal dysfunction.

6.5.5 LRRK2 (PARK 8)

PARK8 is mapped to chromosome 12q12 and encodes for a previously unknown protein named leucine-rich repeat kinase-2 (*LRRK2*), ubiquitously expressed in the CNS. Seven pathogenic *LRRK2* mutations have been found, and are the most frequent genetic cause of familial PD. They account for up to 5 % of sporadic PD in the Caucasian population. In Ashkenazi Jews and North African Berber Arabs, *LRRK2* mutations have been found in up to 20–40 % of both familial and sporadic cases of PD. The most prominent mutation in the Caucasian population is the G2019S substitution. *LRRK2* mutations result in an autosomal-dominant parkinsonism that resembles typical late-onset IPD. Cognitive impairment is usually not a feature. Although the neuropathology associated to *LRRK2* mutations is highly variable, degeneration of substantia nigra neurons has been consistently observed.

6.5.6 Others

Glucocerebrosidase (GBA) gene mutations, when homozygous, cause autosomal recessive Gaucher's disease. Heterozygous carriers are at increased risk of developing parkinsonism that is indistinguishable from IPD. Up to 30 % of Ashkenazi Jews with PD have been found to have this mutation; the mutation causes PD in other ethnic groups as well. Dopa-responsive dystonia may present during adulthood as slowly progressive parkinsonism and tends to responds to low doses of levodopa. Parkinsonism can also be a predominant feature of the Westphal variant of Huntington's disease, although this is usually in juvenile patients and family history should be informative. Some forms of spinocerebellar ataxia (SCA2 and SCA3) can present with a levodopa-responsive parkinsonism with minimal cerebellar features.

Frontotemporal dementia linked to chromosome 17 (FTDP-17) can present with parkinsonism especially the pallido-ponto-nigral degeneration (PPND) variant, which is also associated with insomnia square wave jerks and a supranuclear gaze palsy.

6.6 Clinical Features

6.6.1 Motor

6.6.1.1 Rest Tremor

Rest tremor, typically of 4–5 Hz, is the first symptom recognized in 70 % of patients, but may be absent in 20 %. The classic "pill-rolling" tremor involves the thumb and forefinger and is best seen when the patient is walking. Rest tremor disappears with action but re-emerges after a latent period of seconds as the limbs maintain a posture (*re-emergent tremor*). Tremor increases with walking (a possible early sign), stress or excitement. Tremor is also common in the lips, chin, and tongue but not the head.

6.6.1.2 Bradykinesia with Decrement

Bradykinesia encompasses slowness of movement, difficulty initiating movement and loss of automatic movement. Decrement refers to a reduction in amplitude of movement, particularly with repetitive movements. Often different tactics need to be used by the examiner to bring out bradykinesia that might only be seen during certain actions, such as finger tapping, pronation-suppination movements or opening and closing the fists. The face loses spontaneous expression (*hypomimia*) with decreased frequency of blinking. Speech becomes soft (*hypophonia*), and the voice has a monotonous tone with a lack of inflection (*aprosody*). Some patients do not enunciate clearly (*dysarthria*) and do not separate syllables clearly, thus running the words together (*tachyphemia*) and others stutter (*palilalia*). Bradykinesia of the dominant hand results in small and slow handwriting (*micrographia*). Difficulty rising from a deep chair, getting out of cars and turning in bed are symptoms of truncal bradykinesia. Subtle signs of bradykinesia can be detected by examining for slowness in shrugging the shoulders, smiling, lack of natural gesturing in conversation and decreased blink frequency. Walking is slow, with a shortened stride length and a tendency to shuffle with decreased heel strike; arm swing decreases and eventually is lost.

6.6.1.3 Rigidity

Rigidity is an increase of muscle tone on passive movement and is not velocity dependent as seen with spasticity. Resistance is equal in all directions and usually has a 'cogwheeling' character caused by the underlying tremor even if not visible. Rigidity of the passive limb increases while another limb is engaged in voluntary active movement, also known as the co-activation or facilitation test. Axial rigidity at the neck can similarly be accentuated by asking the patient to open and close both hands. Mild upper limb rigidity can be elicited by standing behind the patient and rocking their shoulders back and forward to produce passive arm swing that will be reduced on the more affected side.

6.6.1.4 Loss of Postural Reflexes
Loss of postural reflexes leads to falling and eventually to an inability to stand unassisted. These reflexes are tested by the pull-test during which the examiner, who stands behind the patient, gives a sudden firm pull on the shoulders after explanation of the procedure, and checks for *retropulsion*. With advance warning, an unaffected person can recover within two steps.

6.6.1.5 Flexed Posture
This commonly begins in the elbows and spreads to involve the entire body. The head is bowed, the trunk is bent forward, the back is kyphotic and the arms are held in front of the body with the elbows, hips, and knees flexed. Walking is marked by *festination*, whereby the patient walks faster and faster with short steps, trying to move the feet forward to be under the flexed body's center of gravity to prevent falling. Deformities of the hands include ulnar deviation, flexion of the metacarpophalangeal joints, and extension of the interphalangeal joints (*striatal hand*). The hallux may be dorsiflexed (*striatal toe*). Lateral tilting of the trunk can develop (*Pisa syndrome*) and extreme flexion of the trunk (*camptocormia*) is sometimes seen which should be abolished when lying flat.

6.6.1.6 Freezing
This manifests as the transient inability to perform active movements. Freezing occurs suddenly and is transient, usually lasting seconds. It will typically occur when the patient begins to walk (*start hesitation*), attempts to turn while walking, approaches a destination, such as a chair in which to sit (*destination hesitation*). Tight spaces can also provoke freezing, such as doorways, as can time-restricted activities such as crossing heavily trafficked streets or answering

the phone. The combination of freezing and loss of postural reflexes is particularly devastating, and a common cause of falls.

6.7 Non-motor Symptoms

Later in the clinical course, non-motor and axial motor symptoms become prominent and account for greater disability, being poorly responsive to dopaminergic treatment (Table 6.4). After 20 years of disease in the Sydney Multicentre Study, falls were experienced by 87 %, moderate dysarthria in 81 %, dementia in 84 %, visual hallucinations in 74 %, postural hypotension in 48 % and urinary incontinence in 71 %. Some non-motor symptoms can be observed as 'pre-motor' phenomena, appearing before typical motor features. These include constipation, rapid-eye-movement (REM) sleep behavior disorder, olfactory impairment and mood disorders. Some of the more troublesome problems and their management are discussed below.

6.7.1 Autonomic Involvement

6.7.1.1 Constipation
Constipation is almost universal in PD and can influence the efficacy of oral therapies by causing erratic absorption. Treatment with a regular stool softener, sometimes combined with a stimulant laxative is usually effective and most patients will require a regular laxative. The use of abdominal plain films can guide the use of laxatives and should be considered in patients whose motor control has deteriorated or where response to levodopa is variable.

6.7.1.2 Dysphagia
Dysphagia is not uncommon. Rarely recurrent aspiration pneumonia can complicate late stages of the disease. Patients benefit from access to a speech and language therapist to teach strategies to improve swallowing. Dysphagia is not typically levodopa-responsive and can deteriorate after deep brain stimulation. A dry oropharyngeal mucous membrane due to anticholinergic agents

Table 6.4 Non-motor symptoms in Parkinson's disease

Neuropsychiatric
Depression
Anxiety, panic attacks
Hallucinations, illusions, delusions
Dementia, mild cognitive impairment
Obsessional, repetitive behaviors[a]
Delirium[a]
Anhedonia
Autonomic symptoms
Orthostatic hypotension
Nocturia, urgency, frequency
Paroxysmal sweating
Seborrhea
Erectile impotence
Xerostomia
Gastrointestinal
Ageusia
Sialorrhea
Nausea and vomiting
Dysphagia
Constipation
Incontinence
Sensory symptoms
Pain (can be pseudoradicular)
Paraesthesia
Olfactory disturbance
Visual blurring
Sleep disorders
REM sleep behavior disorder
Difficulty initiating or returning to sleep, insomnia
Restless legs syndrome
Periodic limb movements in sleep
Vivid dreaming
Nocturnal hallucinations
Excessive daytime somnolence
Others
Fatigue
Seborrhea
Weight loss or gain[a]

[a]May be drug related

is one readily treatable cause of swallowing impairment.

6.7.1.3 Sialorrhea

This is a manifestation of reduced swallow frequency in IPD as opposed to excessive saliva production. Anticholinergics are effective, but most available agents are tertiary amines that enter the CNS and can impair memory or cause hallucinations in older patients. Quaternary amines do not penetrate the CNS and are preferable. Sublingual 1 % atropine can be used with some success. Injections of botulinum toxin into the salivary glands can be attempted. Pharyngeal weakness due to local toxin diffusion is a potential complication but is rarely encountered with dry mouth being a more common side-effect.

6.7.1.4 Orthostatic Hypotension

Orthostatic hypotension (OH) can cause significant morbidity and contributes to the risk of falling. Conservative measures such as increased fluid in-take, additional dietary salt, avoidance of hot baths and large meals and the use of compression stockings can help. More resistant symptoms can respond to the sympathomimetic midodrine, starting with 5 mg and titrating up to three doses of 10 mg a day if necessary. Fludrocortisone can be used, typically starting at 0.1 mg/day but supine hypertension can result from increased salt and mineralcorticoid ingestion. Elevation of the top of the bed to 30° at night may help by reducing renal mineralcorticoid production. OH can be aggravated by dopaminergic therapy (dopamine agonists in particular), dehydration and constipation.

6.7.1.5 Urinary Symptoms

Detrusor hyperreflexia predominates in IPD causing frequency, urge, nocturia and sometimes incontinence. In older male patients the picture may be mixed with prostatism and anticholinergics are ideally prescribed after bladder ultrasound to determine post void residual volume, avoiding exacerbation of pre-existing outflow obstruction. Equally important is the propensity of these agents to cause cognitive impairment in older patients with IPD, in particular the tertiary amines that cross the blood–brain barrier.

Trospium chloride is a quaternary amine that may have a better side effect profile although there is little trial data available addressing this issue. Reduction in late night fluid intake can help nocturia. In patients treated for OH nocturia can occur as a result of nocturnal pressure natri-uresis secondary to supine hypertension.

6.7.1.6 Sexual Dysfunction

Sexual dysfunction is more commonly encoun-tered in IPD than in the general population. Men with erectile dysfunction can be treated with agents such as sildenafil, however this can exac-erbate OH. Female patients may report reduced libido and conversely hypersexuality can occur with dopamine agonist treatment and is particu-larly troublesome if associated with an impulse control disorder (discussed later).

6.7.1.7 Pain

Pain is not uncommon and can vary from uncom-fortable paraesthesias to nonciceptive or neuro-pathic sounding pain. Patients can initially present with pain in a joint on the symptomatic side, typi-cally a shoulder, probably due to hypokinesis and immobility. Adequate treatment and physiother-apy can improve this considerably. Some patients complain of pain down one side of their body or in an apparently radicular distribution, both of which will respond to levodopa suggesting a cen-tral dopamine deficit as the underlying cause. True radiculopathies from nerve root compression can also worsen in the 'off' state. Restless legs syndrome can be seen in association with IPD and can give rise to an aching discomfort in the legs at night that can improve with a low dose of a dopa-mine agonist taken at night.

6.7.1.8 Abnormal Sweating

The pathophysiology of abnormal sweating in IPD is unclear but Lewy body pathology involv-ing the hypothalamus may be contributory. Sympathetic cholinergic fibers are the final com-mon pathway that mediate the sweating response although dopamine would appear to play a role, as excessive sweating of the head and upper body can occur as an 'off' phenomenon, often in bed at night. Sweating can also occur in the context of dyskinesias, but is usually less prominent than the paroxysmal attacks of drenching sweats reported in 'off' periods. Other causes of excessive noctur-nal sweating should be considered including thy-rotoxicosis and latent tuberculosis infection.

6.7.2 Sleep Disturbance and Daytime Somnolence

Sleep disruption is common and multifactorial in IPD. Patients experience difficulty initiating sleep, fragmented sleep, REM sleep behavior disorder (RBD) and inversion of the sleep-wake cycle. RBD can predate the clinical onset of IPD sometimes by up to 10 years. Sleep disruption can exacerbate the excessive daytime somnolence that is both associated with the disease itself and dopaminergics.

Sleep disruption in IPD probably relates to degeneration of brainstem nuclei that regulate the balance between sleeping and waking states. The pedunculopontine and subcoeruleal nuclei are thought to play a role in maintaining the normal muscle atonia of REM that is lost in RBD. Involvement of nondopaminergic nuclei important in maintaining arousal including the raphe nuclei (serotonin), locus coeruleus (nor-adrenaline), the tuberomamillary nucleus (hista-mine) may account for daytime somnolence. The burden on bed-partners can be significant. Factors contributing to sleep disruption and therapies are given in (Table 6.5).

6.7.3 Neuropsychiatric

6.7.3.1 Parkinson's Disease and Dementia

Dementia is not typically an early feature of PD and if evident within 1 year of presentation a diagnosis of dementia with Lewy bodies (DLB) is made, otherwise the term Parkinson's disease and dementia (PD-D) is used. The overall preva-lence of dementia in PD is high at approximately 40 %, increasing in frequency with advancing years. The risk of developing dementia is 2.8 fold greater than controls.

The pathological substrate of dementia in PD remains uncertain. The involvement of subcorti-cal structures, in particular the medial nigra and thalamus may be important but cortical Lewy body burden and co-existent Alzheimer's disease pathology have also been shown to correlate with cognitive impairment. Cholinergic cell loss is

Table 6.5 Causes and treatment of sleep disturbance in Parkinson's disease

Bradykinesia and rigidity	*Can make* it difficult to turn in bed to find a comfortable position. Contribute to difficulty initiating sleep or returning to sleep after an arousal. Some patients overcome this by using satin sheets and nightclothes to facilitate movement
Restless legs syndrome (RLS)	Will respond to dopamine agonists and levodopa preparations given late at night. Treatment can be complicated by augmentation whereby symptoms become longer lasting, more severe and more extensive. It is important to ensure dyskinesias are not the cause of disturbed sleep as increased dopaminergic treatment will exacerbate this. Opioids, such as propoxyphene, can often suppress RLS and not cause augmentation
Periodic limb movements in sleep	Periodic episodes of rhythmic extension of the hallux with dorsiflexion of the ankle, sometimes extending proximally to involve knee and hip flexors. Commonly associated with RLS and can also respond to dopaminergic drugs. Opioids can also be of benefit in resistant cases. Propoxyphene 65 mg late in the day before the onset of symptoms is usually effective. Start with a half-tablet, and titrate up to two tablets if necessary
Nocturia	Common in this age group. Anti-cholinergics can help but may exacerbate vivid dreams or hallucinations. Sometimes responds to dopaminergic treatment. Rule out co-existing pathology with referral to urology for assessment where appropriate
Vivid dreams	Are usually not disruptive to sleep but can be upsetting. Can resolve with a reduction in dopaminergic or anticholinergic drugs taken at night. Can be exacerbated by amphetamine metabolites of selegiline which should be taken early in the day. Low dose quetiapine, starting at 12.5–25 mg at night, can help if required
Nocturnal hallucinations	Are associated with cognitive impairment in IPD and along with vivid dreams can respond to a low dose of quetiapine that can also improve insomnia due to its soporific effects. Donepezil 5–10 mg nocte can also be helpful
REM sleep behavior disorder (RBD)	Semi-purposeful movements in sleep, typically as if kicking or fighting off an attacker. Occurs as a consequence of losing normal physiological paralysis during REM sleep. RBD is typically reported by bed-partners who should be questioned. A small dose of clonazepam, 0.25–1 mg at night, can be very effective. Melatonin, 3–12 mg at night, is an alternative when clonazepam exacerbates daytime somnolence and is generally well tolerated
Insomnia or early morning wakening	Can be markers for underlying depression. Tricyclic antidepressants such as amitriptyline or nortriptyline may have a role in this setting to improve mood and produce a hypnotic effect (use with caution in patients taking an MAO-B inhibitor). Drugs that may be interfering with sleep such as selegiline or modafinil should be withdrawn or taken in the early in the day to minimize their stimulant effect. There is no specific contraindication to the use of benzodiazepines as night sedation although any 'carry-over' into the next day can affect cognition and increase risk of falling
Sleep disordered breathing	Due to sleep apnea and important to consider as treatment with non-invasive ventilatory support at night can be very effective. May not always have the typical body habitus seen in obstructive sleep apnea

more severe than that seen in Alzheimer's disease with severe neuronal loss in the basal nucleus of Meynert. The relative contribution of noradrenergic, dopaminergic and serotonergic neurons to PD-D is unknown.

The hallmark of cognitive impairment in IPD is executive dysfunction with impaired inability to plan, organize or regulate internally generated goal-directed behavior. Memory impairment is not as prominent as in Alzheimer's disease (AD) although responses can be slow (*bradyphrenia*). Memory deficits usually improve with prompting suggesting a problem with memory retrieval rather than encoding. Verbal fluency and visuospatial function may also be affected. Hallucinations are more common than in AD, present in up to 70 % of patients.

Once infectious and drug-related confusional states have been out-ruled, treatment with a cholinesterase inhibitor should be considered. Both rivastigmine and donepezil are effective for cognitive and behavioral symptoms without worsening parkinsonism, although tremor can worsen. Hallucinations can respond to cholinesterase inhibitors, but if antipsychotics are sometimes required clozapine or quetiapine can be used although controlled trials are lacking. Clozapine is associated with a low risk of agranulocytosis (1–2 %) so a baseline full blood count with subsequent monitoring are required; weekly initially for at least 18 weeks with local guidelines being followed thereafter. Treatment is started at 6.25 mg at bedtime and gradually titrated to response to 25–75 mg per day. Quetiapine may be less effective than clozapine although it is generally used first as it is not associated with hematological adverse effects. It is usually started at 12.5–25 mg at bedtime. Other atypical neuroleptics, risperidone, olanzapine and aripiprazole have all been associated with worsening of parkinsonism. There is insufficient evidence to recommend use of the glutamate antagonist memantine in PD-D.

6.7.3.2 Depression

Prevalence data for depression in IPD varies and is dependent on diagnostic criteria. Depressive symptoms often go undiagnosed, with hypophonia, poor sleep pattern and flattened affect being more commonly attributed to parkinsonism. Depression in IPD has a higher prevalence than in other chronic, incapacitating illnesses suggesting an endogenous component. This has been attributed to global monoamine depletion in IPD, in particular that involving noradrenergic neurons. Dopamine receptors are likely to play a role in regulation of mood. SSRI agents reduce dopamine uptake in the prefrontal cortex and chronic treatment leads to changes in D2/D3 receptor sensitivity in the nucleus accumbens.

SSRIs are commonly prescribed for depression in IPD. They are well tolerated but have a theoretical risk of inducing a serotonin syndrome when administered with an MAO-B inhibitor. This does not seem to be relevant with the doses used in clinical practice. Agents targeting dopaminergic and noradrenergic systems may be superior.

The tricyclic antidepressants desipramine (25–50 mg nocte) and nortriptyline (20–40 mg nocte) inhibit noradrenaline uptake and have a better side-effect profile than amitriptyline due to less anticholinergic activity. Nortryptiline was found to be more effective than slow release paroxetine in one randomized double-blinded trial. The dopamine agonists pramipexole and ropinirole have been also shown to be effective. The effect appears to be independent of any effect on motor function and may relate to an effect on limbic D2/D3 receptors.

6.7.3.3 Anxiety

Anxiety is a known preclinical risk factor for IPD suggesting that in at least some patients it is a disease phenomenon and not a reaction to it. Panic attacks can occur in 'off' states and can be managed by minimizing motor fluctuations and 'off' time. It is important to be aware that manic and anxiety states have been reported following dopamine agonist treatment. Some patients benefit from the short-acting benzodiazepines alprazolam (0.25–1 mg TID) and lorazepam (0.5–1.0 mg TID). Tricyclic anti-depressants, or SSRIs are sometimes required where there is additional depression (see section above).

6.7.3.4 Apathy

Apathy is characterized by a reduction in goal-directed behavior and is thought to be related to executive dysfunction in IPD. Disturbance of striato-frontal circuitry may be important. Dopaminergic reward pathways between the midbrain and limbic cortex are affected in IPD. Patients may not report depressive symptoms and typically will not share the frustration of care-givers with respect to their lack of motivation and drive. It is easy to mistake the apathy for depression in a Parkinson's patient. Stimulants such as modafinil are sometimes effective and empirical use of dopaminergics may help. A broader approach increasing monoamine transmission with SSRIs, SNRIs and TCAs can also be used.

6.8 Treatment of Motor Symptoms—Overview

Treatment must be tailored to the individual patient; each with a unique set of symptoms, different functional requirements and responding differently to various treatments. The goal is to maintain independence for as long as possible while attempting to address motor and non-motor symptoms of the disease. Because no treatment has been shown unequivocally to have a neuro-protective effect (discussed later), pharmacological treatment in the early stages is focused on symptomatic management. Levodopa is the most effective oral treatment for bradykinesia and rigidity. Much of the therapeutic effort in advanced disease involves control of the complications associated with chronic levodopa use, namely fluctuations, dyskinesias and increasingly recognized neuropsychiatric aspects. Importance has therefore been placed on the timing of levodopa introduction, particularly in younger patients who have longer to live with dyskinesias should they develop. Advanced IPD is characterized by these treatment complications, non-motor symptoms and motor symptoms that are not levodopa responsive. Non-pharmacological treatments, in particular physiotherapy, have a significant role. Physiotherapy involves patients in their own care, promotes exercise, keeps muscles active, and preserves mobility. This approach is particularly important as IPD advances because many patients will tend to remain sitting and inactive, exacerbating their immobility.

6.8.1 Symptomatic Treatment of Motor Symptoms

6.8.1.1 Levodopa

Dopamine is unable to cross the blood–brain barrier, but its precursor levodopa is and remains the most effective oral therapy. Early concerns that levodopa might be toxic to dopaminergic neurons proved to be unfounded and with respect to the pre-levodopa era, mortality and morbidity rates in PD have fallen. Dopamine has a strong effect on the area postrema, a fourth ventricular structure with high density of dopamine receptors and without protection from the blood–brain barrier. Nausea and vomiting are therefore common side effects.

Levodopa is routinely administered with a dopadecarboxylase inhibitor (carbidopa or benserazide) to prevent its peripheral breakdown to dopamine; these agents do not penetrate the blood–brain barrier. They potentiate the effects of levodopa, allowing about a 4-fold reduction in dose to obtain the same benefit. Approximately 75–100 mg of carbidopa is required to completely suppress peripheral dopadecarboxylase. Some formulations contain additional carbidopa if this is an issue; 'Sinemet Plus' combines 25 mg of carbidopa with 100 mg of levodopa instead of the 10 mg in 'Sinemet 110'. Additional carbidopa can also be prescribed in 25 mg tablets. Domperidone is preferred if an anti-emetic is required. Unlike prochlorperazine and metoclopramide, it does not cross the blood–brain barrier and will not therefore exacerbate parkinsonism. Domperidone is not available in the United States where Trimethobenzamide hydrochloride ('Tigan') can be used instead. Domperidone ('Motilium') should be taken 30 min before each dose and can usually be discontinued gradually within weeks. Other common side effects reported when initiating levodopa treatment include orthostatic hypotension, confusion, hallucinations and sedation.

Levodopa is available in a number of forms and doses that allow treatment to be tailored to the individual needs of each patient. 'Sinemet' (levodopa/carbidopa) is available in strengths of 50/12.5 mg, 100/10 mg, 100/25 mg and 225/50 mg. 'Madopar' (levodopa/benserazide) is only available in Europe and in strengths of 100/25 mg and 50/200 mg. There is also a water-dispersible formulation of Madopar (50/12.5 mg and 100/25 mg) with a more rapid onset and shorter duration of action. In practice, levodopa doses over 1200 mg daily are not often used.

Levodopa, carbidopa and the COMT inhibitor entacapone are available in a single tablet ('Stalevo'). This comes in a number of strengths of levodopa (50, 75, 100, 125, 150, 175 and 200 mg), each combined with 200 mg of entacapone. This reduces the total number of tablets taken daily and reduces 'off' time in patients experiencing the wearing-off phenomenon. Entacapone prolongs the half-life of levodopa from 90 min to approximately 180 min. It was thought that concurrent entacapone may reduce the pulsatile stimulation of dopamine receptors and avoid levodopa-induced dyskinesias, but a clinical trial showed the opposite effect; there were earlier and more severe dyskinesias when concurrent entacapone was utilized when levodopa therapy was started.

Both Sinemet and Madopar are available in modified release formulations that are sometimes used to smooth-out motor fluctuations or for night-time symptoms. Onset of action can be delayed and bioavailability is approximately 75 % of standard release formulations because the entire content of the extended-release formulation is not absorbed before the tablet passes the duodenum and jejunum (the sites where levodopa is absorbed).

6.8.1.2 Dopamine Agonists

Dopamine agonists (DA) directly stimulate dopamine receptors and are not reliant on degenerating striatal nerve terminals for uptake and conversion into an active product. For most patients DA are effective as a monotherapy in the early stage of the disease, allowing later introduction of levodopa and thus delaying motor complications. Dopamine agonists will rarely induce dyskinesia but are less effective for the symptomatic management of IPD; most patients require the addition of levodopa within a few years. Dopamine agonists do not delay the time to onset of dyskinesias once levodopa is added when compared with patients starting on levodopa from the outset.

The earliest DA in use were the ergot derivatives bromocriptine, pergolide, lisuride, and cabergoline. Retroperitoneal, pleural and pericardial fibrosis and restrictive fibrotic valvulopathy were reported with pergolide and cabergoline, attributed to activation of the $5HT_{2B}$ receptor. Pergolide is no longer available in the U.S. Lisuride, a short-acting ergoline agonist given subcutaneously is not associated with fibrotic complications ($5HT_{2B}$ antagonist) but has never been in common usage due to the emergence of apomorphine.

The non-ergoline agonists, pramipexole, ropinirole and rotigotine are currently the most frequently prescribed oral DA. Pramipexole and ropinirole are available in multiple daily dosing formulations and more recently in modified release formulations taken once daily. These formulations may have benefits in improving compliance and nocturnal or early morning symptoms. Rotigotine is administered transdermally, avoiding delays of gastric motility, first-pass metabolism and competition with dietary protein. Skin site reactions are relatively common but mild, occurring in up to 40 % of patients. Typical initiation, maintenance and maximum doses for the non-ergoline DA are given in Table 6.6. The clinical response to pramipexole at doses greater than 0.7 mg TID may not be greater than that at lower doses although side-effects will be more frequent. Conversely, ropinirole is often not titrated quickly enough to an effective treatment dose (minimum of 3 mg TID) due to its low initiation dose. Rotigotine should be titrated straight up to 8 mg/24 h if tolerated whether as a monotherapy or in combination with levodopa. Dose increases are then in 2 mg increments at weekly intervals until a satisfactory response is obtained.

Alternatively prolong release forms of pramipexole (Pramipexole ER), and ropinirole (Requip XL) as a once daily doses, may be used. When switching the patient's medication from the ropinirole immediate-release to the prolong release, patient should be prescribed equivalent dose and if the control is not maintained, ropinirole prolonged release should be titrated (as shown in the table) Typical initiation, maintenance and maximum doses for the long acting DA are given in Table 6.6.

Dopamine agonists have a less favorable side-effect profile than levodopa and are more likely to cause confusion, hallucinations, nausea, postural hypotension and ankle edema. Some patients may idiosyncratically have a better tolerance for one agonist over another. Much attention has been paid to reports of sudden unheralded episodes of sleep or 'sleep attacks' with DA. Daytime somnolence is a common problem in IPD. Further study of this phenomenon suggests that these 'sleep attacks' may represent unintended sleep episodes in individuals with excessive daytime somnolence from disturbed sleep and dopaminergic treatment. Tolerance to the feeling of chronic sleepiness and memory

Table 6.6 Commonly used non-ergot dopamine agonists and typical dose schedules

Dopamine agonist	Start dose (mg)	Week 2 (mg)	Week 3 (mg)	Week 4 (mg)	Therapeutic range mg/24 h	Max dose
Ropinirole	0.25 TID	0.5 TID	0.75 TID	1.0 TID	9.0—12.0	8 mg TID
Pramipexole (salt)	0.88 TID	0.18 TID	0.36 TID	0.7 TID	0.36–0.7	1.08 mg TID
Rotigotine	2	4	6	8	4.0–8.0	16 mg/24 h
Ropinirole prolonged release	2	4	6	8 (further increase by 2–4 mg every 2 weeks)	8–24	24 mg/24 h
Pramipexole extended release (salt)	0.26	052	1.05	Further increase by 0.52 weekly if needed	0.26–3.15	3.15/24 h

impairment may give the impression of sudden 'attacks' of sleep. The soporific effect of dopaminergic therapy would appear to be the same whether dopamine agonist or levodopa is prescribed. Nonetheless, patients on DA who are driving and reporting frequent unintended and reportedly unpredictable episodes of sleep should have their dose reduced and be advised not to drive until there is improvement.

6.8.1.3 Monoamine Oxidase Type B (MAO-B) Inhibitors

Selegiline and rasagiline are irreversible MAO-B inhibitors that have a mild symptomatic effect. MAO-B is an enzyme responsible for the central clearance of dopamine and its inhibition augments the effect of levodopa. Both drugs can be used for management of symptoms in early IPD or as an adjunct to levodopa to reduce 'off' time during motor fluctuations. As a monotherapy selegiline can delay the need for levodopa by an average of 9 months. Selegiline has few adverse effects when given alone. When given concurrently with levodopa, it can increase the dopaminergic effect causing dyskinesias and hallucinations. Selegiline has amphetamine metabolites that can disturb sleep if given late at night. A dose of 5 mg once or twice daily, ideally before midday, is typically used. Above 10 mg selectivity for MAO-B is lost risking a sympathetic crisis. Rasagiline, 1 mg once daily, is a second-generation irreversible MAO-B inhibitor providing a stronger symptomatic effect. It has no amphetamine-like breakdown products and may be associated with less sleep disturbance.

6.8.1.4 Amantadine

Amantadine is a mild indirect dopaminergic agent that augments dopamine release. It also has some anticholinergic and antiglutamatergic properties. Amantadine is now uncommonly used in the treatment of early IPD due to the availability of other symptomatic treatments with better side-effect profiles. In advanced IPD amantadine is used for its anti-dyskinetic effect, possibly as a result of its glutamate antagonism. Unfortunately, patients will often report a fall-off of benefit after several months. Adverse effects include livedo reticularis (a reddish mottling of skin) on the legs, dry mouth, ankle and leg edema, postural hypotension, visual hallucinosis, and nightmares. Amantadine has a long half-life of about 12 h, and if side effects occur, it can be stopped abruptly. The usual dose is 100 mg two times per day, but sometimes a higher dose (up to 200 mg twice daily) may be required for dyskinesias.

6.8.1.5 Anticholinergic (Antimuscarinic) Drugs

Anticholinergic agents are less effective antiparkinsonian agents than are dopaminergic drugs (estimated to improve parkinsonism by about 20 %) but can be a more effective treatment for tremor. Their exact mechanism of action is unknown; they may redress a relative imbalance between cholinergic and dopaminergic transmission in IPD. Trihexyphenidyl is a widely used anticholinergic agent. A common starting dose is 2 mg TID. It can be gradually increased to 15 mg or more per day although doses as high as this are rarely tolerated. Biperedin and procyclidine are alternatives.

Adverse effects are common with many patients reporting poor short-term memory. All patients should have a baseline cognitive assessment performed before starting treatment. These agents are preferably avoided if a patient or relative report prior memory impairment. Occasionally, hallucinations and psychosis occur, particularly in the elderly; these drugs should therefore as a rule be avoided in patients older than 65 years of age, although this is best judged on 'biological age'. In older patients, amitriptyline or diphenhydramine are sometimes beneficial, without the central side effects of more potent anticholinergic agents and can also be used as a hypnotic. Anticholinergics can reduce sialorrhea when tolerated. Peripheral side effects are common, including dry mouth, blurred vision, constipation and urinary retention. One approach is to treat these adverse effects by appropriate antidotes instead of discontinuation. Pilocarpine eye drops can overcome dilated pupils that can cause blurred vision, and can be useful if glaucoma is present. Pyridostigmine, up to 60 mg TID, can help to overcome dry mouth, urinary difficulties and constipation.

6.8.1.6 COMT Inhibitors

When levodopa is administered with a dopa decarboxylase inhibitor, catechol-O-methyltransferase (COMT) then becomes the main enzyme responsible for its breakdown in the periphery. COMT inhibitors prolong the pharmacological effect of levodopa, doubling its elimination half-life and augmenting its peak dose effect. They are useful in managing end of dose deterioration and reducing 'off' time but may exacerbate peak-dose dyskinesias resulting in a need to reduce individual levodopa doses by 15–30 %. Entacapone and tolcapone are approved for use in IPD. Entacapone acts peripherally only and because it has a very short half-life, 200 mg is given with each dose of levodopa. A combined formulation with levodopa and carbidopa (Stalevo) has similar efficacy to these compounds administered separately. Tolcapone acts both

centrally and peripherally. It is initially prescribed at 100 mg TID and is more potent than entacopone. It has been associated with liver enzyme elevations and 3 deaths from hepatic failure occurred in patients not having regular monitoring. It is therefore regarded as a second line agent. Regular monitoring of liver parameters should allow the drug to be used safely with immediate discontinuation if ALT or AST exceed the upper limit of normal.

6.9 Medications on Time Initiative

Taking medications for Parkinson's disease is vital. It may be particularly difficult in a hospital setting, where frequently PD medications are needed outside the routine drug-rounds. It is important to notify the PD Nurse Specialist upon patient's admission, consider self-administration of PD medications by patients, and to share the knowledge about medications on time importance in PD with co-workers.

6.10 Medications to be Avoided in Parkinson's Disease

Some medications should be avoided in Parkinson's disease, upon admission to a hospital medication charts should be carefully reviewed and the names of contraindicated medications inserted in the allergy section of a drug-chart. Assistance of a pharmacist may be needed. Examples of medications which may worsen PD are given below. Worsening of PD by:

6.10.1 Blocking Dopamine Receptors

- Antipsychotics: Chlorpromazine, Fluphenazine, Haloperidol, Loxapine, Thioridazine, Thiothixene, Trifluoperazine, Pimozide, Perphenazine
- *Antiemetics*: Chlorpromazine, Droperidol, Metoclopramide, Prochlorperazine, Promethazine
- Anti-depressants: Amoxapine

6.10.2 Decreasing Dopamine Storages

- Antihypertensives: Reserpine, Methyldopa, Tetrabenazine (may cause parkinsonism itself, but it should be mentioned that according to the most recent studies it may be used with caution for the peak-dose dyskinesias (chorea) in a PD patient, although this indication is uncommon justification for its use in a clinical practice)

Some medications should not be taken with selegiline or rasagiline (MAOI). Other MAO inhibitors should not be used simultaneously with selegiline or rasagiline. Concomitant use with anti-depressants such as mirtazapine, St John's Wort, and analgesics such as tramadol may rarely result in a serotonin syndrome, characterised by autonomic instability, delirium, malignant hyperthermia, coma and death. Other examples of medicines to be avoided include widely used substances in cough medications (pseudoephedrine, phenylephrine, ephedrine) due to a possibility of inducing severe hypertension, and dextromethorphan (also antitussive medication) resulting in episodes of psychosis. (for a full list of contraindicated medications please consult the references given).

Patients with Parkinson's disease should always consult their doctor or a pharmacist before taking any over-the counter medication.

6.11 Neuroprotection

No definitive evidence has been found of neuroprotection using any agent in IPD. There are a number of issues that need to be addressed before neuroprotective strategies in PD can be properly investigated:

1. Timing of neuroprotection: At presentation the majority of nigro-striatal neurons have already been lost, therefore any neuroprotective agent may be too late to be effective.

Studies of at risk asymptomatic carriers of disease causing genes (e.g. LRRK2) may prove useful in teasing out this issue. However, in some cases at least, familial PD may have a different disease mechanism to sporadic disease. Familial cases are also uncommon and age at onset and penetrance are variable making interpretation difficult. The identification of pre-clinical markers in sporadic IPD is therefore of great interest.

2. It is quite possible that IPD represents a heterogeneous group (various PD subtypes) of mechanisms giving rise to a final common phenotype. If this is so, the identification of a single effective neuroprotective agent will be difficult. Clarification of the pathophysiology of IPD will help target specific neuroprotective therapies tailored to one or more responsible mechanisms.

3. Outcome measures that satisfactorily measure neuroprotection are needed. Clinical markers do not necessarily correlate with disease modification, particularly when the agent being studied has symptomatic effects. In IPD the Unified Parkinson's Disease Rating Scale (UPDRS) is commonly used. The patient scores non-motor domains but many non-motor symptoms are not included. These symptoms may be more important in assessing disease modification as they generally are not levodopa-responsive and thus are unmodified by any symptomatic drug effect. The addition of imaging studies to assess striatal dopamine receptor density may be of value as a surrogate of neuronal loss.

4. Trial design is vital to allow interpretation of any findings. A 'wash-out' design allows, in theory, the symptomatic effect of a drug to wear off and thus leaving only a putative neuroprotective effect to account for a group difference. The biological effect of dopaminergic drugs may however last long beyond their pharmacological effect making interpretation difficult. 'Delayed-start' trials have attempted to address this issue by starting one group of patients on a study drug before the other. Failure of the delayed-start group to 'catch

up' with the early start group supports a possible neuroprotective effect of early treatment. This approach also has potential flaws. If a beneficial effect takes a long time to become established the delayed start group may not have had sufficient exposure to the study drug, Also, a strong symptomatic effect can be sufficient to mask any disease modifying effect.

6.11.1 Selected Trials of Interest

- Antioxidants have been investigated because the metabolism of dopamine by MAO-B produces free radicals. The DATATOP trial compared the effects of the MAO-B inhibitor selegiline (10 mg/day) and the antioxidant tocopherol or vitamin E (2000 U/day). Selegiline delayed the requirement of levodopa by a mean of 9 months. Because of an unexpected symptomatic effect of selegiline, disease modification could not be proven. The subsequent trial with selegiline, the BLIND-DATE trial, added selegiline or placebo to patients already taking levodopa. The results showed less clinical worsening of UPDRS scores, less freezing of gait and a lesser increase of additional levodopa in the group taking selegiline compared to the placebo group despite the liberty to take as much levodopa as needed. This supports the possibility of disease modification but doesn't prove it.
- The recent ADAGIO trial attempted to readdress the question by studying a different MAO-B inhibitor, rasagiline (1 or 2 mg), versus placebo using a delayed start protocol. The delayed start group demonstrated significant differences in UPDRS (1.7 points) with respect to the 1 mg dose of rasagiline at the end of 52 weeks. Questions remain however as strangely the findings using a 1 mg dose were not replicated in the group receiving 2 mg.
- Coenzyme Q10, a promising antioxidant and mitochondrial-activeagent, at 1200 mg/day showed some reduction of parkinsonism in a randomized, placebo-controlled, double-blind pilot study of 80 patients not requiring treatment for their disability. The trial met prespecified criteria looking for a linear response between dose and change in UPDRS ($p=0.09$). The placebo group and patient group receiving 1200 mg differed significantly with respect to this change (+11.99 vs. +6.69 respectively). However, recently completed phase III randomized clinical trial was terminated early, after a prespecified futility criterion was reached. The trial has shown the Coenzyme Q10 was safe and well tolerated but showed no evidence of clinical benefit in PD patients.
- The ELLDOPA study was designed to determine if levodopa has a toxic effect on dopaminergic neurons. A placebo group was compared with three groups receiving levodopa at varying doses, 150, 300 and 600 mg per day. All subjects had early PD (less than 3 years). Treatment was for 40 weeks with a 2 week washout period before final assessment. The placebo group UPDRS worsened after 42 weeks while the high dose levodopa group maintained their improvement of −1.4 points with respect to baseline. This result raised the question of a neuroprotective effect of levodopa, however, the improvement could be due to a prolonged symptomatic effect insufficiently washed out over 2 weeks.
- Tozadenant, a selective adenosine A2a receptor antagonist in a dose of 120 or 180 mg twice daily was proven to be effective in reducing the off-time in a recent phase 2b, double blind, randomized trial. While the smaller dose of 60 mg twice daily did not provide a significant reduction of the off-time, the higher 240 mg twice daily dose was associated with markedly increased side effects.
- Cinnamon, a natural spice, improved motor function in MPTP-intoxicated mice in a recent study. Cinnamon expressed a protective effect on dopaminergic neurons by upregulation of Parkin/DJ1 in mice, indicating possible future benefit in PD patients.

6.12 Treatment According to the Stage of Parkinson Disease

6.12.1 When and How Should Treatment Be Started in Early Stage Disease?

In the absence of definitive evidence favoring a disease-modifying drug, authorities in the past have generally agreed that treatment is not necessary when symptoms are not causing disability. This practice was motivated by a desire to avoid unnecessary side effects that might outweigh a small benefit.

With the advent of newer agents that may have a disease-modifying role, some consider that initiation of treatment at the time of diagnosis is warranted to slow degeneration in an already considerably depleted substantia nigra. It is proposed that dopamine depletion in the basal ganglia leads to maladaptive, compensatory changes within basal ganglia circuits that may also put additional metabolic stress on a failing system. Early symptomatic treatment might prevent or delay decomposition by normalizing basal ganglia function. This hypothesis is based on the apparent benefit of early treatment demonstrated in trials with some symptomatic benefit including levodopa, selegiline and rasagiline. This was examined in the recent PROUD study which assessed early versus delayed start pramipexole. No difference was found between early and delayed treatment groups.

Many neurologists will now empirically start with either selegiline or rasagiline monotherapy, providing well tolerated once daily dosing with mild symptomatic benefit before starting more potent dopaminergic drugs or an anticholinergic for tremor predominant disease. The next step is typically the addition of a DA agonist (especially in young patients more prone to develop dyskinesias) due to their low propensity to induce dyskinesias and their ability to provide early symptom control in most patients, but with careful monitoring for side effects such as Impulsive-control disorder.

6.12.2 Stage When Symptoms and Signs Require Treatment with Levodopa

Incremental addition of dopamine follows when symptom control is no longer adequate. Levodopa can be introduced as a first line agent in treatment- naïve patients, but this approach is usually reserved for older patients (>70 years of age for example), patients with cognitive impairment in whom a greater risk of neuropsychiatric complications with DA could be expected or when a patient is at a high risk of injury due to falls.

The conflict exists between the development of dyskinesias after chronic levodopa treatment and its superior efficacy and tolerability when compared to dopamine agonists. After 5 years of levodopa therapy, about 75 % of patients will have some form of motor complication. Those in favor of early levodopa point out the relatively poor tolerability of DA and better quality of life scores with early levodopa compared to those started on an agonist. They also highlight follow-up of these two groups showing that only mild dyskinesias are significantly more frequent in those receiving levodopa ab initio. Furthermore, it is sometimes suggested that earlier levodopa is reasonable with infusional and surgical options now available if dyskinesias become an issue.

Those favoring initial dopamine agonist treatment point out that in young patients having many years of treatment ahead of them, disabling dyskinesias should be avoided for as long as possible if an effective alternative is available. Infusional and surgical options for the management of motor complications are only suitable for some patients and carry their own risks and side effects. It is usually possible to tailor treatment for patients based on individual social and occupational requirements.

The pragmatic approach is to introduce levodopa without undue delay when other antiparkinsonian medications, typically dopamine agonists, at maximum tolerated doses are no longer bringing about satisfactory symptom control or side effects are intolerable. An algorithm giving an overview of treatment options over the natural history of IPD is given in Fig. 6.3.

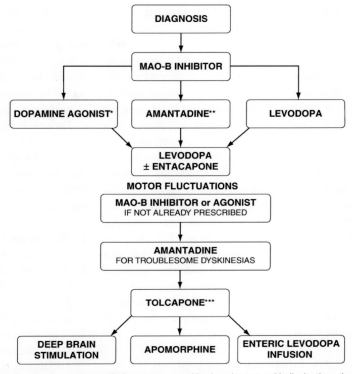

Fig. 6.3 Suggested treatment algorithm in idiopathic Parkinson's disease. Treatment needs to be individually tailored to each patients age, requirement and drug side-effect profiles

DIAGNOSIS

MAO-B INHIBITOR

DOPAMINE AGONIST* AMANTADINE** LEVODOPA

LEVODOPA
± ENTACAPONE

MOTOR FLUCTUATIONS

MAO-B INHIBITOR or AGONIST
IF NOT ALREADY PRESCRIBED

AMANTADINE
FOR TROUBLESOME DYSKINESIAS

TOLCAPONE***

DEEP BRAIN STIMULATION APOMORPHINE ENTERIC LEVODOPA INFUSION

*Dopamine agonists are more likely to cause cognitive impairment and hallucinations than levodopa. Ergot derived agonists are associated with a fibrotic cardiac valvulopathy.
**Amantadine should be avoided where there is pre-existing cognitive impairment or hallucinations.
***Tolcapone is a second line COMT inhibitor after entacapone due to a rare association with hepatic failure. Liver function needs to be regularly followed while on treatment.

6.12.2.1 Initiating Levodopa

Most treatment-naïve patients will tolerate initiation of levodopa/carbidopa at 50/12.5 mg TID. Each dose of 50/12.5 mg can then be gradually replaced by levodopa/carbidopa tablets of 100/10 mg or 100/25 mg until 100 mg of levodopa TID is reached. Many neurologists will initiate treatment using 100 mg doses of levodopa but a more cautious titration can be used in elderly patients and the very young patients as Parkin positive PD is sensitive to levodopa. Nausea is the main side effect in treatment naïve patients and can be treated with domperidone, 10 mg 30 min before or with each dose. The nausea and vomiting will usually settle within 2 weeks. For patients with persistent symptoms the formulation with a higher dose of carbidopa should be used (Sinemet Plus, carbidopa/levodopa 100 mg/25 mg) to

maximize peripheral dopa decarboxylase inhibition or this formulation can be used from the start.

There is no evidence that initiation of levodopa combined with a COMT inhibitor is of any benefit in delaying motor complications. In the early stage of levodopa therapy, before complications have developed, use of extended-release carbidopa/levodopa has no advantage over use of the standard preparation in delaying motor fluctuations. Some patients benefit from use of dispersible levodopa in the morning to achieve faster onset of action providing freedom of movement to get dressed and washed. This approach can be useful for early morning dystonia. Dispersible levodopa can also be used on an 'as required' basis for sudden 'off' periods although subcutaneous apomorphine boluses can prove more practical in this situation.

6.12.3 Management of Advanced Parkinson's Disease

Some patients with longstanding IPD can be effectively managed on oral dopaminergics with occasional adjustments to manage the complications of chronic treatment. Others cannot achieve adequate control despite optimum oral treatment. This group experience dyskinesias, constant swinging between 'off' and 'on' states and unpredictable 'offs'. Options at this stage include subcutaneous apomorphine, jejunal levodopa via gastrojejunostomy (Duodopa) or stereotactic deep brain surgery (DBS). Most patients at this stage have developed additional non-motor features of IPD including cognitive impairment and mood disorders that need to be considered when choosing advanced strategies. Treatment with these advanced therapies usually allows reduction of total dopaminergic drug dose but almost all patients continue to require some oral medication.

6.12.3.1 Infusional Apomorphine

Continuous subcutaneous apomorphine infusion was introduced in the 1980s and is useful in advanced IPD with motor fluctuations refractory to the usual strategies. Symptoms that are not levodopa-responsive will not improve. The drug is delivered via a pump connected to an infusion catheter. The needle sits subcutaneously in the abdominal wall or thigh. The rate of infusion can be adjusted with the ability to deliver bolus doses when required. Most patients require between 50 and 200 mg apomorphine per day. Some patients will take the pump off at night but continuous infusion is possible if nocturnal symptoms are a problem. Total daily levodopa can typically be halved.

The most common side effects with apomorphine are nausea, postural hypotension, daytime somnolence, and psychotoxicity. Patients need to be pre-treated with domperidone for 48 h and this is continued for as long as needed afterwards, usually less than 3 months. Abdominal wall nodules can form at infusion sites. Strict adherence to an aseptic technique during needle placement and regular rotation of sites can limit this problem. Ultrasound therapy and silicone gel patches

can reduce the size of nodules once formed. Coombs positive autoimmune hemolytic anemia is a rare and reversible side effect so a full blood count, reticulocyte count and Coomb's test should be performed intermittently. Patients should be warned that apomorphine can indelibly stain clothing an olive green color.

Patients being considered for an apomorphine infusion first need to be shown to be responsive to and tolerant of an apomorphine challenge as described below. For patients already using intermittent boluses with an apomorphine pen this is not necessary:

1. The patient is pre-treated with domperidone, 20–30 mg TDS for 48 h.
2. Anti-Parkinson medications should not be taken for 4–6 h prior to the challenge. Prolonged release dopaminergics should be omitted the day before.
3. A pre-treatment assessment is performed, typically including the motor subscale of the UPDRS or some other objective test of motor function (e.g. a timed walk).
4. An initial dose of 2 mg is administered. The clinical examination is repeated and the patient is observed for up to 30 min.
5. Increasing doses (in 1–2 mg increments) are given every 45 min until a 20 % improvement is documented or a maximum dose of 10 mg is reached. No response at 7 mg should be considered a negative challenge.
6. The challenge is positive if a 20 % improvement in pre-treatment motor function is observed.

6.12.3.2 Infusional Levodopa via Jejunostomy

Delayed gastric emptying in IPD can lead to erratic and unpredictable delivery of levodopa to the small intestine. Levodopa can be administered in a gel formulation (Duodopa) by infusion through an endoscopically placed gastrostomy with a jejunostomy tube to ensure a more constant and reliable rate of delivery. This method of levodopa administration appears to have similar efficacy to subcutaneous apomorphine, reducing daily 'off' time by up to 80 %.

The total daily dose of Duodopa required can be reduced by 20–30 % with addition of a COMT inhibitor if not already being used. Patients can be treated over 16 h with a break at night or continuously over 24 h for nocturnal symptoms. This form of infusion may be useful for patients intolerant of apomorphine or those with intolerable infusion site complications. Important considerations are the need for the patient or carer to understand how to manage the pump and the relatively high frequency of complications relating to tube placement including hemorrhage, peritonitis and the possibility that tubes can kink, become displaced and require replacement.

6.12.3.3 Surgical Procedures

Prior to the development of levodopa a number of surgical techniques were attempted to treat the motor symptoms of IPD. Thalamotomy emerged as the most effective, particularly for tremor. Surgical options faded from prominence with the miracle of levodopa, however the prevalence of motor complications after long-term levodopa exposure has renewed interest. DBS has replaced ablative procedures as the technique of choice, as it does not destroy brain tissue, it is potentially reversible and adjustments can be made post-operatively. The gait, speech, swallow and cognitive disturbances that are associated with bilateral ablative procedures are also less of a concern as stimulation can be reduced or aborted if required.

DBS does not offer superior control of the cardinal symptoms of IPD compared to levodopa except possibly for tremor. Its role is in the management of motor complications and the management of treatment-refractory tremor. Levodopa-responsive patients with dyskinesias or motor fluctuations affecting their quality of life are the best candidates.

The best results from DBS are seen with younger patients. The presence of cognitive impairment is a relative contraindication as cognition can worsen with any surgical penetration of the brain. However, recent prospectively gathered data from patients undergoing stimulation of the subthalamic nucleus is reassuring. Other adverse effects from DBS include hemorrhage, infection, speech impairment, dystonia and wire breakage. Even in young patients there can be impaired cognition, depression with suicide attempts and an incomplete response. Postoperative follow-up programming of the stimulators is an ongoing process.

Targets for ablative and DBS procedures are discussed below.

- *Thalamotomy and thalamic stimulation*: The target is the ventral intermediate nucleus and best effects are seen for contralateral intractable tremor that can be relieved in at least 70 % of cases. The effect on other parkinsonian features is less impressive. Although a unilateral lesion carries a small risk, bilateral operations result in dysarthria in 15–20 % of patients. Thalamic stimulation seems to be safer than ablation and can be equally effective against tremor.

- *Pallidotomy* and *pallidal stimulation*: The effects of globus pallidus stimulation are broadly similar to pallidotomy. The target is the posterolateral part of the globus pallidus interna (GPi) and outcomes are best treating contralateral dyskinesia with less benefit for bradykinesia and tremor. The target in the GPi is believed to be the site of afferent excitatory glutamatergic fibers coming from the subthalamic nucleus, which is overactive in IPD.

- *Subthalamotomy and subthalamic nucleus (STN) stimulation*: The beneficial effect of targeting this nucleus fits well with observed STN over-activity in IPD. The STN has a central role in the classic model of basal ganglia function, providing excitatory input to the GPi. Subthalamotomy has been infrequently performed in IPD because of the potentially serious side effect of producing contralateral hemiballism. This risk is not present with DBS, which is now the most commonly performed procedure in the treatment of bradykinesia, rigidity and tremor. The antiparkinsonian effect is no better than the best levodopa effect (except for tremor where surgery seems to be superior).

6.12.4 Management of Acute Deterioration in Parkinson's Disease

Sustained functional deterioration in IPD should be investigated thoroughly for a reversible cause. Like many chronic neurological conditions, any systemic illness can cause an acute deterioration from baseline. If treatable, a return to baseline should be expected but this can take weeks after the original insult has resolved. Two causes of acute deterioration worth highlighting are missed medications and inappropriate exposure to dopamine antagonists. Both problems can occur when patients are admitted for surgery, either as an emergency or electively. Involvement of a neurology team in these cases is useful, particularly for patients who are fasting or with advanced disease. Causes of acute deterioration to consider in IPD and their management are given below. In general, an increase in levodopa dose in the setting of one of these precipitants is preferably avoided.

- *Sepsis*: Perform a full septic screen and treat appropriately with advice from microbiology if required.
- *Dehydration*: Rehydrate and correct any electrolyte disturbances.
- *Constipation*: Treat with laxatives and confirm resolution on plain film of abdomen. The aim should be to have at least one normal or soft bowel motion daily.
- *Stress or anxiety*: Treat appropriately with psychiatry advice if required.
- *Missed medication or inappropriate sudden withdrawal of medication*: Reinstate at previous effective dose.
- *Exposure to dopamine antagonists (e.g. prochlorperazine)*: Discontinue drug, use an acceptable alternative.
- *Concurrent, medical or surgical illness*: Supportive care, physiotherapy to maintain mobility and expect slow return to baseline level.
- *Hardware or battery failure if deep brain stimulator in situ*: Immediate neurosurgical referral.

- *Cervical spine injury*: Consider if after a fall there is a deterioration in gait with pyramidal signs in the lower limbs or a history of cervical spondylosis. Compromise of the cervical spine should also be considered in patients with deteriorating mobility despite increasing amounts of levodopa, particularly when resulting dyskinesias are limited to the head and neck region.
- *Serotonin syndrome*: Consider if there has been a recent introduction of an SSRI or TCA; stop any potential causative agent and support acutely.
- *Depression*: Common in PD and may present with somatic symptoms resembling hypophonia and bradyphrenia. Consider an SSRI or tricyclic anti-depressant.

6.13 Long-Term Complications of Treatment

6.13.1 Motor Fluctuations

The pharmacokinetics of levodopa show a peak plasma concentration in about 30 min, and an elimination phase of about 90 min. Despite this, patients typically report no variability in their symptoms initially despite a TID dosing regime. This long-duration benefit may be due to the buffering effect of dopamine storage in surviving nigral nerve terminals and to a long lasting postsynaptic effect, facilitating this early 'honeymoon period'. Ongoing neuronal loss accompanied by functional receptor changes in the striatum may be important in the genesis of motor complications. Over time the clinical response becomes shorter, unpredictable and often inadequate. The long-duration benefit is lost and only the short-duration benefit is seen.

Motor fluctuations typically begin with an end of dose deterioration or *wearing off*, defined as a return of parkinsonian symptoms less than 4 h after the last dose. Patients gradually become aware of increasing contrast between 'on' and 'off' time. Initially, 'off' time will be prior to a scheduled levodopa dose, but unpredictable 'offs' unrelated to the timing of medications may evolve. Patients sometimes report a '*not on*' (dose failures) or '*delayed on*' phenomenon where they get no response or a delayed response to a particular dose. Most dose failures are due to delay in levodopa entering the duodenum where it can be absorbed. Having the patient crush the tablet between his teeth and swallowing with ample amount of water could dissolve levodopa faster and facilitate its entry into the small intestine. Motor 'offs' can be accompanied by non-motor 'offs' with patients reporting anxiety, autonomic symptoms, dysphoria and pain during these periods. Non-motor 'off's' do not always coincide with motor fluctuations and may be difficult to recognize. Patients with non-motor 'offs' tend to take more frequent dosings of levodopa in an effort to avoid these intolerable 'offs.'

Treatment adjustment aiming for continuous dopaminergic stimulation remains a mainstay of treating motor fluctuations. Changes in dosing schedules and the addition of drugs that prolong the life of dopamine at the dopamine receptor can assist in 'smoothing out' the levodopa response. Strategies that are commonly used are given in Table 6.7.

6.13.2 Dyskinesias

These are frequently mild choreic (dance-like) movements that are often unnoticed by the patient and managed with small reductions in levodopa if bothersome. In some cases dyskinesias are disabling and severe, consisting of chorea, ballism, dystonia, or a combination of these. Dyskinesias are more common in young-onset patients, of whom 70 % are affected after 3 years of treatment. Initially patients will spend only a small part of the day in either the 'off' or dyskinetic state with the 'on' period in between representing the target 'therapeutic window' where function is adequate. Over time this window shrinks in duration with patients flipping from the 'off' state to being dyskinetic. Patients at this stage will often prefer to be dyskinetic as it is only when dyskinetic that they can have some freedom of movement. Distressed relatives may not appreciate this functional significance of dyskinesias. Dyskinesias can be

Table 6.7 Management of motor fluctuations in Parkinson's disease

Levodopa should be taken 1 h before or 2 h after eating to enhance passage from stomach to small intestine and to reduce competition against amino acids for large neutral amino acid transporters in the small intestine. This can improve the 'delayed on' or 'no-on' phenomena
Constipation is almost universal in PD. Regular bowel habit can contribute to an overall strategy to make levodopa absorption and motor response more predictable
Additional doses reduce the inter-dose interval and can resolve wearing off. Patients with advanced IPD will commonly require levodopa every 3 h throughout the day
Addition of dopamine agonists which have longer half-lives, particularly modified release formulations of ropinirole, pramipexole or the rotigotine patch, reduce both the frequency and the depth of the "off" states
Addition of selegiline, rasagiline or a COMT inhibitors (entacapone or tolcapone) can improve mild wearing-off. The addition of COMT inhibitors may require a reduction in levodopa dose of 15–30 % as peak-dose dyskinesias can be precipitated or worsen
Slow-release forms of carbidopa/levodopa (Sinemet CR) have been used to improve wearing off although plasma levodopa levels can be erratic and response unpredictable
Patients who have rapid transitions between 'on' and 'off' can benefit from dispersible forms of levodopa (Madopar Dispersible). This speeds up the transit of levodopa to the small intestine giving them a 'kick-start'. Pre-filled apomorphine pen devices delivering bolus doses subcutaneously can also be used for a similar effect
Infusional therapies aim to achieve continuous dopaminergic stimulation to smooth out motor fluctuations. Levodopa in a gel is infused directly into the small intestine (Duodopa), avoiding erratic passage through the stomach. Subcutaneous apomorphine bypasses the gut to provide continuous symptomatic relief although patient selection is important

sub-divided into (1) peak-dose dyskinesias, appearing at the height of antiparkinsonian benefit, 20 min to 2 h after a dose, (2) diphasic dyskinesias, usually affecting the legs, appearing at the beginning and end of the dosing cycle and (3) 'off' dystonia, which can be painful sustained cramping, appear during "off" states and may be seen as early-morning dystonia presenting as foot cramps. Judicious introduction of levodopa with or without

Table 6.8 Strategies for the management of dyskinesias in Parkinson's disease

1. Peak dose dyskinesias can be improved by small reductions in each levodopa dose, facilitated by the addition of a dopamine agonist. COMT and MAO-B inhibitors can be added to facilitate weaning of levodopa that might lead to wearing off, alternatively the inter-dose interval can be reduced

2. Avoid long acting formulations of levodopa that can accumulate over the course of the day leading to dyskinesias that can be prolonged

3. Amantadine can reduce the severity of dyskinesias, but a dose of at least 400 mg/day is usually required and any benefit may not persist. Cognitive impairment, nightmares, hallucinations and myoclonus are not uncommon side-effects and limit its use in older patients

4. Diphasic dyskinesias are more difficult to treat. Increasing the dosage of levodopa can be effective but peak-dose dyskinesia usually ensues. A switch to a dopamine agonist is more effective; low doses of levodopa are used as an adjunctive agent

5. The principle of treating "off dystonia" is to try to keep the patient "on" most of the time. Here again, using a dopamine agonist as the major antiparkinsonian drug, with low doses of levodopa as an adjunct, can often be effective

6. If adjustment of oral medications is ineffective infusional (subcutaneous or jejunal) or surgical options should be explored with good results in appropriately selected patients

dopamine agonists can delay the onset and reduce the severity of dyskinesias, although over time they are inevitable, particularly in younger patients. Treatment strategies are outlined in Table 6.8.

6.13.3 Freezing

Freezing, a sudden inability to move lasting seconds to minutes, can be seen at any stage of PD but typically is seen with motor fluctuations in advanced disease. If early in the illness, think of atypical parkinsonism such as PSP or vascular parkinsonism. Any movement can be involved, but freezing of gait is the most disabling form and can be an important cause of falls where upper body momentum causes loss of balance on freezing when walking or turning. "Off-freezing" must be distinguished from "on-freezing."

Off-freezing was described before the advent of levodopa therapy and therefore is a disease phenomenon and not a complication of treatment; it responds to levodopa. On-freezing remains an enigma; patients can be seen to freeze despite good control of all other symptoms. The etiology is unknown but non-dopaminergic systems are probably involved.

Although rarely successful, reduction of the total amount of 'off' time by increasing dopaminergic medications is the best approach to treating 'off-freezing'. There is no proven treatment for 'on-freezing' but reduction of total levodopa dose can sometimes help, but this can worsen all other levodopa- responsive symptoms. Both on and off-freezing seem to correlate with both the duration of illness and the duration of levodopa therapy. Early use of the MAO-B inhibitors rasagiline and selegiline may reduce the risk of developing the freezing phenomenon. Non-pharmacological approaches include walking aids to reduce the risk of falling. The use of sensory cues takes advantage of *kinesie paradoxale* whereby the inclusion of a sensory stimulus into the motor routine appears to activate a more effective motor program. Examples include the use of a metronome, a bar on a walking cane to step over or internally generated cues such as counting or attempting to walk like a soldier.

New targets for DBS aim to target those motor symptoms not responsive to levodopa, in particular freezing and postural instability. Initial unblinded studies of surgery targeting the pedunculopontine nucleus suggested that stimulation of this mainly cholinergic nucleus might be of benefit in freezing of gait, but this has not been borne out in blinded studies.

6.13.4 Neuropsychiatric

Confusion, agitation, hallucinations, delusions, paranoia, and mania are probably related to activation of dopamine receptors in non-striatal regions although psychosis can be a primary disease phenomenon, especially if the patient has developed dementia. Dopamine agonists more often bring out these complications, particularly at high doses. Early hallucinations or psychosis should prompt the question of underlying Lewy body dementia or concomitant Alzheimer disease. Where possible, reversible causes of any deterioration should be sought before this assumption is made:

1. Eliminate sepsis, dehydration and electrolyte imbalances as a cause of a delirium.
2. Addition of an atypical neuroleptic, preferred for their affinity for D4 more than D2 receptors, such as quetiapine and clozapine.
3. Discontinue any drugs that may be responsible, typically in the following order based on propensity to cause neuropsychiatric side effects—anticholinergics, amantadine, MAO-B inhibitors and dopamine agonists.
4. If discontinuation of the above is ineffective, patients on a high dose of levodopa should have their dose reduced down to the minimal effective dose.

Neuroleptic drugs can induce drowsiness and should therefore be given at bedtime. Start with a dose of 12.5 mg of quetiapine to avoid the biweekly blood counts required with clozapine although it is less effective (see above). If clozapine is not tolerated, other drugs, including small doses of olanzapine, molindone, aripiprazole or pimozide can be used. If the parkinsonism deteriorates, lowering the dosage of levodopa to avoid the psychosis is preferable to maintaining a high dose of the antipsychotic. Levodopa should not be discontinued suddenly; abrupt cessation may induce a neuroleptic malignant-like syndrome, sometimes referred to as parkinsonism-hyperpyrexia syndrome.

6.13.5 Impulse Control Disorders

Impulse control disorders (ICDs) are seen in the general population, but are more common in IPD. ICDs represent an inability to resist a drive or temptation to perform an act harmful to others or oneself. Pathological gambling is most often encountered but hypersexuality, excessive shopping, reckless generosity and hyperphagia are also described. Significant financial, personal and social harm can be done. Young male patients with early-onset disease are at particular risk.

ICDs appear to be specific to treatment with dopamine agonists with a dose–response effect. This may be due to their affinity for D3 receptors of the mesocorticolimbic pathways, stimulation of which is integral to reward and re-enforcement behavior. *Dopa Dysregulation Syndrome* (DDS) is a related phenomenon whereby a patient will take excessive and repeated doses of levodopa or a fast acting agonist such as apomorphine, often despite disabling dyskinesias. Soluble forms of dopamine are often preferred due to their rapid onset of action. *Punding* is repetitive behavior involving purposeless motor tasks such as picking at oneself, taking apart watches, radios, dishwashers and washing machines, sorting and rearranging of common objects, such as lining up pebbles, rocks, or other small objects or more bizarre things such as a patient of ours who cut an expensive leather couch in half to move half of it through the door to a different room.

The management of ICDs involves early recognition and reduction of dopamine agonist doses to a minimum or stopping completely. This approach is effective in the majority of cases. Change to an alternative agonist is of little value and in some cases levodopa will have to be increased to compensate for loss of the agonist. Patients with dopa dysregulation syndrome need to have their levodopa dose reduced to see an improvement. Fast acting water soluble forms should be avoided completely. A difficult aspect of managing ICD and DDS is obtaining a clear history from the patient or family due to embarrassment. Specifically asking for behavioral changes in the spectrum of ICD is therefore vital.

6.14 Recent & Future Developments

6.14.1 New Agonists, Continuous Dopaminergic Stimulation

Continuous dopaminergic stimulation remains a target to achieve sustained control over symptoms without the complications associated with prolonged treatment. A number of treatment options are now available that blunt the peaks and troughs of pulsatile stimulation including direct infusion of levodopa into the small intestine (Duodopa) and transdermal delivery of rotigotine. Some dopamine agonists are now available in a once-daily formulation that may further smooth the response to treatment. New dopamine agonists and delivery methods in the future will need to be potent enough to remain effective without the addition of levodopa since it appears that initial agonist treatment does not prolong the latent period before the onset of levodopa induced dyskinesias.

6.14.2 Dopaminergic Cell Transplantation

To date no double-blind controlled trial has shown a benefit of dopaminergic cell transplantation in IPD. Individual case series have been promising with post-mortem and radiological ([18]flourodopa PET) evidence of functioning graft tissue with some patients enjoying significant and even complete withdrawal of oral therapies. An important adverse effect noted in over 50 % of transplanted patients in one study is so called 'off medication dyskinesias'. This form of dyskinesia can be persistent, lasting for days or weeks. It is also possible that in time transplanted neurons will be susceptible to the same degenerative process that affected native neurons in the first place, however recent observations proved that implanted foetal dopamine neurons remain healthy for up to 15 years post-transplantation. More research is required to determine what immunosuppressive regime, quantity of transplanted cells and target patient group are required to improve outcomes. Importantly, even if eventually successful, dopaminergic cell transplantation may not benefit the disabling non-dopaminergic symptoms of IPD.

6.14.3 Stem Cell Implantation

Stem cell based therapies are an attractive option given the potential of these cells to repair degenerating or injured neural circuits and the ability to generate cell lines in vitro. Stem cells can be derived from pre-implantation human blastocysts. Neural progenitor cells are alternative sources of implantable cell lines, derived from embryonic tissue or post-operative adult specimens. Induced pluripotent stem cells are generated from skin fibroblasts through genetic manipulation and are an exciting proposition in that they avoid the ethical dilemma of using fetal tissue, they are in abundant supply and do not necessitate immunosupression.

No trials to date have evaluated the effect of stem cells in human patients but animal studies are ongoing. Before a human trial can take place the safety profile of implanting stem cells needs to be further evaluated. A major concern has been the development of malignant tumors following the implantation of undifferentiated stem cells in animal studies and in a young boy with ataxia telangiectasia who developed a multifocal glioma derived from transplanted stem cells. Furthermore the ethical issues surrounding stem cell based therapies need to be resolved individually in every jurisdiction. Like dopaminergic cell transplantation, even if successful, stem cell implantation is unlikely to address the many non-motor features of IPD.

6.14.4 Management of Non-dopaminergic Symptoms

Much of the Parkinson's disease research literature has been devoted to management of the complications of long-term levodopa treatment. Infusional dopaminergic treatments and functional neurosurgery have reached a point where motor fluctuations can be addressed to some satisfaction, although more options are needed for patients not suited to current treatment modalities. Attention will increasingly turn to the non-dopaminergic symptoms experienced in advanced PD, in particular dementia, freezing and postural instability. Cholinesterase inhibitors offer limited benefit in the management of dementia in the context of PD. Their general role in mild cognitive impairment is uncertain and many patients with cognitive impairment in PD will only have subtle frontal-dysexecutive features. Safinamide targets dopaminergic and glutaminergic targets and may have neuroprotective properties and a role in cognitive impairment although clinical trials are required.

6.14.5   Gene Therapy

Gene therapy has the potential to restore striatal dopaminergic function to a more physiological level by delivering proteins such as aromatic acid decarboxylase (AADC), 3,4-dihydroxyphenylalanine (DOPA) and glutamic acid decarboxylase (GAD) via an adeno-associated viral vector. Alternatively genes coding for trophic factors delivered to the basal ganglia might preserve or prolong survival of remaining dopaminergic neurons. Phase II clinical trials are currently underway.

6.14.6   Neuroprotection

Because the exact etiology of IPD is unknown it remains difficult to know where the development of a neuroprotective agent should be targeted. A number of potential targets have emerged, including mitochondrial metabolism based upon the study of inherited forms of the disease. Other possibilities include abnormalities in apoptotic and autophagy pathways, excitotoxicity and oxidative stress.

Recent development of a crystal structure of Parkin providing the information about Parkin at atomic level, and insight into its binding site and interaction with possible therapeutic molecules may help in a development of a structure-based novel drug designs.

Although development of a vaccine which will slow or stop PD still remains a challenge, it may be more feasible than previously thought with a phase I clinical trial suggesting in preliminary results that the vaccine may have a neuroprotective effect by reducing the accumulation of alpha-synuclein by inducing the alpha-synuclein-specific antibodies. However this immunotherapeutic approach has failed to date in other neurodegenerative disorders such as Alzheimer's disease.

A combination of factors may be at play with a cumulative effect to produce the parkinsonian 'phenotype'. Identification of genes, which are risk factors for the development of IPD from genome wide association studies, may be informative in the design neuroprotective regimes to target these potential risk factors individually. As stated previously, by the time patients present for treatment the majority of nigro-striatal dopaminergic neurons have been lost. If a disease-modifying agent will need to be introduced as early as possible. To enable this, a reliable biomarker of underlying susceptibility to PD in asymptomatic at risk individuals needs to be identified.

Selected Reading

Braak H, Bohl JR, Muller CM, Rub U, De Vos RAI, Del Tredici K. Stanley Fahn Lecture 2005: the staging procedure for the inclusion body pathology associated with sporadic Parkinson's disease reconsidered. Mov Disord. 2006;21:2042–51.
Brusa L, Orlacchio A, Stefani A, Galati S, Pierantozzi M, Iani C, Biagio Mercuri N. Tetrabenazine improves levodopa-induced peak-dose dyskinesias in patients with Parkinson's disease. Funct Neurol. 2013;28(2): 101–5.

Selected Trials of Interest

Chaudhuri KR, Schapira AH. Non-motor symptoms of Parkinson's disease: dopaminergic pathophysiology and treatment. Lancet Neurol. 2009;8(5):464–74.
Clarke CE, Worth P, Grosset D, Stewart D. Systematic review of apomorphine infusion, levodopa infusion and deep brain stimulation in advanced Parkinson's disease. Parkinsonism Relat Disord. 2009;15(10):728–41.
de Lau LM, Schipper CM, Hofman A, Koudstaal PJ, Breteler MM. Prognosis of Parkinson disease: risk of dementia and mortality: the Rotterdam Study. Arch Neurol. 2005;62:1265–9.
Deuschl G, Schade-Brittinger C, Krack P, Volkmann J, Schäfer H, Bötzel K, Daniels C, Deutschländer A, Dillmann U, Eisner W, Gruber D, Hamel W, Herzog J, Hilker R, Klebe S, Kloss M, Koy J, Krause M, Kupsch A, Lorenz D, Lorenzi S, Mehdorn HM, Moringlane JR, Oertel W, Pinsker MO, Reichmann H, Reuss A, Schneider GH, Schnitzler A, Steude U, Sturm V,

Timmermann L, Tronnier V, Trottenberg T, Wojtecki L, Wolf E, Poewe W, Voges J, German Parkinson Study Group, Neurostimulation Section. A randomised trial of deep-brain stimulation for Parkinson's disease. N Engl J Med. 2006;355(9):896–908.

Dorsey ER, Constantinescu R, Thompson JP, et al. Projected number of people with Parkinson disease in the most populous nations, 2005 through 2030. Neurology. 2007;68(5):384–6.

Fahn S. The freezing phenomenon in parkinsonism. Adv Neurol. 1995;67:53–63.

Fahn S. Parkinson's disease: 10 years of progress, 1997–2007. Mov Disord. 2010;25 Suppl 1:S2–14.

Fahn S, Oakes D, Shoulson I, Kieburtz K, Rudolph A, Lang A, Olanow CW, Tanner C, Marek K, Parkinson Study Group. Levodopa and the progression of Parkinson's disease. N Engl J Med. 2004;351(24):2498–508.

Hallett PJ, Cooper O, Sadi D, Robertson H, Mendez I, Isacson O. Long-term health of dopaminergic neuron transplants in Parkinson's disease patients. Cell Rep. 2014;7:1755–61.

Hauser RA, Rascol O, Korczyn AD, Jon Stoessl A, Watts RL, Poewe W, De Deyn PP, Lang AE. Ten-year follow-up of Parkinson's disease patients randomized to initial therapy with ropinerole or levodopa. Mov Disord. 2007;22(16):2409–17.

Hauser RA, Olanow CW, Kieburtz KD, Pourcher E, Docu-Axelerad A, Lew M, Kozyolkin O, Neale A, Resburg C, Meya U, Kenney C, Bandak S. Tozadenant (SYN115) in patients with Parkinson's disease who have motor fluctuations on levodopa: a phase 2b, double-blind, randomised trial. Lancet Neurol. 2014;13(8):767–76.

Healy DG, Falchi M, O'Sullivan SS, Bonifati V, Durr A, Bressman S, Brice A, Aasly J, Zabetian CP, Goldwurm S, Ferreira JJ, Tolosa E, Kay DM, Klein C, Williams DR, Marras C, Lang AE, Wszolek ZK, Berciano J, Schapira AH, Lynch T, Bhatia KP, Gasser T, Lees AJ, Wood NW, International LRRK2 Consortium. Phenotype, genotype, and worldwide genetic penetrance of LRRK2-associated Parkinson's disease: a case–control study. Lancet Neurol. 2008;7(7):583–90.

Hely MA, Reid WGJ, Adena MA, Halliday GM, Morris JGL. The Sydney multicentre study of Parkinson's disease: the inevitability of dementia at 20 years. Mov Disord. 2008;23(6):837–44.

Horn JR, Hansten PD. Preventing rasagiline drug interactions. Pharm Times. 2007. www.pharmacytimes.com/publications/issue/2007/2007-01/2007-01-6227.

Khasnavis S, Pahan K. Cinnamon treatment upregulates neuroprotective proteins Parkin and DJ-1 and protects dopaminergic neurons in a mouse model of Parkinson's disease. J Neuroimmune Pharmacol. 2014;9(4):569–81.

Lang AE. When and how should treatment be started in Parkinson disease? Neurology. 2009;72 Suppl 2:S39–43.

Lees AJ, Katzenschlager R, Head J, Ben-Shlomo Y. Ten-year follow-up of three different initial treatments in do-novo PD: a randomised trial. Neurology. 2001;57:1687–94.

Lippa CF, Duda JE, Grossman M, Hurtig HI, Aarsland D, Boeve BF, Brooks DJ, Dickson DW, Dubois B, Emre

M, Fahn S, Farmer JM, Galasko D, Galvin JE, Goetz CG, Growdon JH, Gwinn-Hardy KA, Hardy J, Heutink P, Iwatsubo T, Kosaka K, Lee VM, Leverenz JB, Masliah E, McKeith IG, Nussbaum RL, Olanow CW, Ravina BM, Singleton AB, Tnner CM, Trojanowski JQ, Wszolek ZK, DLB/PDD Working Group. DLB and PDD boundary issues: diagnosis, treatment, molecular pathology, and biomarkers. Neurology. 2007;68(11):812–9.

Lucking CB, Durr A, Bonifati V, Vaughan J, De Michele G, Gasser T, Harhangi BS, Meco G, Denèfle P, Wood NW, Agid Y, Brice A, French Parkinson's Disease Genetics Study Group; European Consortium on Genetic Susceptibility in Parkinson's Disease. Association between early-onset Parkinson's disease and mutations in the parkin gene. N Engl J Med. 2000;342:1560–7.

Marder K, Tang MX, Mejia H, Alfaro B, Côté L, Louis E, Groves J, Mayeux R. Risk of Parkinson's disease among first-degree relatives: a community based study. Neurology. 1996;47(1):155–60.

Marras C, Lang A. Parkinson's disease subtypes lost in translation? J Neurol Neurosurg Psychiatry. 2013;84(4):409–15.

O'Dowd S, Murray B, Roberts K, Cummins G, Magennis B, Lynch T. Pallidopontonigral degeneration: a deceptive familial tauopathy. Mov Disord. 2012;27(7):817–9.

Olanow CW, Goetz CG, Kordower JH, Stoessi AJ, Sossi V, Brin MF, Shannon KM, Nauert GM, Perl DP, Godbold J, Freeman TB. A double-blind controlled trial of bilateral fetal nigral transplantation in Parkinson's disease. Ann Neurol. 2003;54:403–14.

Olanow CW, Rascol O, Hauser R, Feigin PD, Jankovic J, Lang A, Langston W, Melamed E, Poewe W, Stocchi F, Tolosa E, ADAGIO Study Investigators. A double-blind, delayed-start trial of rasagaline in Parkinson's disease. N Engl J Med. 2009;361(13):1268–78.

Olesena J, Gustavssonb A, Svenssond M, et al. The economic cost of brain disorders in Europe. Eur J Neurol. 2012;19:155–62.

Parkinson Study Group QE3 Investigators, Beal MF, Oakes D, Shoulson I, Henchcliffe C, Galpern WR, Haas R, Juncos JL, Nutt JG, Voss TS, Ravina B, Shults CM, Helles K, Snively V, Lew MF, Griebner B, Watts A, Gao S, Pourcher E, Bond L, Kompoliti K, Agarwal P, Sia C, Jog M, Cole L, Sultana M, Kurlan R, Richard I, Deeley C, Waters CH, Figueroa A, Arkun A, Brodsky M, Ondo WG, Hunter CB, Jimenez-Shahed J, Palao A, Miyasaki JM, So J, Tetrud J, Reys L, Smith K, Singer C, Blenke A, Russell DS, Cotto C, Friedman JH, Lannon M, Zhang L, Drasby E, Kumar R, Subramanian T, Ford DS, Grimes DA, Cote D, Conway J, Siderowf AD, Evatt ML, Sommerfeld B, Lieberman AN, Okun MS, Rodriguez RL, Merritt S, Swartz CL, Martin WR, King P, Stover N, Guthrie S, Watts RL, Ahmed A, Fernandez HH, Winters A, Mari Z, Dawson TM, Dunlop B, Feigin AS, Shannon B, Nirenberg MJ, Ogg M, Ellias SA, Thomas CA, Frei K, Bodis-Wollner I, Glazman S, Mayer T, Hauser RA, Pahwa R,

Langhammer A, Ranawaya R, Derwent L, Sethi KD, Farrow B, Prakash R, Litvan I, Robinson A, Sahay A, Gartner M, Hinson VK, Markind S, Pelikan M, Perlmutter JS, Hartlein J, Molho E, Evans S, Adler CH, Duffy A, Lind M, Elmer L, Davis K, Spears J, Wilson S, Leehey MA, Hermanowicz N, Niswonger S, Shill HA, Obradov S, Rajput A, Cowper M, Lessig S, Song D, Fontaine D, Zadikoff C, Williams K, Blindauer KA, Bergholte J, Propsom CS, Stacy MA, Field J, Mihaila D, Chilton M, Uc EY, Sieren J, Simon DK, Kraics L, Silver A, Boyd JT, Hamill RW, Ingvoldstad C, Young J, Thomas K, Kostyk SK, Wojcieszek J, Pfeiffer RF, Panisset M, Beland M, Reich SG, Cines M, Zappala N, Rivest J, Zweig R, Lumina LP, Hilliard CL, Grill S, Kellermann M, Tuite P, Rolandelli S, Kang UJ, Young J, Rao J, Cook MM, Severt L, Boyar K. A randomized clinical trial of high-dosage coenzyme Q10 in early Parkinson disease: no evidence of benefit. JAMA Neurol. 2014;71(5):543–52.

Polymeropoulos MH, Lavedan C, Leroy E, Ide SE, Dehejia A, Dutra A, Pike B, Root H, Rubenstein J, Boyer R, Stenroos ES, Chandrasekharappa S, Athanassiadou A, Papapetropoulos T, Johnson WG, Lazzarini AM, Duvoisin RC, Di Iorio G, Golbe LI, Nussbaum RL. Mutation in the alpha-synuclein gene identified in families with Parkinson's disease. Science. 1997;276(5321):2045–7.

Riley BE, Lougheed JC, Callaway K, et al. Structure and function of Parkin E3 ubiquitin ligase reveals aspects of RING and HECT ligases. Nat Commun. 2013;4:1982.

Schapira AH. Neuroprotection in Parkinson's disease. Parkinsonism Relat Disord. 2009;15 Suppl 4:S41–3.

Schapira AH, Obeso J. Timing of treatment initiation in Parkinson's disease. A need for reappraisal? Ann Neurol. 2006;59:559–62.

Schwarz ST, Afzal M, Morgan PS, Bajaj N, Gowland PA, et al. The swallow tail appearance of the healthy nigrosome-a new accurate test of Parkinson's disease: a case–control and retrospective cross-sectional MRI study at 3T. PLoS One. 2014;9(4), E93814.

Shoulson I, Oakes D, Fahn S, Lang A, Langston JW, LeWitt P, Olanow CW, Penney JB, Tanner C, Kieburtz K, Rudolph A, Parkinson Study Group. Impact of sustained deprenyl (selegiline) in levodopa-treated Parkinson's disease: a randomized placebo-controlled extension of the deprenyl and tocopherol antioxidative therapy of parkinsonism trial. Ann Neurol. 2002;51(5):604–12.

Szewczyk-Krolikowski K, Menke RA, Rolinski M, Duff E, Salimi-Khorshidi G, Filippini N, Zamboni G, Hu MT, Mackay CE. Functional connectivity in the basal ganglia network differentiates PD patients from controls. Neurology. 2014;83(3):208–14.

Thenganatt MA, Jankovic J. Parkinson disease subtypes-review. JAMA Neurol. 2014;71(4):499–504.

Fronto-Temporal Dementia (FTD)

Marwa Elamin, Taha Omer, Siobhan Hutchinson, Colin P. Doherty, and Thomas H. Bak

7.1 Introduction

The terms "Frontotemporal dementia" or "Frontotemporal lobar degeneration" are often used interchangeably to describe a clinically and pathologically heterogeneous group of disorders characterized by degeneration of the frontal and temporal lobes. This disorder is comprised of multiple clinical variants. These include the "frontal" or "behavioural" variant which is characterised by decline in behaviour and several

M. Elamin • T. Omer
Academic Unit of Neurology, Trinity Biomedical Sciences Institute, Dublin, Ireland
e-mail: marwaelamin08@gmail.com; eldoory@hotmail.com

S. Hutchinson
Cognitive Neurology Clinic, St. James's Hospital, Dublin, Ireland
e-mail: SHutchinson@STJAMES.IE

C.P. Doherty (✉)
Academic Unit of Neurology, Trinity Biomedical Sciences Institute, Dublin, Ireland

Department of Neurology, St. James's Hospital, Dublin, Ireland
e-mail: colinpdoherty@gmail.com

T.H. Bak
The Anne Rowling Regenerative Neurology Clinic, Centre for Clinical Brain Sciences (CCBS), University of Edinburgh, Edinburgh, UK
e-mail: thomas.bak@ed.ac.uk

language variants where the clinical presentations is with language difficulties. Neary et al. use the umbrella term Frontotemporal Lobar Degeneration (FTLD) for all of the above and reserved the term "Frontotemporal dementia" to refer specifically to the "frontal" / "behavioural" variant. In contrast, McKhann et al. 2001 used the term Frontotemporal dementia (FTD) to refer to all of the above presentations. For the purposes of this chapter we use the term Frontotemporal dementia (FTD) in the general sense of McKhann et al. In addition, the term "behavioural" variant FTD is currently preferred to the tem "frontal" as it addresses the behavioural syndrome rather the presumed anatomical localisation and is thus more comparable to the terms used for the language variants. The description of the FTD language variants in this chapter is guided the most recent classification of primary progressive aphasia (PPA) syndromes and includes progressive non-fluent aphasia or nfvPPA (previously PNFA), the semantic variant or svPPA (previously called semantic dementia) and the recently described logopenic variant or lvPPA.

7.2 History

Arnold Pick (1892) is credited with the first description of a progressive disorder of behaviour and language associated with circumscribed atrophy of the frontal and temporal lobes. Later,

© Springer International Publishing Switzerland 2016
O. Hardiman, C.P. Doherty (eds.), *Neurodegenerative Disorders: A Clinical Guide*,
DOI 10.1007/978-3-319-23309-3_7

Alois Alzheimer (1911) described the classical histological changes associated with "Pick's disease" that of inter-neuronal inclusions and ballooned neurons. In the 1980's, two groups in Lund, Sweden and Manchester, United Kingdom published separately large series of patients with frontotemporal atrophy and dementia with prominent behaviour and language difficulties. They noted that Pick-type histology was only one of three main histological changes seen and they came up with the first consensus criteria for frontotemporal dementia. At the same time Mesulam described a series of patients with a progressive language disorder with sparing of other cognitive domains and non-Alzheimer's pathology, which he termed primary progressive aphasia (PPA).

Over the subsequent decade further clinical, imaging and pathological studies prompted the consensus group to refine the criteria in 1998. They separated the language variants from the behavioural disorder. The separation of these syndromes has led research focused on different clinical variants. This has resulted in significant advances in our understanding of the genetics and molecular pathology underlying these variants. However, overlap between the clinical syndromes is still apparent. Indeed, in familial FTD each of the different clinical syndromes can be seen in the same kindred. Also, in later stages of each syndrome, patients will often have a mixed clinical picture of behaviour and language difficulties.

7.3 Epidemiology and Demographics

Age of onset of FTD is typically younger than other forms of dementia being between 45 and 65 years, though cases are reported outside this range. FTD is the third most common form of cortical dementia after Alzheimer's disease (AD) and Dementia with Lewy Bodies (DLB) and the second most common cause of young-onset dementia after AD.

Studies in the UK and U.S.A suggest that the prevalence of FTD in 45–64 age group is 15–22 per 100,000 with incidence estimates for the same age group ranging from 2.7 to 4.1 per 100,000 person-years. A population-based study

in the Netherlands reported lower prevalence rates of 3–4 per 100,000 in the 45–64 age group, 9.4 per 100,000 for the 60–69 age group, and 3.8 per 100,000 at 70–79 age group. Although this supports that concept that FTD is not a dementia of old age, a recent study based on the Swedish Registry for Dementia, reported that 70 % of FTD cases were 65 years or older at the time of diagnosis. Both FTD and AD displayed an increased incidence with age in that study, with FTD incidence in the 80–84 years reaching 6.04 per 100,000 person-years.

Data from UK registry suggest a male predominance (14:3), several studies from Italy suggest a female predominance (1: 1.3–2), while other reports suggested equal sex distribution.

The duration of illness from onset to death has a range from 2 to 20 years with a mean of 6 to 8 years. Behavioural variant FTD (bvFTD) is the most common FTD syndrome affecting 55 % of all cases, while non-fluent progressive aphasia (nfvPPA) accounts for 25 %, and the semantic variant (svPPA) for 20 %. Demography does differ between the syndromes: For example, svPPA has a later age of onset (though still younger than typical AD patients) and a slower rate of progression with a median survival of about 12 years. Patients with bvFTD have the earliest age of onset and generally more rapid progression with a survival of about 9 years. The presence of co-morbid motor involvement in the form of amyotrophic lateral scleroses (FTD with co-morbid ALS or FTD-ALS) is associated with shortest survival (2–5 years).

7.4 Clinical Features

As with other forms of cortical dementia, symptoms are gradual in onset and progressive over time. Below is a description of the most common FTD variants.

7.4.1 Behavioural Variant FTD (bv-FTD)

The hallmark of bvFTD is gradual onset deterioration in behaviour and inter-personal conduct. Patients often lack insight into their abnormal behaviour. This often leads to delay in seeking medical attention. Thus detailed semi-structured interviews with family members focused on behavioural changes are an essential component of evaluating patients with suspected bvFTD. It is important to note that the patient's family and friends often excuse some or all the personality changes, at least initially, as part of "mid-life crisis". Thus, the interviews should include a mixture of open questions (e.g. "have you noticed any change in personality/behaviour?") and direct questions about the specific behavioural changes that can be encountered in this condition.

It is usually socially inappropriate interpersonal behaviour that is noted initially due to impulsivity and disinhibition of verbal, physical or sexual impulses. Difficulties with interpersonal conduct are not only due to disinhibition but also due to deficits in emotional processing, social awareness and social cognitive skills. These deficits can lead to inability to express and recognize facial or vocal expressions of emotion and/or inferring the mental states and intentions of others from social cues. These abilities form part of the so called "theory of mind". This results in problematic social interactions, loss of empathy and a reduced concern for others. These behaviours are often perceived by the caregiver as 'out of character' and constitute a significant change in personality. It is important to note that for these reasons distress is common among the caregivers of bvFTD patients, compared with caregivers of other forms of cortical dementia.

In tandem with the decline in interpersonal conduct, there is often a change in personal conduct, usually in form of loss of drive/motivation or apathy and rarely hyperactivity. Apathy is often noted by caregivers and can be mistaken for depression. It is one of the factors that contribute to the loss in previous hobbies and social activities and the decline in personal hygiene and grooming that is frequently reported.

Other behavioural symptoms that have been reported in bvFTD patients include perseverative and stereotyped (ritualistic/compulsive) behaviour and speech patterns. This can include simple behaviours such as humming, or tapping, as well as complex behaviours such as constant checking of door locks or light switches. Preservative

speech patterns includes repeating the same catchphrases and repeating what others say (echolalia). Patients may also develop hyper-orality, over-eating or bingeing, and change in food preference (usually developing a "sweet tooth"). Utilization behaviour, the act of compulsively grasping and using objects within one's visual field, has also been described and seems to be particularity frequent in bvFTD patients from Asia.

The cognitive symptoms experienced are due to executive dysfunction – therefore patients have difficulties in planning, problem solving, organization, attention and mental flexibility. These are symptoms that are not easily identified either by the caregiver or history taker but important clues include decline in performance at work and home ("activities of daily living") and adherence to a rigid routine or way of doing things. Notably, cognitive function can be intact early in the disease even in the context of marked behavioural changes.

Cummings et al. have suggested three distinct bvFTD syndromes based on the predominance of disinhibition, apathy or dysexecutive behaviour. In contrast, Snowden et al. suggested that bvFTD can be subdivided into apathetic variant, disinhibited variant and a variant of stereotyped-compulsive syndromes. These syndromic sub-classifications are supported by anatomic and radiological correlations. Apathetic behaviour has been associated with changes in medial frontal cortex, anterior cingulate and superior frontal gyrus, particularly on the right. Disorders of self-regulation and disinhibition as associated with changes in the ventromedial prefrontal cortex (VMPC), the anterior temporal lobe, the amygdala, and the orbito-frontal cortical subcortical circuit. Dorsolateral prefrontal (DLPC) changes are linked to a dysexecutive syndrome. Overall involvement of the right hemisphere is associated with more severe behavioural changes. However, in practice these symptoms frequently co-occur, and the clinical usefulness of these distinctions is limited.

7.4.2 Language Variants of bv-FTD

Patients with the language variants of FTD are generally more aware of their deficits compared

Table 7.1 Examples of spoken and written language from patients with non-fluent/agrammatic aphasia

Examples of speech
"We are looking for one hor....like we...are just saying...I should not have done...I didn't realize it, like I say.......... I used to be very ..... I had just first thing I do....here is what she says is ...I am giving her problems....... It is me making something I don't think about."
Till a few years ago...... I had business.... for saying... because things going wrong because I was dealing people in the house......... I could not get the word. ....Just had to stop.

Examples from written description of the Cookie-Theft Picture test
Boy trying to get cookies. Boy folling of chair. Mother wiping plate. Water overflow. Mother not taken much notice about water on floor.
Cook. Jar Dishis Flood Sink Di Stool

All patients are native English speakers

to bvFTD patients and they will frequently complain, "I've forgotten the words for things". However, the presentation can still be delayed as their difficulties are often put down as normal aging.

In progressive non-fluent aphasia (nfvPPA) there is breakdown in spontaneous speech. The core changes in nfvPPA are reduced fluency leading to effortful halting speech and deficits in grammar. The later deficits often lead to simplification, distorted word order as well as omissions of function words such articles and propositions (see Table 7.1 for examples).

Anomia is common due to difficulties in word retrieval but object knowledge remains intact. Thus although the patient cannot name an object, they may be able to pick the correct name from choice and will be able to match the object with other objects that semantically linked to it.

Comprehension for single words in usually intact but impaired comprehension of syntactically complex sentences is often an early feature. In addition, these patients have difficulties in speech production due to speech apraxia leading to word sound distortions.

The semantic variant (svPPA, previously semantic dementia) is the second FTD language variant. The hallmark of svPPA is loss of semantic knowledge. This manifests as severe naming and word comprehension impairment in the context of fluent, effortless, and grammatically correct speech output. Semantic paraphasias are common. Words are often substituted by a semantically related but more frequent object (e.g. "horse" for "zebra") or a more general categorical term (e.g. "animal" for "cow").

Due to the loss of semantic knowledge, patients have difficulties in single word comprehension and are unable to match the object with semantically similar objects or pick an object from description of its use. Knowledge loss affects initially the less frequent or atypical exemplars of category (e.g. first "hamster", then 'rabbit', then 'animal'). Knowledge of more personally relevant objects is more resistant. Of note, episodic memory remains intact and patients often remain oriented, are able to keep appointments, and to learn and recall visuospatial information.

Repetition is not impaired in svPPA and patients can repeat multi-syllable words without difficulty. In contrast writing and reading relies exclusively on phonological (letter by letter) reading/writing as patients have no access to previously learned word knowledge, which includes the correct way to read irregular words (such as "yacht" or "cough"). This leads regularisation errors when reading or writing. This is termed as "surface alexia/dyslexia" and "surface agraphia/dysgraphia" respectively.

The above described svPPA phenotype is usually associated with predominant involvement of the dominant hemisphere. A rarer form of svPPA is seen where the disease process affects mainly the non-dominant hemisphere. The phenotype in this form usually includes agnosia (a failure to recognise objects or people) and more prominent behavioural changes.

The logopenic variant of progressive aphasia (lvPPA) is the third type of primary progressive aphasia syndrome. This variant has been recognised only recently and its exact syndromic classification remains controversial. Unlike the other language variants of PPA, the most common pathology underlying this disorder is that of Alzheimer's type pathology. However, recent evidence suggests that 23 % of lvPPA patient have FTD pathology on autopsy.

lvPPA is characterised by fluctuating interruptions of fluency due to word finding difficulties, with intact grammar and sound production. There is often impaired repetition and comprehension, particularly for long improbable phrases, an observation in line with the hypotheses that episodic memory impairment plays a central role in this condition.

Finally, it is worth noting that while the most salient complaints in language variants of FTD are by definition language related, there are often associated behavioural changes, particularly in svPPA patients. The pattern of behavioural changes in language variant FTD may be different from that of bvFTD. Some reports suggest that apathy, lack of empathy and hyper-orality are more common in bvFTD while compulsive and complex stereotypic behaviours, mental rigidity anxiety, repetitive themes, and sleep disorders may be more common in svPPA.

7.5   Associated Syndromes

7.5.1   Syndromes That Overlap and Mimic FTD

Research has shown the significant pathological and molecular overlap between FTD and other neurodegenerative disorders and hence the crossover in clinical features. Table 7.2 summarizes the syndrome that overlap.

On the other hand, there are a range of clinical disorders that have no pathological overlap but whose clinical phenotype can mimic those of FTD. Table 7.3 summarises the syndrome that mimic FTD.

7.6   Clinical Assessment

The first part of the clinical assessment in FTD patients is obtaining a detailed history, emphasising any changes in behaviour, language and other cognitive domains and their impact on the patient's ability to function at home and at work and to maintain inter-personal relationships. The history should also include a detailed family history and clues suggesting overlap or mimic syndromes (see Table 7.2 and Fig. 7.1). The examination should cover both cognitive functions and motor signs.

Cognitive assessment should focus on identifying the cognitive deficits specific to each syndrome in addition to noting which cognitive domains are spared. The most affected domains are executive functions and (in the language variants) language function. In contrast, orientation, calculation, visuospatial skills should be relatively well preserved early in FTD. Although early memory impairment is generally considered to exclude a diagnoses of FTD, recent

Table 7.2 Clinical syndromes known to display clinical overlap with FTD

Amyotrophic Lateral Scleroses (ALS)	The association between ALS and dementia has been described for over a century. It is now recognised that 13–15 % of FTD patients have evidence of co-morbid ALS (FTD-ALS). Up to 50 % of ALS may have cognitive or behavioural abnormalities on neuropsychological testing which in about 13 % are severe enough to fulfil the criteria for FTD, most frequently bvFTD.
Corticobasal syndrome (CBS)	This is a progressive disorder characterized by asymmetrical motor and sensory cortical and extrapyramidal dysfunction. It is classically associated with tau pathology though recent evidence suggests that AD pathology underlie many cases. There are two main clinical presentations. In the first one, the patient presents to movement disorders clinic with a "useless arm" due to unilateral rigidity, bradykinesia, apraxia, tremor, and dystonia. In the second, cognitive symptoms, in particular nonfluent progressive aphasia, are the presenting feature.
Progressive supranuclear palsy (PSP):	This is a rapidly progressing disorders characterized by supranuclear gaze palsy, an akinetic rigid syndrome with pronounced axial rigidity, postural instability causing falls, (mainly backwards), and bulbar symptoms (dysarthria and dysphasia). It is classically associated with PSP pathology.

Table 7.3 This is a summary of conditions that can mimic FTD

FTD-Phenocopy Syndrome	There are recent reports of patients who have a typical clinical presentation of FTD (sometimes associated with executive dysfunction and impaired activities of daily living) but they display extremely slow or no progression over time and have normal imaging. The underlying pathology in these patients is yet to be established. It has been suggested that such cases might constitute pathological but stable personality variants
Psychiatric illness:	Behavioural changes can be interpreted by family and medical professionals as a psychological reaction or psychiatric disorder. For example, apathy may be interpreted as depression and irritability or disinhibition as a midlife personality change. In addition, the negative symptoms characterizing some types of schizophrenia (such as schizophrenia simplex) can be very similar to the behavioural changes of bvFTD, particularly if they are not associated with florid "positive symptomatology". On the other hand, positive psychotic symptoms such as hallucinations and delusions, though rare have been described in *C9orf72* related FTD. Association with other symptoms of FTD and the time course of "insidious onset and gradual progression" can help differentiate FTD
Alzheimer's disease (AD)	AD is characterized by early and prominent deficit in episodic memory, and is thus easy to differentiate from FTD. However, atypical variants of AD can be characterized by more prominent involvement of behaviour and language (the so called frontal and language variants) and therefore can pose diagnostic challenges. On the other hand, FTD can also be associated with prominent amnestic features. Notably, attention, orientation, visuospatial skills tend to be preserved in early FTD and impaired in AD.
Other neurodegenerative disorders	FTD symptoms such apathy irritability and stereotypic behaviour can also be associated with other neurodegenerative disorders affecting the fronto-striatal circuits such as Parkinson's disease (PD), Huntington's disease (HD), Wilson's disease, and Multiple system atrophy (MSA). Olivopontocerebellar atrophy (*OPCA*) can also present with a range of symptoms reminiscent of FTD. These disorders should have distinguishable features with differing collections of symptoms e.g. tremor in PD, cerebellar ataxia and autonomic failure in MSA and chorea in HD.
Vascular dementia (VD)	Apathy, executive dysfunction, frontal release signs, and parkinsonian features can occur in VD. However, the stepwise time course and presence of cortico-spinal tract signs would suggest VD over FTD. MRI may be helpful, indicating FTD if there is focal lobar atrophy and VD if there is diffuse white matter changes

evidence suggest that memory changes in FTD are common, especially in younger patients. Occasionally, memory dysfunction occasionally can be as severe as that observed in AD patients. In fact, severe amnesia can be the presenting feature in some patients. However, typically memory function in FTD affects free recall to a higher degree than recognition or cued recall while in AD the impairment extends to all three aspects of episodic memory.

A variety of rapid screening tests have been designed specifically for the purpose of discriminating FTD from non-FTD dementias such as the third version Addenbrooke's Cognitive Examination (*ACE-III*, Hsieh 2013) which is the most updated version of the ACE (Mathuranath 2000), the *Executive Interview* (Royall, Mahurin

RK, and Gray, 1992), and the Frontal Assessment Battery (FAB, Dubois, Slachevsky, Litvan and Pillon B, 2000), and *The Montreal Cognitive Assessment* (*MoCA*, Nasreddine et al. 2005). If feasible, the patient can be referred to a clinical psychologist for a more detailed neuropsychological evaluation.

The motor examination should focus on the presence of motor signs suggesting disease mimics (e.g. stroke) and disorders that overlap with FTD such as corticobasal syndrome (CBS), Progressive Supranuclear Palsy (PSP), and amyotrophic form of Motor Neuron Disease (FTD-ALS). Thus presence of extra-pyramidal signs, muscle wasting, fasciculations or unilateral apraxia add to the behavioural and cognitive profile in characterizing the syndrome (Fig. 7.1).

Fig. 7.1 Clinical crossover of
frontotemporal dementia,
corticobasal degeneration, and
progressive supranuclear palsy
(Courtesy of Dr. B. Murray,
Hermitage Hospital, Dublin)

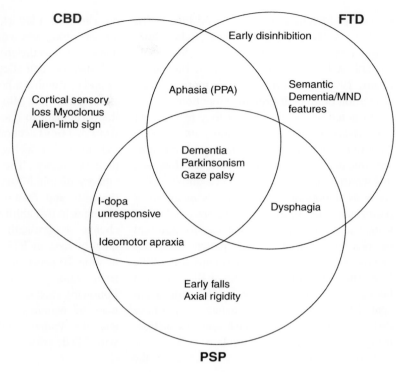

7.7   Neuropsychological Assessment

Given the wide variability of presentations in
FTD and the fact that there are a number of other
overlapping conditions, a comprehensive neuropsychological assessment can greatly contribute
to differential diagnosis. However, as FTD can
frequently present with alterations in behaviour
and personality one should not over-rely on cognitive testing per se. Depending on the locus of
pathology patients may do extremely poorly on
conventional "frontal lobe" tests (such as the
Wisconsin Card Sorting Test, Trail Making Test,
verbal fluency etc.), or they may in fact perform
normally, yet still show major impairment in self-
and social regulation. Therefore it is essential to
conduct a detailed evaluation of behaviour.

Behavioural evaluation should include direct
observation of the patient as well as collateral
information from informants using semi-
structured interviews and preferably a suitably
designed behavioural instrument. One such

instrument is the Frontal Systems Behaviour
Scale (FrSBe, Grace & Molloy 2001) which was
designed based on Cummings' neuroanatomical
model to provide self and informant based ratings
of apathy, disinhibition, and executive dysfunction both pre-morbidly and currently. In addition
to permitting age and gender graded interpretation of behaviour change, the self- and informant-
based ratings can be compared to evaluate the
degree of insight or lack thereof. Other commonly used behavioural instruments include the
Cambridge   Behavioural   Inventory   (CBI,
Wedderburn et al. 2008) and the Neuropsychiatric
Inventory Questionnaire (NPI-*Q*, Kaufer et al.
2000).

The typical pattern of cognitive change
reported in FTD patients is impairment of executive functions. There are purpose designed comprehensive batteries to evaluate a broad range of
cognitive processes encompassed within the term
executive function, the majority of which are
dependent on the integrity of the frontal lobes.
Notable examples include the Delis-Kaplan

Executive Function System (D-KEFS, Delis, Kaplan, & Kramer, 2001) and Behavioural Assessment of the Dysexecutive Syndrome (BADS, Wilson, Alderman, Burgess, Emslie, & Evans, 1996), (see Chap. 3 for a more detailed discussion of tasks of executive functions).

As noted above, the patient may or may not have associated significant memory impairment. Attention, orientation and visuo-spatial functions are typically preserved in FTD patients. However, it is worth noting that *qualitative* cognitive analysis is as important as the patient's *quantitative* performance on the different neuropsychological tests. Patients can fail the same tests for different reasons. For example, an AD patient could fail visuo-construction tasks such as copy trial of the Rey Osterrieth Complex Figure or Block Design because of memory problems and/or poor visuo-spatial functions while FTD patients might have difficulties with the same task due to constructional praxis and planning problems.

Patients with an early disease focused in the orbitofrontal-ventromedial prefrontal cortex, may perform normally on tests traditionally considered sensitive to frontal lobe/executive dysfunction but have a profound deficit in everyday decision making and social regulation. To address this issue novel batteries have been developed to focus on emotional decision making and social cognitive skills. Many tasks intend to mimic every day functioning and as such maybe more sensitive to cognitive changes in early bv-FTD.

One such battery is the Executive and Social Cognitive Battery (ESCB, Torralva 2009) which includes the Iowa Gambling Task (IGT, Bechara et al. 1994), the Multiple Errands Task (MET, Shallice & Burgess, 1991), the Hotel task (HOT, Manly et al. 2002), the Mind in the Eyes task (Baron-Cohen et al. 2001), and the Faux Pas test (Stone et al. 1998). The IGT evaluates decision making and learning in high and low risk situations. During the task healthy individuals learn to avoid the risky choices while those with FTD continue to make high risk choices which results in an overall net loss. The MET and the HOT are both designed to mirror everyday tasks. The MET involves the participant running "real life" errands such as purchasing three items (a soda, a

postcard and a letter), using the internal phone, and obtaining and writing down pieces of information such as the area code of a city. The Hotel task involves activities that are often undertaken as part of running a hotel such as sorting bills by client name. The Mind in the Eyes task requires the participant to choose from four options the word that most accurately describes how a set of individuals are feeling based on photographs of their eye region. The Faux Pas test is based on "theory of mind" (the ability to infer another's thoughts and feelings based on social cues). Changes in this ability may underlie some of the changes in personality and social functioning frequently seen in FTD patients. The task entails hearing 20 short stories, 10 of which contain a social faux pas and 10 of which are neutral. Following each story, questions are asked to evaluate the patient's social awareness and understanding. Patients with bvFTD, but not patients with AD do poorly on this test.

7.8   Neuropathology

The neuropathology associated with the clinical entities of FTD is heterogeneous with the unifying feature being a relatively selective and impressive atrophy of the frontal and/or temporal lobes on macroscopic examination of the brain. The pattern of atrophy in FTD is linked to the clinical phenotype: mainly left hemispheric atrophy in nfvPPA, bilateral (often asymmetrical) atrophy of the middle and inferior temporal lobes in svPPA, while in bv-FTD there is usually early bilateral orbito-mesial atrophy, followed by atrophy of the dorsolateral frontal cortex, temporal pole, hippocampal formation, and the basal ganglia.

Importantly, the lack of macroscopic atrophy does not exclude microscopic evidence of FTD pathology. Crucial also is the observation that microscopic neuropathological changes in FTD do not map onto clinical features in a one-to-one manner. The association of a highly specific constellation of symptoms and signs with more than one neuropathological signature may seem paradoxical but it may be understood in terms of systems neurodegeneration i.e. degeneration of neuronal populations that are connected structurally and functionally.

The microscopic appearance of the cortex in FTD patients includes neuronal loss, widespread spongiosis and astrocytosis obscuring normal pathology. In addition, as in other neurodegenerative conditions, FTD is characterised by specific kinds of intracellular protein inclusions. In 1911 Alois Alzheimer described round silver-impregnated inclusions and swollen neuronal perikarya (cell bodies) in cases of dementia with prominent language and behavioural symptoms, first described clinically by Arnold Pick in 1892. The inclusions would become known as "Pick Bodies", the defining histopathological lesion of Pick's disease.

In the last 30 years there has been significant progress in the neuropathology of FTD. This prompted the Midwest Consortium for Frontotemporal (Lobar) Degeneration and other groups to review the existing neuropathological diagnostic criteria for FTD. Currently, the heterogeneous group of disorders referred to under the umbrella term of FTD are categorized pathologically based on the biochemical composition of the observed protein inclusions.

7.8.1 Tau

Tau is a phosphorylated protein expressed predominantly in neurons. The phosphorylation of tau is believed to be critical to its ability to bind and stabilize neuronal microtubules which are cytoskeletal structures of axonal transport.

Tauopathies are characterized by deposits of tau protein and represent approximately 40–50 % of sporadic FTD cases. A tauopathy is almost always observed in post mortem studies of patients with nfvPPA, FTD with Pick bodies (Pick's disease), and patients with BVFTD and parkinsonism linked to mutations in the microtubule-associated protein tau (MAPT) on chromosome 17 (FTDP17, see Sect. 7.9 below). Behavioural or language variant FTD patients who exhibit extrapyramidal signs often have tau pathology. Other tauopathies include cortico-basal degeneration (CBD), progressive supranu-clear palsy (PSP), argyrophilic grain disease, and neurofibrillary tangle dementia (Tangle-only dementia). Although tau pathology is also present in AD, this disease is usually not referred to "tauopathy" since it always associated with co-existing amyloid pathology.

Pick bodies as originally described by Alzheimer are now known to be spherical cytoplasmic inclusions that are tau positive. Pick bodies are typically found in the cingulated gyrus, insula, inferior parietal lobule and inferior temporal gyri. They are also found in the mesial structures particularly the granule cells of the dentate fascia. White matter pick bodies are more common in CBD and PSP but can be found in FTD. Pick bodies may also be found in the basal ganglia and substantia nigra.

7.8.2 TDP-43

Many FTD cases are tau negative. Until recently, ubiquitin immunohistochemistry was the only method to detect the abnormal protein inclusions in the vast majority of these cases, prompting the term frontotemporal dementias with ubiquitin inclusions (FTLD-U), which is thought to represent about 60 % of FTD cases.

A major discovery in 2006 by Neumann and colleagues revealed that the main constituent of ubiquitin inclusions in up to 90 % of FTLD-U cases is a protein called trans-activating responsive DNA-binding protein 43 (TDP-43). It is now recognized that almost all svPPA and FTD-ALS patients as well as 50–60 % of bvFTD patients are TDP-43 positive. Of note, the vast majority of patients with sporadic amyotrophic lateral sclerosis (ALS) and some familial ALS patients are also positive for TDP-43 pathology. This discovery was a major milestone in understanding the degree of overlap between ALS and FTD and led to the emergence of a new family of neurodegenerative disorders, the so called TDP-43 proteinopathies, which includes ALS as well as FTLD-U with and without ALS.

TDP-43 is a ubiquitously expressed protein encoded by the *TARDBP* gene on chromosome one. It is a nuclear protein, but it shuttles between

Table 7.4 This table provides a summary of the harmonised classification (Mackenzie 2011) of pathological subtypes within the family of TDP-43 proteinopathies

Subtype Mackenzie 2011	Characteristic Pathology		Previous Nomenclature	
	Inclusions/Cellular changes	Cortical distribution	Mackenzie	Sampathu
Sub-type A	NCIs Abundant NCIs ± Moderate numbers of lentiform NIIs Many crescentic or oval DNs	Mainly layer II of cortex	Type 1	Type 3
Sub-type B	Moderate NCIs Occasional NIs DNs rare	Affects all cortical layers	Type 3	Type 2
Sub-type C	Very Few NCIs Abundant long DNs	Mainly layer II of cortex	Type 2	Type 1
Sub-type D	Rare NCIs, Abundant lentiform NIIs Abundant short DNs	Affects all cortical layers	Type 4	Type 4

Reproduced and modified with permission of Springer from Mackenzie (2011)

the nucleus and the cytoplasm with normally low concentrations in the cytoplasm. Both the structure and cellular distribution of TDP-43 is abnormal in TDP-43 proteinopathies. TDP-43 loses its nuclear position and aggregates mainly in cytoplasm. The TDP-43 protein itself is truncated at the N-terminus while the remaining C-terminus fragment is abnormally phosphorylated to form insoluble cytoplasmic protein deposits observed in the brain and spinal cord in FTLD-U and sporadic ALS.

Brains with TDP-43 pathology can display neuronal *cytoplasmic* inclusions (NCIs), neuronal *nuclear* inclusions (NNIs) and/or dystrophic neurites (DNs). These changes have been described in the neocortex and hippocampus and the lower motor neurons in both FTLD-U and ALS. On other hand, TDP-43 positive glial inclusions (GI) were mainly considered a feature of ALS, but have been described in FTLD-U.

There is pathological heterogeneity within the TDP-43 proteinopathy family with more than one classification proposed. The harmonized classification system, recently published by Mackenzie et al. in 2011, described four main subtypes of TDP-43 pathology (see Table 7.4).

The pathological subtypes summarized in Table 7.4 have distinct clinical and genetic correlations. In subtype A, the clinical presentation is usually bvFTD or nfvPPA (rarely svPPA) with high prevalence (up to 50 %) of familial disease. This subtype is consistently reported in patients with *GRN* gene mutations and has recently been reported in *C9orf72* gene mutations.

Subtype B is associated a clinical picture of FTD-ALS or bvFTD and is associated with generally poor prognoses. Genetically, subtype B is linked to mutations in the *C9orf72* gene.

Subtype C is associated with the svPPA variant of FTD and less commonly bvFTD but there are no genetic associations to date.

Subtype D is associated with familial Inclusion body myopathy with Paget Disease of Bone and frontotemporal dementia (IBMPFD) which is due to mutations in the valosin-containing protein (*VCP)* gene.

Detailed discussions of these gene mutations are included in the Sect. 7.9 below.

Of note, the authors of the new classification highlighted its limitations which include failure to incorporate sub-cortical changes or describe the TDP-43 pathology recently reported in normal aging population, in the Guam Parkinson Dementia Complex patients, in about 20 % of AD patients, and up to 70 % of patients with hippocampal scleroses with and without AD as demonstrated by Amador-Ortiz et al. (2007).

7.8.3 FUS

Up to 10 % of FTLD-U patients are not only tau negative but also TDP43 negative. In addition, 15 % of ALS-FTD cases do not belong to the

FTLD-U subtype and do not stain with ubiquitin or TDP-43. Interestingly, most cases of familial ALS associated with mutations in the superoxide mutase gene are also TDP-43 negative.

In 2009, the inclusions in some TDP-43 negative FTLD-U cases and some familial ALS cases are found to be positive for Fused in Sarcoma (FUS) protein. FTLD-U patients who are positive for FUS protein are termed FTD-FUS.

FUS is a protein involved in RNA processing and is strikingly similar to TDP43 in in structure and function. Nuclear FUS is believed to play an essential role in regulation of transcription and pre-mRNA splicing while in the cytoplasmic FUS is likely to be involved mRNA transport.

All reported cases of FTLD-FUS have been associated with a clinical diagnosis of bvFTD (with or without the signs of MND).

7.8.4   Rare Subtypes

A small number of tau negative FTLD-U cases are negative for TDP-43 and FUS. These are referred to as FTLD- ubiquitin proteasome system (FTLD-UPS).

Other rare types of FTD pathology include basophilic inclusion body and neuronal intermediate filament inclusion disease.

There are also FTD cases that are negative for tau as well as ubiquitin. They form a rare and controversial entity referred to a Dementia lacking distinctive histopathology (DLDH). This previously large group of identified pathology has been gradually replaced by newly identified pathological variants (Fig. 7.2).

7.8.5   Clinical Phenotype and Neuropathology

As noted in the beginning of this section, the clinical presentation in FTD does not map in a one-to-one manner with the clinical phenotypes. The exceptions to this general rule are FTD-ALS which is generally positive for TDP-43. In a recent study by Chare and colleagues (2014) the newly proposed clinical classifications of FTD were retrospectively applied to 135 autopsy ascertained FTD cases from the Cambridge Brain Bank (UK) and the Sydney Brain Bank (Australia). The brain pathology underlying different FTD syndromes in that cohort was as follows:

- *bvFTD patients* :42 % FTLD-Tauopathy, 30 % FTLD-TDP-43 proteinopathy, 13 % FTLD-FUS, 9 % Alzheimer's type pathology, and 6 % other rare FTLD pathologies;
- *svFTD* : 68 % FTLD-TDP-43 proteinopathy while both FTLD-tauopathy and AD type pathology were responsible for 16 % of cases each;
- *nfvPPA*: 50 % FTLD-tauopathy, 31 % AD type pathology, and 19 % TDP43-proteinopathy; and
- *lvPPA:* 77 % AD type pathology, 14 % TDP-43 proteinopathy and 9 % FTLD-tauopathy.

7.9   Genetics

The progress in this area, moribund for decades despite the recognition of the important of heritability since the 1920s, has been rapid and ever-expanding in the last two decades. The traditional disease dichotomy of 'sporadic' versus 'genetic' is still used but is increasingly difficult to support, due to the likely polygenic factors influencing sporadic FTD. Nevertheless, the first step in determining whether there is a genetic influence in a disorder is to establish the frequency of a family history of the disorder.

The earliest well documented large pedigree was first reported in 1939 by Sanders and Colleagues who described an autosomal dominant dementing disorder with behavioural and cognitive disturbances with relatively preserved memory affecting a Dutch Kindred. However, the earliest estimates of the frequency of family history came from the Lund and Manchester clinico-pathological series, which estimated that up to 50 % of patients with FTD had a first degree relative with dementia. More recent studies have confirmed that about 30–50 % of FTD patients have family histories of dementia. However, the accuracy of ascertainment of familial disease is

Fig. 7.2 Microscopic staining in FTD. (**a**) Tau-positive staining in FTD17-T (*arrow*) (Courtesy Prof. Michael Farrell); (**b**) TDP-43 staining in FTD-U/ALS (*arrow*) (Courtesy Prof. Ian R. A. Mackenzie)

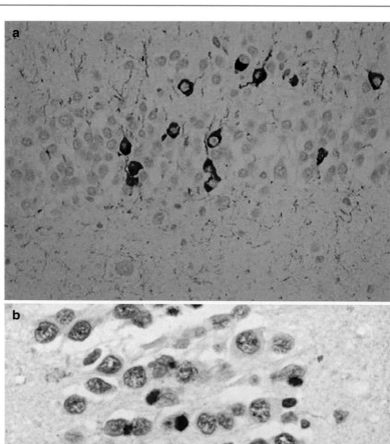

confounded by informant reliability, the late onset of the disease, the possibility of death before disease expression, and the fact that informants often report a vague history of "dementia" of unknown type in elderly relatives. It is also worth noting that the variable phenotype of FTD seems to have a direct effect of reported rates of familial disease with highest rates reported in FTD with co-morbid ALS (up to 60 %) and lowest rates reported in svPPA variants of FTD (20 % or less).

The main genes are associated with familial FTD are listed here in chronological order of discovery

1. **MAPT gene** on chromosome 17, (1998),
2. **VCP gene** on chromosome 9, (2004),
3. **CHMP2B gene** on chromosome 3, (2005),
4. **GRN (or PGRN) gene** on chromosome 17 (2006),
5. **TARDBP gene** on chromosome 1, (2008),
6. **C9orf72 gene** on chromosome 17, (2011),
7. **SQSTM1 gene** on chromosome 5 (2012).

Mutations in *GRN, MAPT* and *C9ORF72* together account for the majority of cases, with the *C9orf72* repeat expansion reported to account for up to half familial cases in some populations. On the other hand, mutations in *VCP, CHMP2B, SQSTM1* and *TARDBP* genes are rare, each explaining less than 1–5 % of the familial FTLD. We provide below a brief summary of the phenotypic and neuropathological profile reported with each of these gene mutations.

7.9.1 MAPT Gene Mutations

In 1994, Wilhelmson et al. described a large Irish and American Kindred with a genetic locus linked to 17q21-22 where the tau gene is located. The disease, originally known as Disinhibition-Dementia-Parkinsonism-Amyotrophy Complex or DDPAC, was reported to have a highly variable phenotype. In 1998, the MAPT gene was identified and the disease was subsequently termed FTD with Parkinsonism linked to chromosome 17 or "FTDP-17".

The age of onset in patients with this disease is between 30 and 65 years. The clinical spectrum encompasses behavioural and cognitive changes typical of bvFTD with memory and praxis relatively preserved. By definition most patients have prominent parkinsonian features while amyotrophy is less common. Most recently, it has become clear that such widely varying clinical syndromes such as PSP, CBS and FTD can co-exist within families with MAPT mutations. At autopsy *MAPT* positive patients are usually positive for the microtubule-associated protein Tau.

Tau has six known isoforms of tau protein which are produced by alternative splicing of exons 2, 3, and 10. Alternative splicing of exon 10, results in tau isoforms with either three or four amino acids repeats in the C-terminus microtubule binding domain (3R and 4R isoforms respectively). More or less equal amounts of the 3R and 4R isoforms are produced in normal circumstances. Pathogenic *MAPT* mutations are thought to alter the splicing processes in a manner that promote an increase in the production of 4R isoforms. The proposed effects of this change are reduced binding to microtubules, formation of neurotoxic aggregates and abnormal axonal transport.

7.9.2 VCP Gene Mutation

In 2004, mutations in the valosin-containing protein (VCP) gene located on chromosome 9p13.3 were identified. The protein product of this gene is a ubiquitously expressed, highly abundant, multi-function ATPase which has been reported to play a role in the assembly of the endoplasmic reticulum and Golgi body, protein breakdown, inhibition of protein aggregation as well as DNA replication. Pathogenic mutations are believed to cause loss of function leading to disruption of the ubiquitin-proteasome mediated protein degradation system, autophagy, and/or ATP production within the cell.

Clinically *VCP* mutations are associated with inclusion body myopathy with Paget's disease of bone and frontotemporal dementia (IBMPFD). This condition usually presents with a disabling myopathy starting in the proximal muscles then spreading to involve the distal muscles, as well as the heart and respiratory muscles. Muscle biopsy show sarcoplasmic inclusion bodies reactive with ubiquitin and TDP-43. Osteolytic bone lesions and FTD usually emerge later in the course of the disease. On autopsy, brain pathology is usually consistent with FTLD-TDP subtype D (see the Sect. 7.8).

7.9.3 CHMP2B Gene Mutation

In 1984 a researcher came across a very large family in Jutland in Denmark with an unusual dementia. There were over 27 affected individuals with a very wide range of clinical variability. In 1995 genetic linkage to chromosome 3 was established. In 2005 mutations in the gene encoding the chromatin modifying protein 2B (*CHMP2B*) at chromosome 3p11.2 was identified.

The *CHMP2B* gene protein product is a heteromeric ESCRT-III complex expressed by neurons and is believed to play an essential role in endosomal-lysosomal function, protein breakdown, and neuronal survival. Mutations usually result in aberrant splicing affecting the C-terminus of the protein.

To date, *CHMP2B* gene mutations have only been reported in Danish Kindreds manifesting clinically as familial FTD with autosomal dominant mode of inheritance. Pathology is usually ubiquitin positive FTD (FTLD-U) that is not only tau negative but also TDP-43 negative.

7.9.4 GRN Gene Mutations

In 2006, only 1.7 M nucleotides centromeric to the *MAPT* gene, a mutated gene located on chromosome 17q21.31 was identified. The GRN gene codes for progranulin, a precursor of granulin, a ubiquitously expressed growth factor. Following translation, splicing and processing in the Golgi body and endoplasmic reticulum (including aspargine-linked glycosylation and enzymatic cleavage) the mature glycoprotein (granulin) is secreted. Granulin is believed to be a neurotropic factor involved in a wide range of functions including tissue repair, inflammation, neuronal growth, and tumorigenesis. The vast majority of reported pathogenic mutations reported to date cause reduced protein expression by disrupting either translation or splicing.

GRN gene mutations are responsible for 10–20 % of familial FTD and are associated with an autosomal dominant mode of inheritance. Pathologically *GRN* mutations have been linked to often to severe, often asymmetrical, frontal atrophy that can extend to the basal ganglia with Mackenzie et al. in 2006 reporting changes in the caudate and substantia nigra. Microscopically *GRN* mutations are consistently associated with FTD-TDP43 Type A pathology (see Sect. 7.8 above).

Phenotypic expression is less consistent. The clinical presentation is predominantly bvFTD but nfvPPA and rarely ALS-FTD kindreds have been reported. A possible explanation for this heterogeneity in phenotypic expression was proposed by Rogalski et al. The authors observed that dyslexia was overrepresented in patients with PPA and their first degree relatives when compared to controls and AD patients. This led to the interesting proposal that the phenotypic expression may be a function of a latent vulnerability within the kindred as it becomes "the locus of least resistance".

7.9.5 TARDBP Gene Mutations

In 2006 TDP-43 was identified as the major constituent of vast majority of ubiquitin positive inclusions in both FTD and ALS. In 2008 mutation in the transactive response-DNA binding protein (*TARDBP*) gene on chromosome 1 was identified as a cause of ALS. Since then more than 30 mutations in the *TARDBP* gene have been reported. Almost all reported *TARDP* mutations are in exon 6 affecting the highly conserved C-terminus of the TDP-43 protein known to be involved in RNA recognition.

Mutations have been reported primarily in familial and occasionally sporadic ALS or ALS-FTD, but recently the phenotype has been extended to include patients with bvFTD without motor involvement. Yet the current literature suggests that *TARDBP* mutations are rare, accounting for less than 1 % of FTD cases. A recent Italian study suggested that *TARDBP* related FTD may be associated with a predominance of svPPA variants and temporal atrophy on imaging.

7.9.6 C9ORF72 Hexanucleotide Gene Mutations

Since 1991, linkage studies of ALS-FTD and FTD kindreds suggested a locus on chromosome 9p.21. In 2011 two different groups identified the genetic mutation at that locus as a substantial expansion of GGGGCC hexanucleotide repeats in a non-coding region of the *C9orf72* gene (DeJesus-Hernandez et al. 2011; Renton et al. 2011). Affected individuals had 60–1600 repeats, whereas normal individuals have less than 23–25 repeats.

The gene is known to have three transcripts. The function of the final protein product is not confirmed but there is evidence to support a role in in endocytic and autophagic pathways as well as motor function. Some evidence supports loss of function as the main pathomechanism underlying the *C9orf72* gene mutation as it is associated with reduced expression of gene's three major transcripts. However, toxic gain of function is also possible in the context of the presence of brain aggregates of both aberrant protein and abnormal repeat RNA. The latter aggregates are termed RNA foci and form core of the 'toxic RNA' hypothesis.

The current data suggests that the *C9orf72* repeat expansion accounts for 40–50 % of cases of familial ALS, 20–25 % of FTD cases, and 0–7 % of the sporadic cases in white Americans, Europeans and Australians, with recent evidence raising the possibility of a single founder in Europe. Reported rates are much lower in non-white populations including the Chinese and the Japanese populations. Inheritance follows an autosomal dominant pattern with incomplete penetrance.

Studies published to date confirm that the most common clinical presentation associated with the *C9orf72* repeat expansion is behavioural variant FTD and/or ALS. Other characteristics, including younger age at onset, florid psychotic symptoms, anxiety, poor memory, and poor outcome have been reported but are not consistent Clinical observations predating the discovery of the *C9orf72* gene mutation suggested the presence of delusional ideation in younger bvFTD patients with tau negative pathology, though the anatomic substrate was not fully understood. It is conceivable that these patients might have been positive for the *C9orf72* repeat expansion.

C9orf72 associated disease also has a distinct radiological and pathological signature. There is symmetrical fronto-temporal atrophy but changes often extend to involve the parieto-occiptal cortex and the cerebellum. The pathological hallmark of *C9orf72* related disease is TDP-43 inclusions (predominantely subtype B) and ubiquitin-binding protein p62/sequestosome 1 inclusions. The latter inclusions are considered highly specific to the *C9orf72* gene mutation as they are rare in non-*C9orf72* FTD. The p62/sequestosome 1 inclusions can occur with and without co-existing TDP-43 and have been observed in the frontal neocortex, cerebellum and hippocampus.

It is important to note that *C9orf72* gene mutations have been reported in patients presenting with the clinical picture of AD, cortico-basal syndrome (CBS), dementia with lewy bodies (DLB), and Huntington disease (HD).

7.9.7 SQSTM1 Gene

The sequestosome 1 (SQSTM1) gene, located on 5q35, encodes p62 protein adapter protein which is involved in multiple functions including autophagy, oxidative stress response, and cell signalling. As noted above, neuronal p62-positive inclusions have been shown to be abundant in both FTD and ALS patients, particularly disease associated with the *C9orf72* gene mutation. In addition, an increase in p62 immuno-reactivity has also been reported in AD, DLB, Parkinson's disease and HD.

Mutations in the SQSTM1 gene were initially thought to cause only Paget's disease of the bone, but in 2011 mutations in this gene were also reported in patients with ALS. In 2012, Rubino and colleagues from the TODEM study group screened for this mutations 170 unrelated FTD patients (138 bvFTD, 6 svPPA, and 19 nfvPPA), 124 ALS patients, 288 patients with Paget's disease and 145 healthy controls. Noncoding SQSTM1 mutations were found in three patients presenting with bvFTD. Aggressiveness, mood lability, and social withdrawal were prominent behaviours in these patients. In the same study mutations were also found in three patients presenting with bulbar ALS but not in patients with Paget's disease or healthy controls.

A recent French series reported SQSTM1 missense mutations in 4 unrelated families with FTD out of 188 suggesting that this mutation is responsible for only about 2 % of familial cases of FTD. Of note, co-morbid parkinsonian signs were observed in 2 families, 1 family had coexisting clinical symptoms of Paget disease of bone, and 1 family had clinical symptoms of FTD-ALS.

7.9.8 Other Mutations

As discussed is the Pathology section FUS protein was identified in many TDP-43 negative FTLD-U cases. Recently, mutations in the Fused in Sarcoma (FUS) gene have been reported. Although the clinical phenotype associated with FTLD-FUS pathology is invariably FTD (with or without MND), the vast majority of cases of reported FUS gene mutations had ALS or ALS-FTD with very rare reports of pure FTD (Van Langenhove et al. 2010).

A few families with FTD have been shown to have mutations in Presenilin1 a gene usually associated with familial AD. This finding confirms the notion of convergence amongst mechanisms of neurodegeneration and is reciprocal to recent finding of MAPT polymorphisms in large AD cohorts. The exact role of presenilin in FTD is unclear but the mutations appear to be novel.

Prion protein (PRNP) gene mutations have also recently been associated with clinical pictures resembling FTD. In addition, there is a single reported case of FTD related to UBQLN2 gene mutation which is a recognized but rare cause of ALS.

7.10 Biomarkers

In FTD, a number of biomarkers are being used clinically and in a research capacity including brain imaging, neurophysiology and biological markers.

7.10.1 Brain Imaging

Brain imaging is an essential and routine examination in any dementia to exclude non-neurodegenerative (e.g. neoplastic or vascular) pathology and aid in the diagnostic process. Advances in brain imaging have grown at a remarkable pace in the last 10 years. Specific patterns of lobar atrophy can now be reliably mapped to clinical phenotypes. In this section, imaging in FTD will be discussed in the context of MRI-based techniques, non-MRI based functional

imaging and other techniques worth noting including those that are in the experimental phase.

7.10.1.1 MRI-Based Techniques

Structural MRI

T1 weighted MRI is the method of choice for evaluation of structural changes in the brain. In particular, the addition of coronal imaging to the standard axial slicing allows for the detection of visually obvious atrophy in frontal and temporal regions. T2 weighted imaging usually using fluid attenuated sequences (FLAIR) allows for the evaluation pathology that might exclude FTD or point to a mimic syndrome such as vascular related white matter pathology.

Quantitative MRI remains generally a research tool and embodies three main techniques; volumetric analysis of specific brain regions, Voxel Based Morphometry (VBM), and serial co-registration.

The aim of structural MRI brain imaging in FTD is to exclude other pathologies and to document the presence and pattern of brain atrophy. Brain atrophy is one of the cardinal features of all neurodegenerative processes, even if it occurs at variable rates and by vastly different and sometimes convoluted processes. The most convincing hypothesis underlying the atrophic process suggests that we can no longer think of this as a generalized shrinkage but more along the lines of a Wallerian degeneration constrained by neuronal and functional networks. The process often starts focally and spreads along these networks whose predictability gives us the clinical phenotypes we know.

Brain atrophy on structural MR imaging is the most reproducible feature of all FTD subtypes. The presence of true focal atrophy has a high positive predicative value for clinical dementia. On the other hand the absence of atrophy has been noted increasingly in cases deemed to have all clinical, behavioural and neuropsychological features of bvFTD. This raises the question of either a behavioural phenocopy of FTD or else cases where atrophy is either negligible or will occur later in the disorder.

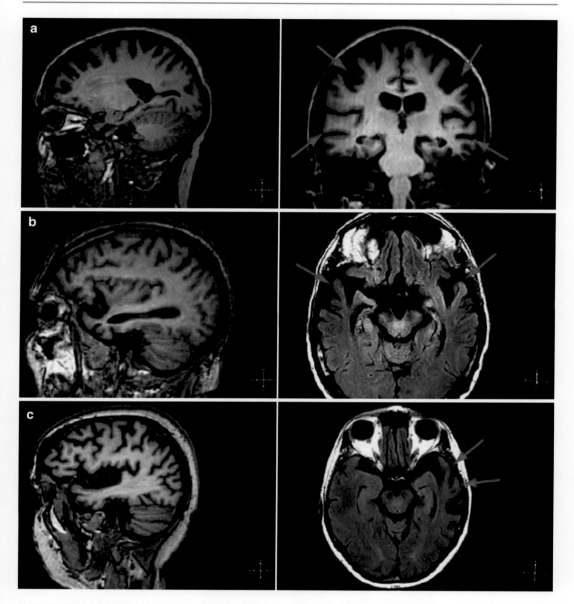

Fig. 7.3 (**a**) Behavioural variant FTD. Note generalized atrophy in frontal and temporal regions (*arrows*) with slight asymmetry favouring more atrophy on the left. (**b**) Semantic dementia. Note anterior temporal tip atrophy bilaterally (*arrows*). (**c**) Progressive non-fluent aphasia. Note asymmetric atrophy favouring the left temporal lobe (*arrows*)

The pattern of brain atrophy on standard MRI predicts FTD clinical subtype. Focal asymmetrical frontal lobe atrophy with or without temporal atrophy is the best predictor of the bvFTD subtype (see Fig. 7.3a). Recent research indicates that the process starts in the orbitofrontal and cingulate regions and spreads to insular cortex and thence to the basal ganglia.

Recent VBM data suggests that even within the bvFTD group there are several distinct subgroups. One study described four subgroups based on patterns of grey matter loss. Two of these displayed temporal lobe atrophy, either in isolation ("temporal-dominant subtype") or in combination with frontal and parietal lobe involvement ("temporo-fronto-parietal subtype"). The other two subtypes were characterized by predominance of frontal lobe atrophy with or without temporal lobe involvement ("fronto-temporal subtype" and "frontal-dominant subtype" respectively). Interestingly, while these radiological subtypes did not differ with regard to the severity of behavioural impairment, they did display significant correlations with cognitive performance as well as genetic and pathological diagnoses (which were available in about half the cohort).

Other VBM studies attempted to correlate patterns of atrophy in bvFTD to specific behavioural manifestations and reported correlations include those with apathy (frontal pole), disinhibition (subcallosal region), and abnormal motor control (dorsal medial atrophy).

MRI findings in svFTD tend to be more consistent showing atrophy of the polar regions of the temporal lobe along with the fusiform gyrus (see Fig. 7.3b). Patients typically have focal anterior temporal pole atrophy with involvement of the inferior surface (especially the fusiform gyrus) more than superior. The atrophy is usually bilateral but asymmetrical, with predominant left-sided atrophy being more common than predominant right-sided atrophy. There is still a considerable debate whether this left sided dominance of svFTD reflects biological differences or a differential pattern of referrals in which patients with a predominantly right sided atrophy presenting with a clinical picture dominated by behavioural changes are referred to psychiatric rather than neurological services.

A variable amount of frontal atrophy is almost always found in svFTD. It is clear that while atrophy maybe wide spread in both frontal and temporal lobes as in other cases of FTD, it is the predominance of the anterior and inferior temporal lobe atrophy that appear to correlate with the main clinical findings in svFTD. Loss of ability to form semantic word associations correlates most strongly with damage in Brodmann's areas 37 and 38 which include the fusiform gyrus and inferior temporal gyrus and the anterior temporal pole respectively (for a more detailed discussion refer to the Chap. 3).

Imaging findings in nfvFTD and lvFTD are less reliable than in either bvFTD or svFTD. However, most MRI studies report predominant involvement of the left hemisphere. In nfvFTD, VBM studies found atrophy in the region of the including the pars opercularis of inferior frontal lobe (Broca's area), upper part of the temporal pole, the lentiform nucleus, middle frontal gyrus (see Fig. 7.3c). Atrophy of anterior insula and basal ganglia has also been described in this variant.

In lvFTD, the variant most commonly associated with AD rather than FTD pathology, VBM findings have shown more posterior abnormalities with the angular and supramarginal gyrus and other posterior perisylvian regions involved.

Although most MRI studies focused on the differences between FTD clinical variants, Whitewell et al. examined the pattern of atrophy in different genetic sub-groups suggesting specific radiological signatures in these subgroups: symmetrical anteromedial temporal atrophy in *MAPT*-related FTD; symmetric frontal atrophy with variable involvement of other brain regions including the cerebellum in *C9orf2*-related FTD; and asymmetrical inferior frontal and temporoparietal atrophy in *GRN*-related disease.

Diffusion Tensor Imaging (DTI)

While the above mentioned studies examined pattern of grey matter loss, DTI is a MRI-based technique that examines white matter integrity. Several DTI studies have reported widespread white matter injury in FTD patients most prominent in the white matter tracts underlying the frontotemporal cortex. Recent evidence suggests that DTI may be superior to volumetric grey matter analyses in differentiating FTD-tau and FTD-TDP-43.

Agosta and colleagues descried bilateral and widespread white matter damage in bvFTD including frontal and temporal areas such as the anterior superior and inferior longitudinal fasciculus, the inferior fronto-occipital fasciculus, the anterior cingulate, and parts of the corpus callosum. DTI changes in FTD language variants tended to be more focal and asymmetrical (more on the left). The best predictors svPPA were involvement of the left uncinate and inferior longitudinal fasciculus, while nfvPPA was associated with changes in the left arcuate fasciculus and superior longitudinal fasciculus.

Notably, a large study of FTD gene carriers (*MAPT* or *GRN*) with no clinical evidence of the disease showed changes in the right uncinate fasciculus compared to controls suggesting that this technique may play a role in detection of early and pre-symptomatic FTD patients.

Functional MRI (fMRI)

Functional MRI (fMRI) is a recent technique employed to investigate regional activation during specific tasks (activation fMRI) and functional connectivity between brain regions as measure neural network integrity (resting state or functional connectivity fMRI). The latter endeavour is of particular interest to FTD researchers in the context of the emerging hypotheses of preferential targeting of specific brain networks in different in neurodegenerative disorders.

The two main networks examined in FTD studies are the "Default Mode Network" (DMN) and the "Salience Network" (SN). The DMN is believed to be associated introspective cognitive processes e.g. strategy making, daydreaming, memory retrieval, contemplating the motives of other individuals etc. Thus the DMN is activated during wakeful rest and deactivated during cognitive tasks requiring redirection of attention to the external goal-directed behaviour. Brain regions associated with the DMN include the memory centres in the medial temporal lobe, medial prefrontal cortex (one of the core regions involved in theory of mind), the posterior cingulate cortex, the ventral precuneus and the medial, lateral and inferior parietal cortex. Decreased resting-state functional connectivity among DMN regions has been consistently shown in AD patients including patients with early or pre-symptomatic disease.

The SN, on the other hand, is linked to processing and adapting to salient emotional and external stimuli and goal-oriented behaviour. Components of the SN include the anterior cingulate, anterior insula, amygdala, and dorsal striatum.

Using fMRI findings, Zhou and colleagues proposed preferential damage to the SN in FTD (akin to the preferential damage of DMN in AD). This postulate was supported by decreased connectivity of the SN and increased connectivity

of the DMN. As the SN may play a role in modulating the activity of other networks to ensure optimum performance during goal-directed behaviour, the damage to the SN may be connected to the observed lack of deactivation of the DMN. A combined index of DMN and SN activity differentiated FTD and AD cases with high levels of accuracy approaching 100 % in genetically and pathologically confirmed cases. Decreased SN activity would be expected to lead to poor emotional processing and decline in executive control of goal oriented tasks. An overactive DMN would facilitate excessive reliance on self-generated narratives and over-learnt behaviour and a reduced ability to adapt to external social and environmental stimuli.

Subsequent work by Farb et al. demonstrated correlations between changes in connectivity and both FTD subtypes and specific behavioural manifestations. Disrupted fronto-limbic connectivity and increased local connectivity within the prefrontal cortex was demonstrated in both bvFTD and svPPA. Prefrontal hyperconnectivity was more diffuse in bvFTD and was associated in this subgroup with higher apathy and disinhibition scores. Increased DMN connectivity in the right angular gyrus was associated with stereotypic and apathetic behaviours, a finding that was also exclusive to bvFTD.

More recent work showed within the bvFTD variant, different genetic subgroups (such as patients with and without the pathogenic *c9orf72* repeat) display similar patterns of network connectivity (diminished SN activity and heightened DMN activity) despite differences in patterns of cortical atrophy on structural MRI. Moreover, the connectivity changes correlated with the severity of reported behavioural abnormalities.

Finally, there is evidence suggesting that alterations in DMN activity in FTD gene carriers may predate the emergence of clinical symptoms and cortical atrophy, which supports a potential role in pre-symptomatic screening.

7.10.1.2 Non-MRI Based Functional Imaging

[^{99}mTc]-hexamethylpropyleneamine oxime single-photon emission computed tomography (SPECT) and [^{18}F]-fluorodeoxyglucose (FDG)-PET are increasingly being used to help with the diagnosis of FTD, mainly by detecting regional hypometabolism in cases where there is no evidence of focal atrophy of structural imaging.

Changes in frontal regions extending to the anterior temporal regions on SPECT and FDG-PET have been shown to be sensitive but not specific for bvFTD. However, specificity increases in individual cases where asymmetrical frontal abnormalities are demonstrated in the context of little or no atrophy MR imaging. PET changes can be widespread but are most significant in the mesial frontal regions, consistent with the focal onset of many bvFTD patients.

The value of functional imaging in svFTD patients in the setting of typical clinical and radiological findings is limited. There is usually dramatic bilateral hypometabolism in the anterior temporal lobes, cortical regions that are universally affected by regional atrophy in this condition. In nfvPPA, functional imaging may show widespread abnormalities but the focus is usually left posterior fronto-insular regions. The imaging of lvPPA shows changes in the left posterior perisylvian, lateral temporal and parietal cortex.

Functional imaging, particularly FDG-PET can be regarded as an established imaging tool in FTD and changes in FDG-PET and SPECT are now incorporated in recent diagnostic criteria for FTD syndromes (see Sect. 7.11 below).

7.10.1.3 Other Techniques

Amyloid-PET neuroimaging, using amyloid-β-detecting ^{11}C-Pittsburgh compound B (PiB), is a sensitive and specific marker for underlying Aβ amyloid deposition. Amyloid deposition is an early event in AD while it is rare in FTD. As such there is increasing evidence that Amyloid-PET has a promising role in diagnosing AD even in early or pre-manifest stages and in differentiating it from FTD. However, the use of amyloid PET is restricted by its prohibitive costs and logistics which largely relate to the short half-life of PiB, the most established ligand in the market. Newly developed 18 F-labelled tracers with longer half-lives are increasingly gaining FDA approval and may result in wider use of this technology in a clinical context. Clinicians using this technology

to exclude FTD must be aware of the rare patients reported in the literature with mixed FTD and AD pathology.

Other advances in neuroimaging include techniques designed to identify protein aggregates in vivo including ligands that bind to tau and to TDP-43. As these techniques are still in progress with only a handful in-human studies, their potential utility in a clinical context is yet to be established.

7.10.2 Neurophysiology

7.10.2.1 Electroencephalography (EEG)

The use of EEG in dementia was more widespread before the advent of brain imaging though even then its clinical and diagnostic use was limited. There is a tendency for the background organization features of the EEG to be preserved in FTD whereas in AD the emergence of background slowing is common as the disease progresses. The reasons for such preservation in FTD are unclear but the observation may be related to the relatively rare association between FTD and seizures compared to AD.

In the research lab, quantitative EEG (qEEG), which is a digital algorithm of the different wave frequencies, has tended to confirm the preservation of resting alpha rhythm but the loss of some faster frequencies in the Beta range. Further work in this area is required before qEEG is to be considered a useful biomarker.

7.10.2.2 Nerve Conduction Studies and Electromyography (NCS/EMG)

Because of the co-existence of ALS and FTD, NCS and EMG studies have become an important diagnostic tool in FTD patients who have associated motor or swallowing difficulties (See Chap. 8). Limited data suggests the presence of motor neuron dysfunction in FTD patients on the neurophysiological evaluations in the context of minimal or absent clinical signs or symptoms. As yet, the status of EMG as a biomarker is unclear, since the use of EMG in unselected FTD cohort is not likely to be either cost-effective or clinically valuable.

7.10.2.3 Transcranial Magnetic Stimulation (TMS)

TMS is a promising non-invasive neurophysiological tool that examines cortical networks by testing excitatory and inhibitory properties of the cortex, conduction in the cortico-spinal tracts, and functional integrity of cortical structures including the corpus callosum. Advances in TMS have enabled in vivo investigations of the cortical cholinergic, glutaminergic and GABAergic circuits.

Although TMS investigation in FTD is still in its early stages, the available data provide fascinating insights into the disease such as the presence of motor circuit abnormalities in the absence of clinical evidence of pyramidal involvement. Limited data also suggest that TMS may have a potential role in disease therapeutics as evidenced by improved language function in PPA patients following high frequency TMS over the dorsolateral prefrontal cortical region. Further research is needed to confirm or refute the applicability of TMS to FTD clinical care.

7.10.3 Proteomics

The identification of a reliable protein biomarker in the cerebrospinal fluid (CSF) or serum facilitates in depth investigation of disease proteomics during life (as opposed to neuropathological examinations on autopsy). In addition, such a biomarker would potentially be useful in diagnoses of atypical, early stage, and or even pre-symptomatic patients as well as monitoring of disease progression and/or response to therapeutic agent. In general, CSF biomarkers have attracted more interest in neurodegenerative conditions as they are more likely to mirror the pathological processes taking place in the CNS.

The progress in CSF biomarkers (tau and abeta-42) in AD has been a major milestone in AD research, and these biomarkers have already been incorporated in the updated AD diagnostic criteria (see Chap. 4). The identification of reliable CSF (or serum) biomarkers in FTD remains elusive.

The detection of low or high levels of tau, progranulin, or TDP-43 are considered to be the "holy grail" of biomarker research in FTD since they would be conforming with key elements of what is already known about its molecular pathogenesis. The most obvious reason our failure to find such a biomarker lies in the pathological heterogeneity of FTD compared to AD. For example, measuring tau is less likely to be of value in tau negative FTD. This is complicated by the overlap between clinical and pathological phenotypes which means that a group of patients belonging the same FTD variant could eventually prove to have either tau-positive, or ubiquitin positive, or even occasionally AD pathology. Moreover, there is the problem of FTD phenocopy syndrome, which may include normal brains.

7.10.3.1 Tau and aBeta1-42

By far, the most investigated CSF biomarkers in FTD are tau and aBeta1-42, mainly in the context of studies evaluating the use of these biomarkers in differentiating FTD from AD.

Studies of CSF tau in FTD have yielded contradictory results (normal or high). It is important to note that CSF tau does not necessarily reflect brain pathology, as normal tau levels have been documented in Tau positive FTD patients (e.g. *MAPT*-related FTD).

Levels of CSF aBeta1-42 in FTD have been shown to be more consistently, though not universally, low in FTD. However, this observation is not useful in differentiating FTD from AD, which is also associated with low level of the same biomarker. Interestingly, other amyloid Beta1 sub-species have also been reported to be low in FTD, with data suggesting that a reduction in aBeta1-38 may be more specific to FTD and that levels of some species (e.g. aBeta1-37) vary in different FTD variants. Further research is needed to elucidate the role of abeta1 protein as a disease biomarker in FTD.

7.10.3.2 TDP-43

Studies of CSF TDP-43 in FTD have also been inconclusive. Some studies showed similar levels to controls. Other studies reported TDP-43 levels that were significantly higher than those of controls, but not significantly higher than the respective serum levels, raising the possibility that the identified protein was blood-derived.

More promising is the attempt to focus on more CNS specific isoforms of the protein, such as abnormally phosphorylated TDP-43 which is the main constituent of protein aggregates in TDP-43 proteinopathies. A recent study documented that FTD patients with likely TDP-43 pathology (positive gene mutations in *C9orf72* or *GRN*) had higher serum and CSF levels of phosphorylated TDP-43 compared to other FTD patients and controls, though in case of controls only the differences in serum levels reached statistical significance.

7.10.3.3 Progranulin
Serum prograulin has been shown to low in FTD patents with null pathogenic mutations of the *GRN* gene including those in the pre-symptomatic stage. However, proganulin levels are normal in FTD patients without these mutations, limiting the usefulness of this biomarker to clinical trials targeting *GRN*-related FTD.

7.10.3.4 Ubiquitin
Ubiquitin is another major constituent of abnormal protein aggregates in FTLD-U. CSF ubiquitin levels in FTD patients have been reported to be significantly higher than those in AD patients, but not significantly different from that of healthy controls. This suggests a potential role for CSF ubiquitin in differentiating AD and FTD, but further research is needed to replicate these findings.

7.10.3.5 Other Biomarkers
Neurofilaments (NFH), often in phosphorylated isoforms, constitute an integral part of the axonal cytoskeleton. The high levels of NFH in neurons have led to an interest in investigating their CSF levels in several neurodegenerative disorders as a surrogate marker of neuronal degeneration and loss. Several studies have shown remarkably high CSF levels of both light chain and hyperphosphorylated heavy chain neurofilaments in FTD. The degree of NFH phosphorylation is increased in FTD compared to both AD and

controls. Of note, levels were normal in gene carriers with pre-manifest disease. The pathological significance of these neurofilaments remains to be determined.

Less established is the role of pro-inflammatory cytokines (e.g. TNF-alpha and IL6) as biomarkers in FTD as the few studies conducted in this area arrived at contradictory conclusions.

Finally, several recent studies employed advanced mass-spectrometric techniques to simultaneously examine multiple analytes simultaneously (15 to more than 2000) in an attempt to identify a reliable biomarker in FTD. Candidates proteins proposed to date (alone or in combination) include the neurosecretory protein VGF, transthyretin, S-cysteinylated transthyretin, truncated cystatin C and a fragment of chromogranin B. However, there is still a considerable journey ahead prior to the translation of these efforts into a biomarker of practical value in research or clinical setting.

7.11 Diagnostic Criteria

The diagnostic criteria in FTD have been subject to a number of changes over the years. The first set of criteria was devised at a consensus meeting in 1996 (Neary et al. 1998) where it was decided to separate the three clinical syndromes in FTD (bvFTD, progressive non-fluent aphasia and semantic dementia) and criteria were devised for each. Core diagnostic features thought to be integral to each syndrome had to be present to make the diagnoses. Supportive diagnostic features were not considered necessary for a diagnosis but were considered characteristic of the syndrome and "added more weight" to the diagnosis. Exclusion criteria were listed to prevent the inclusion of other forms of cortical dementia, specifically AD and psychiatric disorders. All must be absent in order to make a diagnosis.

Some researchers (McKhann et al. 2001) have suggested simplifying the clinical criteria into either behaviour or language presentation of FTD and then qualifying this classification further with a neuropathological diagnosis when and if a patient comes to autopsy. However, most researchers of the language variants of FTD would view svPPA and nfvPPA as distinct and separate entities. The risk of combining these syndromes is that important clinical findings, including potential biomarkers are missed because the population studied is heterogeneous.

Indeed, the tripartite division of FTD (bvFTD, svFTD, nfvFTD) have been preserved in the new diagnostic criteria, published by Rascovsky in 2011 (Table 7.5). However, the inclusion criteria have been substantially modified. In the same year, a separate revision of the diagnostic criteria and of classification the

language syndromes has been agreed upon and published by Gorno-Tempini et al. (2011). The proposed criteria create a four step diagnostic framework. The first step is the diagnoses of PPA as condition where the earliest, most salient and most disabling feature of the condition, at least in the initial stages, is decline in language function. The symptoms must also not be better accounted for by a non-neurodegenerative or a medical condition, The subsequent steps of the diagnostic framework aim to identify the different variants of PPA with increasing levels of certainty (see table 7.6).

Table 7.5 The diagnostic criteria for behavioural variant FTD (bvFTD) proposed by Rascovski et al. in 2011

I –Presence of dementia	The following symptom **must** be present to meet criteria for bvFTD
	Shows progressive deterioration of behaviour and/or cognition by observation or history (as provided by a knowledgeable informant).
II- Possible bvFTD	At least 3 of the following behavioural/cognitive symptoms (A–F) **must** be present to meet criteria.[a]
	A. Early behavioural disinhibition [
	A.1. Socially inappropriate behaviour
	A.2. Loss of manners or decorum
	A.3. Impulsive, rash or careless actions
	B. Early apathy or inertia must be present]:
	B.1. Apathy
	B.2. Inertia
	C. Early loss of sympathy or empathy
	C.1. Diminished response to other people's needs and feelings
	C.2. Diminished social interest, interrelatedness or personal warmth
	D. Early perseverative, stereotyped or compulsive/ritualistic behaviour
	D.1. Simple repetitive movements
	D.2. Complex, compulsive or ritualistic behaviours
	D.3. Stereotypy of speech
	E. Hyperorality and dietary changes [
	E.1. Altered food preferences
	E.2. Binge eating, increased consumption of alcohol or cigarettes
	E.3. Oral exploration or consumption of inedible objects
	F. Neuropsychological profile:
	F.1. Deficits in executive tasks
	F.2. Relative sparing of episodic memory
	F.3. Relative sparing of visuospatial skills
III. Probable bvFTD	All of the following (A–C) must be present to meet criteria.
	A. Meets criteria for possible bvFTD
	B. Exhibits significant functional decline (by caregiver report or as evidenced by Clinical Dementia Rating Scale or Functional Activities Questionnaire scores)
	C. Imaging results consistent with frontal and/or anterior temporal involvement (on MRI, CT, PET or SPECT)

(continued)

Table 7.5 (continued)

IV. Bv FTD with definite FTLD Pathology	Criterion A + either criterion B or C must be present to meet criteria
	A. Meets criteria for possible or probable bvFTD
	B. Histopathological evidence of FTLD on biopsy or at post-mortem
	C. Presence of a known pathogenic mutation
V. Exclusionary criteria for bvFTD	Criteria A and B must be answered negatively for any bvFTD diagnosis.
	Criterion C can be positive for possible bvFTD but must be negative for probable bvFTD.
	A. Pattern of deficits is better accounted for by other non-degenerative nervous system or medical disorders
	B. Behavioural disturbance is better accounted for by a psychiatric diagnosis
	C. Biomarkers strongly indicative of Alzheimer's disease or other neurodegenerative process.

Reproduced and modified with permission of OUP from Rascovski et al. (2011)

[a]For a patients to have one of the behavioural symptoms (A–E) he/she must have at least 1 of sub-symptoms (e.g. section A these are symptoms listed in A-1, A-2, OR A-3) in a persistent or recurrent, rather than single or rare events. For the cognitive symptoms (Section F) the patient must fulfil all criteria (F1 to F3)

Table 7.6 The diagnostic criteria for primary progressive aphasia (PPA) syndromes proposed by Gorno-Tempini et al. in 2011

		Nonfluent/agrammatic variant PPA	Semantic variant	Logopenic variant
Step 2: Clinical Diagnoses of PPA variant	*Core criteria*	*(at least 1 required)* 1. Agrammatism in language production 2. Effortful, halting speech within consistent speech sound errors and distortions (apraxia of speech)	*(both must present)* 1. Impaired confrontation naming 2. Impaired single-word comprehension	*Core criteria (both must present)* 1. Impaired single-word retrieval in spontaneous speech and naming 2. Impaired repetition of sentences and phrases
	Other features	*At least 2 must be present)* 1. Impaired comprehension of syntactically complex sentences 2. Spared single-word comprehension 3. Spared object knowledge	*At least 3 must be present* 1. Impaired object knowledge, particularly for low-frequency or low-familiarity items 2. Surface dyslexia or dysgraphia 3. Spared repetition 4. Spared speech production (grammar and motor speech)	*At least 3 must be present)* 1. Speech(phonologic) errors in spontaneous speech and naming 2. Spared single-word comprehension and object knowledge 3. Spared motor speech 4. Absence of frank agrammatism
Step 3. Imaging Supported Diagnoses of PPA variant		Both criteria must be present 1. Clinical diagnosis of nonfluent/agrammatic PPA variant 2. Imaging (MRI, SPECT or PET) much show predominant involvement of the left posterior fronto-insular region.	Both criteria must be present 1. Clinical diagnosis of semantic variant 2. Imaging (MRI, SPECT or PET) much show predominant involvement of the anterior temporal lobe	Both criteria must be present 1. Clinical diagnosis of logopenic variant 2. Imaging (MRI, SPECT or PET) much show predominant involvement of the left posterior perisylvian or parietal region
Step 4 Definite Diagnoses of PPA variant		Clinical diagnoses Plus one of the following 1. Histopathological evidence of a specific Neurodegenerative pathology (e.g. FTLD-tau, FTLD-TDP43, AD, other) 2. Presence of a known pathogenic mutation		

Reproduced and modified from Gorno-Tempini et al. (2011) with permission from Wolters Kluwer Health

7.12   Therapy

Before the treatment, comes the diagnosis. Indeed, appropriate care of FTD patients starts with communicating the diagnoses. The diagnoses and its implications should be explained to patients, families and caregivers in lay terms and in a sensitive manner. This should be carried out in a specialist environment with an understanding of the unique features of FTD such as the personality changes, loss of empathy and socially embarrassing behaviours. Multidisciplinary support should be offered.

7.12.1 Disease Modifying Therapy

Currently there are no FDA approved disease modifying therapies for FTD.

However, preclinical and early clinical phase trials of true disease modifying therapies are underway. The main targets are protein pathways known to be integral to the pathological process in FTD including tau, progranulin, and TDP-43 (described in the Sect. 7.8). This approach has produced several promising candidates. However, the logistic difficulties intrinsic to a disease such as FTD are significant. The first clinical trial for a disease modifying therapy in bvFTD was initiated in 2013. This involved TRx0237 (also called LMTX™) which acts by reducing levels of aggregated or misfolded tau protein. Many patients had to be excluded because of lack of supportive MRI changes and/or diagnostic uncertainty raising the possibility of "FTD phenocopies". Others displayed advanced cognitive impairment, lack of interest and/or inability to give informed consent. Other challenges included the reduced ability of bvFTD patients to wait for prolonged periods or to tolerate MRI scanning. The patients' behavioural changes posed significant challenges to untrained staff. Of the first 275 potential subjects who were pre-screened, 55 progressed to formal screening, and only 20 patients proceeded to the randomisation. The results of the trial are still pending.

Granulin, the product of the *GRN* gene, displays low levels in FTD patients with this mutation. Granulin is a growth factor believed to play a role in multiple essential biological processes like regulating inflammatory reactions, energy and protein homeostasis, neurite outgrowth, and neuronal survival. Several new therapies are being developed to increase granulin including PTC124-a new chemical entity that selectively induces ribosomal read through premature but not normal termination codons. Early trials have demonstrated safety in healthy volunteers is in preclinical trials for *GRN* related FTD.

Davunetide is an intranasal neuropeptide therapy derived from a growth factor called activity-dependent neurotrophic protein and is believed to have neuroprotective effects. Despite early promising Phase II trials in MCI and AD patients, a more recent trial in FTD with predicted tau pathology (which included CBS and PSP) was halted following a large multicentre trial involving PSP patients reporting negative results in all outcome measures.

Preclinical studies are also investigating the therapeutic value of immune therapy or efforts to block cleavage in removing abnormal TDP-43.

7.13   Symptomatic Treatment

There are no FDA approved therapies for symptomatic treatment of the cognitive or behavioural difficulties in FTD. A few small randomised controlled clinical trials have been undertaken in FTD including those for memantine, paroxetine, trazadone, oxytocin, methylphenidate, and galantamine. These largely yielded negative results, though a few reported modest improvements in behavioural symptoms (e.g. nasally administered oxytocin, methylphenidate, trazadone, paroxetine in 1 of 2 trials).

Current therapeutic management of FTD involves the off-label use of medications based on efficacy in treating other neurodegenerative or psychiatric disorders with similar behavioural problems. Selective serotonin reuptake inhibitors or serotonin-norepinephrine reuptake inhibitors are now considered first line treatments to help control the behavioural symptoms in FTD particularly disinhibition and poor impulse control. This is based on open label studies as case controlled randomised trials have produced mixed results. A meta-analyses of trazadone and SSRIs studies suggest that the use of these medications may indeed be helpful in ameliorating behavioural changes in FTD. Case reports suggest that atypical antipsychotic agents such as quetiapine and anti-epileptics may be considered for treatment of agitation, delusions and aggression.

No drug to date has been shown to have any significant benefit on cognitive function in FTD. In some cases (e.g. paroxetine) the drugs had a negative effect on cognitive performance. There is some evidence suggesting that intranasal oxytocin may have a beneficial effect of recognition of facial emotions, but it has no effect on other measures of cognitive function including executive functions.

Limitations of most FTD trials published to date include small sample size and in many cases poor selection of cognitive measures.

Supportive therapy remains the cornerstone of treatment in FTD. A multidisciplinary approach is essential to tackle the range of behaviour and neuropsychiatric manifestations bvFTD. Neuropsychological strategies can help patients and caregivers cope with the worst effects of the cognitive and behavioural impairment.

Sleep disturbances should be managed by maintaining a regular sleep regime and may be aided by the use of the sedating anti-depressant e.g. Trazadone.

Speech and language therapy including the utilization of communication aids by carers .may offer some benefit to PPA patients early in the course of the illness,

Parkinsonism and amyotrophy are the most common motor manifestations of advanced FTD. Multidisciplinary care including physiotherapy, occupational therapy and speech language therapy are the cornerstone of treating motor symptoms. Riluzole in the only FDA approved treatment for motor system degeneration associated ALS. Although the parkinsonian symptoms in FTD rarely respond to dopamine replacement therapies, it is worth noting that a small proportion of these patients do report some benefit from these therapies. More detailed

discussion of these disorders can be found in the relevant chapters.

Prominence of early bladder difficulty should give rise to suspicion of disorders of autonomic control such as PSP rather than FTD. However early involvement of the medial frontal lobe in both bvFTD and CBD can lead to incontinence which should be managed with intermittent catheterization, indwelling catheters, and the use of a leg bag or in some cased urinary diversion. The use of anti-cholinergic must be tempered by the possibility of increasing confusion.

The inexorable decline in function and quality of life that currently follows a diagnosis of FTD should always be met with a plan for palliation and appropriate end of life care. There has been significant improvement in the knowledge and understanding of this process amongst palliative care specialists. For further discussion see Chap. 17.

Supportive care should always include the patient's carer. It has been recognized that carers of patients with FTD report significant distress and depression even when compared to carers of patients with other forms of dementia. This is most likely due to the FTD patient's behavioural dysfunction and poor social cognition. The multidisciplinary team should be aware of these stressors on the carer. Support to the carer can be provided through advice and instruction on how to manage disruptive behaviour and the availability of respite care.

Conclusion

FTD researchers world-wide are working on translating the progress made over the last decade in furthering our understanding of FTD molecular pathology and proteomic into clinically relevant disease biomarkers and potentially targeted disease modifying therapy. However, until then the corner stone of caring for FTD patients continues to be the use of symptomatic pharmacological therapy and comprehensive multidisciplinary care that includes the expertise of neurologists with a special interest in cognitive neurology, clinical nurse specialists, clinical psychologists, speech therapist, physiotherapists, and palliative care specialists along with social workers.

Further Reading

Amador-Ortiz C, Lin WL, Ahmed Z, Personett D, Davies P, Duara R, Graff-Radford NR, Hutton ML, Dickson DW. TDP-43 immunoreactivity in hippocampal sclerosis and Alzheimer's disease. Ann Neurol. 2007;61(5): 435–45.

Cairns NJ, Bigio EH, Mackenzie IR, Neumann M, Lee VM, Hatanpaa KJ, White 3rd CL, Schneider JA, Grinberg LT, Halliday G, Duyckaerts C, Lowe JS, Holm IE, Tolnay M, Okamoto K, Yokoo H, Murayama S, Woulfe J, Munoz DG, Dickson DW, Ince PG, Trojanowski JQ, Mann DM, Consortium for Frontotemporal Lobar Degeneration. Neuropathologic diagnostic and nosologic criteria for frontotemporal lobar degeneration: consensus of the Consortium for Frontotemporal Lobar Degeneration. Acta Neuropathol. 2007;114(1):5–22.

Chare L, Hodges JR, Leyton CE, McGinley C, Tan RH, Kril JJ, Halliday GM. New criteria for frontotemporal dementia syndromes: clinical and pathological diagnostic implications. J Neurol Neurosurg Psychiatry. 2014;85(8):865–70.

Cummings JL. Frontal-subcortical circuits and human behaviour. Arch Neurol. 1993;50:873–80.

Diehl-Schmid J, Onur OA, Kuhn J, Gruppe T, Drzezga A. Imaging frontotemporal lobar degeneration. Curr Neurol Neurosci Rep. 2014;14:489.

Hodges JR, editor. Frontotemporal dementia syndromes. Cambridge: Cambridge University Press; 2007.

Mackenzie IR, Neumann M, Baborie A, Sampathu DM, Du Plessis D, Jaros E, Perry RH, Trojanowski JQ, Mann DM, Lee VM. A harmonized classification system for FTLD-TDP pathology. Acta Neuropathol. 2011;122(1):111–3.

McKhann GM, et al. Clinical and pathological diagnosis of frontotemporal dementia. Arch Neurol. 2001;58:1803–9.

Neary D, et al. Frontotemporal lobar degeneration. A consensus on clinical diagnostic criteria. Neurology. 1998;51:1546–54.

Neumann M, Sampathu DM, Kwong LK, Truax AC, Micsenyi MC, Chou TT, Bruce J, Schuck T, Grossman M, Clark CM, McCluskey LF, Miller BL, Masliah E, Mackenzie IR, Feldman H, Feiden W, Kretzschmar HA, Trojanowski JQ, Lee VM. Ubiquitinated TDP-43 in frontotemporal lobar degeneration and amyotrophic lateral sclerosis. Science. 2006;314(5796):130–3.

Nilsson C, Landqvist Waldö M, Nilsson K, Santillo A, Vestberg S. Age-related incidence and family history in frontotemporal dementia: data from the Swedish Dementia Registry. PLoS One. 2014;9(4), e94901.

Onyike CU, Diehl-Schmid J. The epidemiology of frontotemporal dementia. Int Rev Psychiatry. 2013;25(2):130–7.

Piguet O, et al. Sensitivity of current criteria for the diagnosis of behavioural variant frontotemporal dementia. Neurology. 2009;72:732–7.

Rascovsky K, Hodges JR, Knopman D, Mendez MF, Kramer JH, Neuhaus J, van Swieten JC, Seelaar H, Dopper EG, Onyike CU, Hillis AE, Josephs KA, Boeve BF, Kertesz A, Seeley WW, Rankin KP, Johnson JK, Gorno-Tempini ML, Rosen H, Prioleau-Latham CE, Lee A, Kipps CM, Lillo P, Piguet O, Rohrer JD, Rossor MN, Warren JD, Fox NC, Galasko D, Salmon DP, Black SE, Mesulam M, Weintraub S, Dickerson BC, Diehl-Schmid J, Pasquier F, Deramecourt V, Lebert F, Pijnenburg Y, Chow TW, Manes F, Grafman J, Cappa SF, Freedman M, Grossman M, Miller BL. Sensitivity of revised diagnostic criteria for the behavioural variant of frontotemporal dementia. Brain. 2011;134(Pt 9): 2456–77.

Snowden JS, Bathgate D, Varma A, Blackshaw A, Gibbons ZC, Neary D. Distinct behavioural profiles in frontotemporal dementia and semantic dementia. J Neurol Neurosurg Psychiatry. 2001;70(3):323–32.

Vossel KA, Miller BL. New approaches to the treatment of frontotemporal lobar degeneration. Cur Opin Neurol. 2008;21(6):708–16.

Weintraub S, Mesulam M. With or without FUS, it is the anatomy that dictates the dementia phenotype. Brain. 2009;132:2906–8.

Whitwell JL, Weigand S, Boeve BF, Senjem ML, Gunter JL, DeJesus-Hernandez M, Rutherford NJ, Baker M, Knopman DS, Wszolek ZK, Parisi JE, Dickson DW, Petersen RC, Rademakers R, Jack Jr CR, Josephs KA. Neuroimaging signatures of frontotemporal dementia genetics: C9orf72, tau, progranulin and sporadics. Brain. 2012;135:794–806.

Whitwell JL, Przybelski SA, Weigand SD, Ivnik RJ, Vemuri P, Gunter JL, Senjem ML, Shiung MM, Boeve BF, Knopman DS, Parisi JE, Dickson DW, Petersen RC, Jack Jr CR, Josephs KA. Distinct anatomical subtypes of the behavioural variant of frontotemporal dementia: a cluster analysis study. Brain. 2009;132(Pt 11): 2932–46.

Amyotrophic Lateral Sclerosis

Orla Hardiman, Matthew C. Kiernan,
and Leonard H. van den Berg

8.1   Introduction

Amyotrophic Lateral Sclerosis (ALS), also known as motor neuron disease (MND) is the commonest neurodegenerative condition of the young and middle aged. The disease is characterised by progressive upper and lower motor neuron degeneration. Mean life expectancy is 3–5 years from first symptom. Although primarily a disorder of the motor system, ALS also has non-motor features and overlaps clinically and pathologically with other neurodegenerative conditions including fronto-temporal dementia (FTD). Up to 13 % of incident patients have evidence of behavioural variant frontotemporal dementia on presentation, and a further 30–40 % have evidence of cognitive/behavioural impairment, including deficits in social cognition. Once symptoms develop, the course of ALS is progressive, and death is usually from respiratory failure. Although treatment options are limited, multidisciplinary management can preserve quality of life and interventions such as aggressive secretion management and non-invasive ventilation can improve survival.

8.2   Clinical Features

The clinical onset of ALS is usually asymmetric. The first symptom may be a gait disturbance (e.g. tripping, dragging one leg) or difficulty with fine movements in the upper extremities e.g. fastening buttons. As motor neurons are affected segmentally, clinical presentation depends on where in the neuroaxis the disease is first manifest. Up to 25 % of patients present with bulbar symptoms such as dysarthria and dysphagia and 1–5 % present with respiratory failure. The site of disease onset is of prognostic significance, as limb onset carries a better prognosis than bulbar onset, and lower limb onset carries a better prognosis than upper limb onset. Respiratory onset disease carries the worst prognosis.

People with ALS almost never describe fasciculations as key part of their presenting symptomatology, and fasciculations in the absence of muscle weakness or other neurologic signs are extremely rare as a first presentation of ALS. The clinical hallmark of ALS on neurological

O. Hardiman (✉)
Academic Unit of Neurology,
Trinity Biomedical Sciences Institute,
Dublin, Ireland
e-mail: orla@hardiman.net

M.C. Kiernan
Brain and Mind Centre, Sydney Medical School,
University of Sydnes, Royal Prince Alfred Hospital,
Camperdown, NSW, Australia
e-mail: M.Kiernan@unsw.edu.au

L.H. van den Berg
Department of Neurology, University Medical
Center Utrecht, Utrecht, The Netherlands
e-mail: L.H.vandenBerg@umcutrecht.nl

© Springer International Publishing Switzerland 2016
O. Hardiman, C.P. Doherty (eds.), *Neurodegenerative Disorders: A Clinical Guide*,
DOI 10.1007/978-3-319-23309-3_8

examination is the presence of both upper and lower motor neuron signs that are not attributable to other causes. A combination of upper and lower motor signs occurring concomitantly at the same spinal level s (e.g., brisk reflexes in a weak, fasciculating limb) should raise a differential diagnosis of ALS, although cervical spondylotic myelopathy could also produce this clinical picture. Bladder function is not usually impaired in the early stages of the disease, but is often involved in later stages of the illness. Up to one quarter of patients complain of minor sensory symptoms, however formal sensory examination is generally normal.

The time from symptom onset to diagnosis is usually in the order of 9–15 months. Many people will have seen two or three other specialists before they are correctly diagnosed.

Behavioural variant frontotemporal dementia (FTD) occurs in up to 13 % of incident patients with ALS. This is characterized by personality change, irritability, obsessions, poor insight and pervasive deficits on frontal executive tests. A milder form of cognitive impairment occurs in up to 50 % of patients with ALS, and can include subtle executive deficits, apathy, verbal fluency deficits and changes in memory. Behavioral change may also be reported by a spouse or relative and may not be apparent during formal clinical interview. Deficits in social cognition are common and frequently under-reported. Cognitive dysfunction can precede or follow the onset of motor symptoms.

A number of screening tests for cognitive impairment in ALS have been generated. The most widely used is the Edinburgh Cognitive and Behavioural ALS Screen (ECAS) (http://hdl.handle.net/1842/6592). This 15 min screening tool has been validated and is the preferred cognitive screening tool used by the European ALS Consortium (ENCALS). Within a clinic setting, verbal fluency can be a sensitive marker of cognitive impairment in ALS, and a simple 2-min word-generation test can help to identify patients in whom more detailed neuropsychological evaluation may be required. Patients with severe deficits in verbal fluency are more likely to exhibit frontal and executive deficits on more formal testing although these tests are also predicated on pre-morbid intellectual ability. Short batteries of tests, such as the MMSE, are not sensitive to frontotemporal syndromes and should not be used for diagnostic purposes.

In patients with features of frontotemporal dementia, behavioural change can be assessed using carer-based instruments such as The Neuropsychiatric Inventory or Frontal Systems Behavioural Scale, or more recently developed disease specific scales such as the Beaumont Behavioural inventory. These questionnaires are completed by caregivers and can convey how the patient functions on a day-to-day basis compared with his or her premorbid status.

Once symptoms and signs of ALS develop, the condition progresses. Functional decline can be measured using the revised ALS Functional Rating Scale (ALSFRS-R) (Table 8.1).Up to 70 % patients die within 3 years of their first symptom. Approximately 10 % of patients experience a more protracted disease course, and may live for up to 10 years from the time of first symptom.

Variants of ALS include primary lateral sclerosis (PLS), in which clinical signs are confined to upper motor neurons, and progressive muscle atrophy, in which signs are confined to the lower motor neuron. Diagnostic criteria for PLS require the presence of signs for a minimum of 3 years. These ALS variants can be difficult to diagnose in the early stages, and prognosis is generally better than in typical ALS.

Restricted forms of ALS have also been described including flail arm and flail leg syndromes, and monomelic disease. The former two are more common in men, and may carry a better prognosis that typical ALS.

Other variants include bulbospinal muscular atrophy (Kennedy's disease). This X-linked disorder is due to an expansion of trinucleotide repeats in the androgen receptor. The clinical features include slowly progressive lower motor neuron signs in bulbar and proximal limbs. Up to 50 % of cases have gynaecomastia; Progression is usually slower than in typical ALS. Nerve conduction studies can be helpful as, in contrast to ALS, the sensory nerve action potentials may be absent in Kennedy's disease (Table 8.2).

Table 8.1 ALS FRS—revised

1. Speech	
4	Normal speech
3	Detectable disturbance
2	Intelligible without repeating
1	Speech with non-verbal communication
0	Loss of useful speech
2. Salivation	
4	Normal
3	Slight but definite excess of saliva
2	Moderate excessive saliva, minimal drooling
1	Marked excessive of saliva, some drooling
0	Marked drooling, requires constant tissue
3. Swallowing	
4	Normal eating habits
3	Early eating problems, occasional choking
2	Dietary consistency changes
1	Needs supplemental tube feeding
0	Nil orally
4. Handwriting	
4	Normal
3	Slow or sloppy, all words legible
2	Not all words legible
1	Able to grip pen but cannot write
0	Unable to grip pen
5. Cutting food & handling utensils	
4	Normal
3	Slow & clumsy but no help needed
2	Can cut most foods, although clumsy & needs some help
1	Food must be cut by someone else
0	Needs to be fed
6. Dressing & hygiene	
4	Normal
3	Independent but decreased efficiency
2	Some help with closures & fasteners
1	Provides minimal assistance to caregiver
0	Unable to perform any task
7. Turning in bed	
4	Normal
3	Slow & clumsy
2	Can turn alone with difficulty
1	Can initiate but cannot turn or adjust sheets
0	Total dependence
8. Walking	
4	Normal
3	Early ambulation difficulties
2	Walks with assistance

(continued)

Table 8.1 (continued)

1	Non ambulatory, functional movement
0	No purposeful leg movement
9. Climbing stairs	
4	Normal
3	Slow
2	Mild unsteadiness/fatigue
1	Needs assistance
0	Cannot do
10. Dyspnea	
4	None
3	Occurs when walking
2	Occurs when eating, bathing or dressing
1	Occurs at rest
0	Considerable difficulty
11. Orthopnea	
4	None
3	Some difficulty, does not routinely use more than two pillows
2	Needs extra pillows to sleep
1	Only sleeps sitting up
0	Unable to sleep
12. Respiratory insufficiency	
4	None
3	Intermittent use of non invasive ventilation
2	Continuous use of non invasive ventilation at night
1	Continuous use of non invasive ventilation day & night
0	Mechanical ventilation via tracheostomy

The majority of ALS patients die from respiratory failure. Prognostic indicators include time from first symptom to diagnosis (longer duration carries a better prognosis), presence of executive impairment (poorer prognosis), bulbar or respiratory onset disease (poorer prognosis) older age of onset (poorer prognosis), marked weight loss (poorer prognosis) and presence of pure upper or pure lower motor syndromes (better prognosis) (Table 8.3).

8.2.1 Discussing the Diagnosis

Once the diagnosis has been established, the patient should formally meet with an experienced doctor who has been involved in the care, to

Table 8.2 Variants of ALS/MND

Disease	Clinical features	Other comments	Median survival
ALS	Both upper and motor neurone signs in multiple spinal segments	Most common adult-onset form of motor neuron disease	Three to five years
Primary lateral sclerosis	Upper motor neuron signs only	Many patients eventually develop clinical or electrophysiological signs of LMN involvement. ALS develops in up to 77 % within 3–4 years	For those who remain with a diagnosis of PLS, median survival = 20 years or more
Progressive muscular atrophy	Lower motor neuron signs only	Variable evolution to ALS	Five years. A subset survive 20 years or more
Progressive bulbar palsy	Speech and swallowing affected initially due to LMN involvement of CN IX, X, XII	Symptoms include dysarthria, dysphagia, and dysphonia. Aspiration pneumonia is usually the terminal event	Two to three years
Bulbospinal Muscle atrophy (Kennedy's disease)	Speech and swallowing affected, proximal limbs	X-linked recessive inheritance pattern Pure lower motor neuron condition due to trinucleotide repeat in androgen receptor	Ten years or more

CN cranial nerves, *UPM* upper motor neuron, *LMN* lower motor neuron

Table 8.3 Prognostic indicators

Poor prognostic indicators
Short interval between first symptom & diagnosis
Bulbar onset disease
Respiratory onset disease Malnutrition
Rapidly progressive decline in ALSFRS
Presence of executive impairment
Familial disease (some SOD1 mutations) Hyperlipidemia Increased homocysteine
Vital capacity <50 % of normal
Sniff nasal inspiratory pressure <40 cm H_2O
Good prognostic indicators
Long interval between first symptom and diagnosis
Lower limb onset
Flail arm/flail leg syndrome
Upper motor neuron predominant disease
Lower motor predominant disease
Familial disease (some SOD1 mutations)
Age of onset <50 years

discuss the outcome of the investigations. Specific techniques should be used as outlined in Table 8.4, including the provision of a quiet space and adequate time to discuss the diagnosis. The patient should be accompanied by a close friend or family member. The level of information the patient has about the disease should be explored. Some patients have specific concerns including a fear of choking to death; reassurance can be provided about these and other anxieties relating to the progress of the disease. Despite the inevitable decline associated with the condition, it is important to convey hope when disclosing the diagnosis. Positive prognostic aspects of the disease can be emphasized, and the likelihood of new therapeutics in the form of future clinical trials discussed. Patients should be provided with a follow up appointment within 2–4 weeks of diagnosis. Some patients seek a second opinion. This should be facilitated.

8.3 Epidemiology

The incidence of ALS/MND in Europe is approximately 2 per 100,000 and the overall lifetime risk is approximately 1:350. In populations of non-European or mixed ethnicity, current evidence suggests that the frequency of ALS is lower. While the reasons for this difference

Table 8.4 How should a physician tell the patient that they have ALS

Task	Recommendations
Location	Off the ward, in a quiet room
	Not as an outpatient clinic
Participants	Senior clinician
	Patient
	Family member
	Nursing staff
Breaking the news	Ask what the patient/family knows about their condition
	Approach the diagnosis with sensitivity
	Use diagrams to help explain the concept of upper & lower motor neurons
	Be honest about prognosis
	Acknowledge the distress that the diagnosis causes
	Allow plenty of time for questions
	Allow time for reflection
Hope and reassurance	Provide hope: up to 10 % of patients survive for >10 years
	Identify positive prognostic indicators
	Explain that support is available, and that the patient and family are not alone
	Reassure that as the condition progresses, interventions can help to maintain independence, quality of life and dignity
	Reassure that decline occurs gradually
	Provide information about voluntary organizations
	Discuss likely opportunities to participate in research and clinical trials
Honesty	Be honest but empathic
Communication	Simple language, no jargon

remain unclear, preliminary evidence suggests that genetic admixture may be protective. Careful evaluation of populations over a long period of time has indicated that the adjusted age-specific incidence of the disease is not increasing.

ALS is more common in males than females by a ratio of 1.2–1.5 to 1. This disparity is mostly due to the increased frequency of spinal onset alS in men. In contrast to Parkinson's disease and Alzheimer's disease, the risk of developing ALS peaks between the ages of 50–75, and declines thereafter. This suggests that ALS is not a disease of ageing, but a disease for which age is one of a number of risk factors.

As ALS is a rare disease, environmental factors that confer increased risk have been difficult to identify. Case controlled studies seeking to establish exposure risks are often inadequately powered and confounded by methodological errors. High incidences of ALS in Guam and the Kii Penninsula in Japan have been associated with cyanobacterial neurotoxins including BMAA, although definitive evidence in this regard is lacking, and more recent evidence from Kii also suggests the presence of a genetic founder effect. Clustering of ALS has been identified in certain occupations including Italian soccer players. The factors that lead to this apparent increased risk remain to be determined. Other environmental factors that have been associated with ALS have included smoking, exposure to pesticides and organic toxins, and electromagnetic radiation. With the exception of smoking, definitive evidence of risk remains to be established and will require large unbiased population-based case controlled studies for confirmation.

8.4   Genetics

ALS is frequently described as being either familial or sporadic. A total of 22 genes and loci of major effect have been identified, (Table 8.5) and the majority of these are autosomal dominant in inheritance pattern. Of these, the hexnucleotide repeat expansion in C9orf72 accounts for over 50 % of known familial ALS in populations of European extraction, and up to 8 % of apparently sporadic disease. This variant is rare in other populations. The C9orf72 repeat expansion is associated with a distinct ALS phenotype with prominent cognitive and behavioural impairment, and with higher rates of neuropsychiatric conditions in kindreds of those affected. The pathogenesis of C9orf72 repeat related disease

Table 8.5 Known genes associated with ALS

Gene	Functional significance
Oxidative stress	
SOD1	Cytoplasmic Antioxidant Soluble form may become neurotoxic
HFE	Regulator of iron metabolism
Cytoskeleton, microtubule, axonal transport	
MAPT	Microtubule protein disruption Involved in other neurodegenerative diseases
NEFH	Neurofilament protein, mutations alter axonal transport
PRPH	Intermediate filament, transgenic mice develop motor neuron degeneration
Prophillin	Cytoskeleton dynamics
TubA4A	Microtubular function
Peripherin	
DCT1	Disruption in dynein/dynactin complex alter axonal transport, produce phenotype in mice
KIFAP3	Kinesin associated protein, modulates survival
Metabolism	
PON 1–3	Paroxonases are important detoxifying enzymes. Association in five different populations, but different haplotypes implicated in different ancestral populations
Progranulin	Gene of major effect in FTD. Coding variations associated with ALS in some populations, similar in function to angiogenin
DNA/RNA repair	
ANG	RNA ribonuclease and hypoxia responsive agent; overlap in function with VEGF & progranulin
APEX FUS	RNA regulation
SMN1, SMN2	Affects RNA splicing, gene of major effect in spinal muscular atrophy
TDP-43	RNA regulator
ELP 3	RNA polymerase
C9orf-72	RNA regulation, RNA transcription
TAF 15 EWSR1 Senetaxin	RNA processing

Table 8.5 (continued)

Gene	Functional significance
Excitotoxicity	
UNC13A	FTD
Proteostatic	
VCP CHMPT2	
Ubiquilin 2	Autophagy
Optineurin (OPTN)	Vesicular transport
Sequestosome (SQSTM)	Vesicular transport

has not been established, but is thought to relate in part to aberrant RNA transcription with accumulation of sense and antisense RNA foci, coupled with proteins expressed by repeat-associated non-ATG (RAN) translation. Sense and antisense RNAs are thought to accumulate in nuclear foci, and RAN proteins are thought to form cytoplasmic aggregates in neurons.

Mutations in superoxide dismuatase (SOD1) account for up to 15 % of familial ALS, and up to 5 % of apparently sporadic disease in some populations. However as is the case for the C9orf72 variant, mutations in SOD1 are population specific, occurring with low frequency in familial and sporadic disease in The Netherlands and Ireland, and with higher frequency in Italy and the USA.

Mutations in two different DNA/RNA binding proteins, TDP-43 and FUS/TLS account for a further 10–15 % of familial ALS in some populations. Both TDP-43 and FUS code for proteins involved in gene regulation including transcription, RNA splicing, RNA transport, and translation, and in the regulation and processing of small regulatory RNAS (microRNAs). Of the currently known genes, only C9orf-72 SOD1, TDP-43, and FUS mutations occur with sufficiently high frequency in European populations to warrant diagnostic testing. The remainder have been described in small numbers of kindreds are often associated with unusual phenotypes.

While there is currently no accepted definition of familial ALS, up to 85 % percent of people diagnosed with ALS have no family history and are classified as having sporadic disease. The frequency of familial disease can be under-estimated by the late onset of disease phenotype, incomplete penetrance, and small kindreds. Moreover, family aggregation studies have identified an overlap between ALS, FTD and other neurodegenerative and neuropsychiatric conditions. While a proportion of these families are associated with the repeat expansion on C90rf72, some repeat-negative kindreds also exhibit prominent aggregation of neuropsychiatric disease, suggesting the presence of other gene variants with phenotypic pleotropy.

Population-based studies of "at risk" genes that increase disease susceptibility suggest that up to 17 % of those with ALS carry an "at risk" variant, although the relative contribution of each identified gene rarely exceeds an odds ratio of 2.0, and in most cases the mechanism by which the risk is conferred remains to be elucidated.

Genome-wide association studies (GWAS) in ALS have been relatively disappointing to date, primarily because of small sample size (5000 patients, 15,000 controls). Increasing the sample size to over 15,000 patients have shown to increase the number of 'hits' substantially in other diseases such as Parkinson's disease, Alzheimer's disease, Multiple Sclerosis and Schizophrenia. A combined GWAS for ALS has included over 16,000 patients and 25,000 controls is being analysed. However increased international collaboration coupled with the combination of detailed clinical phenotyping with next generation whole genome sequencing and bioinformatics technology is likely to provide a wealth of new information about ALS pathophysiology (www.ProjectMine.com). This in turn will provide exciting new avenues for developments in disease therapeutics.

8.4.1 Genetic Testing

Because most ALS is thought to be non-familial, there is currently little advantage in testing sporadic individual patients for known gene mutations, with the possible exception of the C9orf72 repeat expansion. In general, genetic testing should only be undertaken in known familial disease, where the presence of mutations in known

genes might accelerate the diagnostic process. Expert genetic counseling is recommended prior to testing. Presymptomatic genetic testing should only be performed in first degree adult bloodrelatives of patients with a known gene mutation. As many mutations in ALS are incompletely penetrant, the identification of a mutation in an asymptomatic relative cannot accurately predict development of the disease. Testing should be performed on a strictly volunteer basis and should following extensive genetic counseling. However, with the advent of new therapeutics including anti-sense therapies for SOD1 – and C9orf72 – related disease, there may be a case in future for identifying pre-symptomatic carriers of known pathogenic variants.

8.5 Overlap Syndromes

Up to 13 % of patients with ALS have frontotemporal dementia (FTD), and up to 30 % of those with FTD have neurophysiologic evidence of anterior horn cell degeneration (see Chap. 6). A smaller percentage (2–5 %) of patients with ALS have evidence of other forms of dementia including features of Alzheimer's disease. Patients with ALS are more likely to have a family history of neurodegenerative disease – this is driven in part by the C9orf72 repeat expansion. Occasional patients with extrapyramidal syndromes and anterior horn cell degeneration have been reported and a small minority of ALS patients are ataxic. Rarely, Huntington's disease can present with amytrophy (see Chap. 8).

8.6 Diagnostic Criteria

Formal diagnosis of ALS is based upon clinical criteria that include the presence of upper motor neuron (UMN) and lower motor neuron (LMN) signs, progression of disease, and the absence of an alternative explanation. There is no single diagnostic test that can confirm or entirely exclude the diagnosis of motor neuron disease.

The *El Escorial* criteria were developed in 1990 by the World Federation of Neurology

Table 8.6 EL Escorial and Airlie house criteria for diagnosis of ALS

The presence of:
(a) Evidence of LMND degeneration by clinical, electrophysiological or neuropathological examination
(b) Evidence of UMN degeneration by clinical examination; and
(c) Progression of the motor syndrome within a region or to other regions, as determined by history or examination;
and:
The absence of:
(a) Electrophysiological and pathological evidence of other disease processes that might explain the signs of LMN or UMN degeneration; and,
(b) Neuroimaging evidence of other disease processes that might explain the observed clinical and electrophysiological signs.
El Escorial criteria
Definite ALS: UMN and LMN signs in three regions
Probable ALS: UMN & LMN signs in at least two regions with UMN signs rostral to (above) LMN signs
Possible ALS: UMN & LMN signs in one region, UMN signs alone in two or more regions, or LMN signs above UMN signs
Suspected ALS: LMN signs only in two or more regions
Airlie house (modified) criteria
Clinically definite ALS: clinical evidence alone of UMN & LMN signs in three regions
Clinically probable ALS: clinical evidence alone of UMN and LMN signs in at least two regions with some UMN signs rostral to (above) the LMN signs
Clinically probable—laboratory-supported ALS: clinical signs of UMN and LMN dysfunction are in only one region, or UMN signs alone in one region with LMN signs defined by EMG criteria in at least two limbs, together with proper application of neuroimaging and clinical laboratory protocols to exclude other causes
Possible ALS: clinical signs of UMN and LMN dysfunction in only one region, or UMN signs alone in two or more regions; or LMN signs rostral to UMN signs and the diagnosis of clinically probable—lab-supported ALS cannot be proven
Suspected ALS: this category is deleted from the revised El Escorial criteria

(WFN) for research and clinical trial purposes. These guidelines were subsequently revised in Airlie House in April 1998 (Table 8.6).

Both sets of criteria are based on the degree of certainty of diagnosis, which in turn is based on clinical assessment and the presence of upper and lower motor neuron signs together in the same topographical anatomic region in the brainstem, cervical, thoracic, or lumbosacral spinal cord. Although not validated at the time of inception, a number of inter-rater reliability studies have shown that among experts, the criteria are in general uniformly applied and reproducible. Notwithstanding, the criteria have been criticized as being too restrictive, as up to 10 % of patients with ALS remain within the "possible" category at the time of death and are thus excluded from most clinical trials, which require a diagnosis of "probable" "or "definite" ALS. Moreover, the criteria were developed prior to the recognition of the cognitive domain associated with ALS. The *El Escorial* and Airlie House criteria are not considered helpful in day-to-day management of ALS and should be reserved for classification of patients for research purposes.

8.7 Differential Diagnosis of ALS

Some conditions can closely resemble ALS and should be actively considered in the differential diagnosis. Consideration of the "mimic syndromes" is important, as the diagnosis of ALS is based primarily on clinical examination, supported by a series of laboratory investigations to exclude other conditions.

The majority of likely mimic syndromes are listed in Table 8.7. In practice, the most frequent conditions mistaken for ALS are multifocal motor neuropathy with conduction block and cervical spondylotic myelopathy.

Based on these studies, factors that should lead to revision of the diagnosis of ALS can be divided into two broad categories:

Failure of symptom progression
In general, patients with common mimic syndromes do not progress as rapidly as those with ALS, and tend to survive for longer periods.
Atypical history or symptoms
Common clinical features that lead to a reconsideration of the diagnosis of ALS include the

Table 8.7 Differential diagnosis of MND

Hereditary	Kennedy's disease
	Hereditary spastic paraparesis
	Acid maltase deficiency
	Facioscapulohumeral muscular dystrophy
	Adrenomyeloneuropathy
	Huntington's disease
	Hexosaminidase deficiency
Metabolic/toxic	Hyperthyroidism
	Hyperparathyroidism
	Heavy metal intoxication
	Lathyrism
	Organophosphate toxicity
Immune/ inflammatory	Multifocal motor neuropathy with conduction block
	Chronic inflammatory demyelinating Polyneuropathy
	Myasthenia gravis
	Inclusion body myositis
	Polymyositis
	Multiple sclerosis
	Paraneoplastic disorders
Structural	Cervical spondylotic myelopathy
	Syringomyelia/bulbia
	Post-irradiation myelopathy/ plexopathy
	Tumor
	Cerebrovascular disease
Other neurodegenerative diseases	Corticobasal degeneration
	Multiple system atrophy
	Progressive supranuclear palsy
	Parkinson's disease
	Huntington's disease
Other motor neuron diseases	Primary lateral sclerosis
	Progressive muscular atrophy
	Spinal muscular atrophy
	Post polio spinal muscle atrophy
	Benign fasciculation syndrome
	Hirayama disease

Table 8.8 Clinical features that should prompt a search for mimic syndromes

History of poliomyelitis
Family history with no affected females and no male to male transmission
Symmetrical signs
Pure upper or pure lower motor neuron syndrome
Upper motor signs caudal to lower motor neuron signs, with no bulbar involvement
Development of sensory signs
Development of sphincter disturbances

presence of isolated upper or isolated lower motor neuron signs (leading to possible diagnoses of hereditary spastic paraparesis, multiple sclerosis and motor neuropathy respectively); the development of sensory complaints or bladder involvement (leading to diagnoses of myelopathy or demyelinating disease); the absence of upper motor neuron signs rostral to lower motor neuron signs; or the absence of bulbar signs in patients with prominent spinal signs (leading to a diagnosis of cervical myelopathy); and a family history of males only affected, and no male to male transmission (suggesting X-linked bulbospinal muscle atrophy (Kennedy's disease) . The presence of asymmetric weakness and wasting in a C8 T1 distribution in a young man should raise the possibility of Hirayama disease (Table 8.8).

8.8 Diagnostic Tests

There is no definitive diagnostic test for ALS. The combination of suggestive clinical signs with negative laboratory and imaging studies supports the diagnosis. Progression of the condition is a prerequisite for diagnosis (Fig. 8.1).

8.9 Essential Investigations

Routine laboratory investigation of a patient with apparently "typical" ALS should include ESR, serum and urine protein electrophoresis, thyroid function tests and serum calcium and phosphate (Table 8.9).

CSF analysis may be considered. CSF protein levels above 80 mg% are unusual and should prompt a search for other pathology, particularly for the presence of an associated lymphoproliferative disease. Heavy metal screen should be performed in those with a potential history of

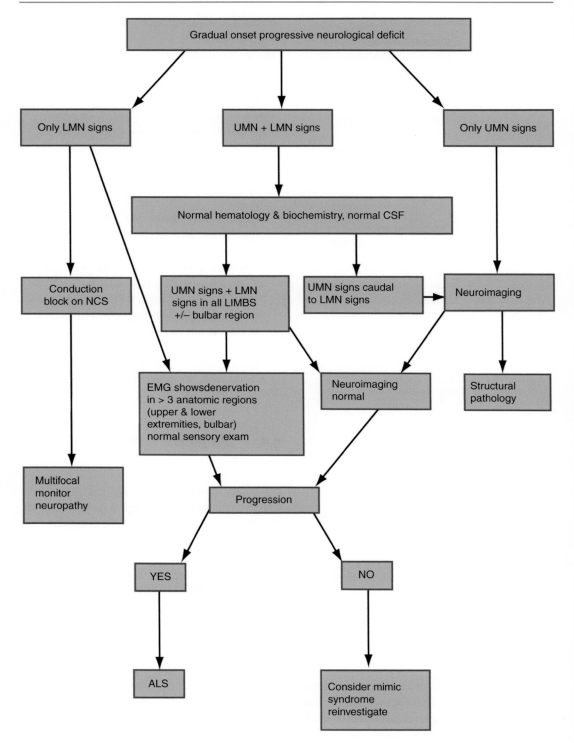

Fig. 8.1 Diagnostic algorithm for ALS. *UMN* upper motor neuron, *LMN* lower motor neuron, *NCS* nerve conduction studies

Table 8.9 Essential investigations

Blood erythrocyte sedimentation rate (ESR)
C-reactive protein (CRP)
Hematological screen
ASAT, ALAT, LDH
TSH, FT4, FT3 hormone assays
Vitamins B12 and folate
Serum protein electrophoresis
Serum immunoelectrophoresis
Creatine kinase (CK)
Creatinine
Electrolytes ((Na$^+$, K$^+$, Cl), (Ca2$^+$, Phosphate))
Glucose
Hexoaminidase A and B assay (where clinically indicated)
Ganglioside GM-1 antibodies (where clinically indicated)
Serology (Borrelia, virus including HIV) (where clinically indicated)
CSF cell count, protein, glucose
Neurophysiology: EMG, nerve conduction velocity
Radiology MRI/CAT (head/cervical, thoracic, lumbar)
Chest x-ray

exposure. Hexosaminidase A and B activity should be tested in patients of Ashkenazi Jewish extraction.

Neurophysiologic studies can assist in the diagnosis by demonstrating ongoing denervation (fibrillation potentials and positive sharp waves) and re-innervation (large-amplitude, long duration, polyphasic units) in affected and clinically unaffected limbs, with normal sensation, and normal or near-normal motor nerve conduction velocities. For corroboration of diagnosis, the distribution of denervation-associated changes on EMG should be outside the anatomic territories of peripheral nerves and roots. At least two proximal and two distal muscles in each of the four limbs should be sampled by EMG. These EMG changes may be evident sub-clinically, thereby enabling an earlier diagnosis of ALS. Widespread fasciculations, especially when evident in bulbar muscles, are specific for ALS, as are findings of a higher fasciculation firing rate and increased frequency of double fasciculations. With disease progression, fasciculations may develop a complex morphology reflecting remodeling of the underlying motor unit. At a molecular level,

upregulation of persistent sodium conductances combined with reduced potassium currents, appear to underlie the development of fasciculations in ALS.

The presence of conduction block should suggest an alternative diagnosis, such as multifocal motor neuropathy, while prolonged F-wave responses may suggest an inflammatory, demyelinating process. Sensory nerve action potentials (SNAPs) are preserved in ALS. Abnormalities in SNAPs should prompt a search for an alternate diagnosis. In males, the possibility of Kennedy's disease should be considered.

Electrophysiological results should be evaluated in conjunction with the clinical and other ancillary findings. A recent algorithm to enhance the electrophyiologic criteria for ALS diagnosis (The Awaji Algorithm) has been published by de Carvehlo et al. (See Suggested Reading at the end of this chapter). Less conventional neurophysiological techniques for establishing LMN dysfunction in ALS include motor unit number estimation, electrode impedance myography, axonal excitability and neurophysiological index, although these are not routinely applicable.

At present, there are no validated, reliable and accessible neurophysiologic investigations to establish the presence of upper motor neuron dysfunction, although a number of recent studies using transcortical magnetic stimulation have suggested increase cortical excitability in ALS.

Neuroimaging studies should be used to exclude other conditions that may cause UMN and/or LMN signs.

Advances in neuroimaging technology are likely to provide further anatomic definition of ALS . Although not currently suitable in primary diagnosis of ALS, detailed neuroimaging using modern scanners has potential as a research tool to further characterize the neuroanatomic substrates of ALS.

8.10 Biomarkers in ALS

There is a growing interest in identifying biomarkers for diagnosis, progression and prognosis in ALS. To date, no biomarker has been of sufficient sensitivity and specificity to incorporate into clinical practice. Although protein profiling in CSF

Table 8.10a A staging systems

Milan-torino staging system				
MITOS domain	ALSFRS-R item	ALSFRS-R score		MITOS score
Breathing	10 Dyspnoea	4 none 3 occurs when walking 2 occurs with one or more of: eating, bathing, dressing	*Or*	0
		1 occurs at rest, difficulty breathing when either sitting or lying 0 loss of useful speech		1
	12 Respiratory insufficiency	4 none 3 intermittent use of NIPPV		0
		2 continuous use of NIPPV during the night 1 continuous use of NIPPV during the night and day 0 invasive mechanical ventilation by intubation or tracheostomy		1

MITOS score		
ALS-MITOS	Stage	Functional domains lost
	0	None
	1	One domain
	2	Two domains
	3	Three domains
	4	Four domains
	5	Death

[a]The MITOS score 1 for *Breathing* should be recorded if either Dyspnoea or Respiratory Insufficiency are scored 1

has yielded findings that are of interest, standardized handling of spinal fluid will be required to ensure reproducibility of results. Neuroimaging and quantitative neurophysiological techniques such as motor unit number estimation (MUNE) and motor unit index (MUNIX) are considered to have potential. Disease signatures may also be possible using transcriptomics and metabolomics. However, it is likely that further sub-categorization based on clinical phenotype will be necessary to generate reproducible biomarkers.

8.11 Staging

Two staging systems have been developed for ALS (Tables 8.10a and 8.10b) At present, neither system incorporates the presence or absence of cognitive impairment.

The Kings system was developed as a universal and objective measure of disease stage based on easy to identify clinical milestones which reflect disease course and progression. This system represents the course of the illness across four stages: Stage 1, functional involvement of one central nervous system region (bulbar, upper limb, lower limb); Stage 2, functional involvement of two regions; 3, functional involvement of three regions; and 4, respiratory or swallowing involvement requiring intervention. It has been shown that stages occur at distinct times (0, 40, 60 and 80 %) through the disease course. A separate system (ALS-Milano-Torino) is based on loss of independence in four key domains on the ALS Functional Rating Scale (ALSFRS): swallowing, walking/self-care, communicating and breathing.

Table 8.10b King's college ALS staging (May 2014)

This procedure takes the form of a semi-structured interview. It is hierarchical and is not therefore a functional scale. In all cases, if involvement of a region is obvious to an untrained observer it should be counted as involved. Only findings related to ALS should be scored

KCL stage definition	Details
Stage 4 has been reached if advanced disease requiring intervention (If gastrostomy or NIV are recommended but the intervention is *refused* by the patient, Stage 4 has still been reached)	1. Weight loss more than 10 % of baseline 2. SNIP <40 cm H_2O or a decrease >10 cm H_2O over 3 months 3. Patient responded *Yes* to any of the questions regarding breathing involvement <u>AND</u> SNIP is <65 cm H_2O (for men) or <55 cm H_2O (for women) 4. FVC: <50 % of predicted FVC 5. Patient has responding *Yes* to any of the questions regarding breathing involvement <u>AND</u> FVC <80 % of predicted FVC 6. SpO$_2$ on oximetry is ≤94 % AND either pCO$_2$ >6 kPa <u>OR</u> Overnight oximetry shows ≥5 dips/h below 80 %
To assess earlier stages the bulbar, upper limb, and lower limb regions are considered and the number of regions involved defines the stage: | Involvement	Stage
One region involved	1
Two regions involved	2
Three regions involved	3		*Symptoms/signs signifying involvement by region are a follows*: **Bulbar**: *Symptoms*: slurred speech, dysphonia, problems swallowing liquids, choking. and/or *Signs*: tongue atrophy, fasciculation, slowness of movement or a pathologically brisk jaw jerk reflex is acceptable as an alternative if no symptoms are reported **Upper limbs**: Symptoms e.g. trouble with keys, doors, buttons, zips or carrying bags, reported by the patient Signs: wasting of the first dorsal interosseus, pectoral reflexes or Hoffman's sign is acceptable as an alternative if no symptoms are reported. (A clinician may examine any reflexes and draw their own conclusion) **Lower limbs**: *Symptoms*: stiffness, spasm or cramping, falls, or the foot catching on walking *Signs*: gait stiffness or foot drop, crossed adductor reflexes, pathologically brisk patellar reflexes or ankle clonus is acceptable as an alternative if no symptoms are reported. (A clinician may examine any reflexes and draw their own conclusion). Extensor plantar responses are *not* acceptable as suggesting of involvement

Notes

Any deep tendon reflexes may be examined at the time of interview if the interviewer is clinically trained, or they can be taken from the most recent clinical examination. If an appropriate recent clinical examination is not available, the following abnormal signs can be tested by a suitably trained non-clinical examiner: a pathologically brisk jaw jerk, pectoral reflexes, Hoffman's sign, crossed adductor reflexes, pathologically brisk patellar reflexes or ankle clonus

The following examples of clinical findings which do <u>not</u> meet staging criteria for involvement:

1. Extensor plantar reflexes with no other lower limb involvement do not satisfy criteria for involvement of the lower limbs

2. Dysphagia not secondary to ALS or without weight loss greater than the 10 % threshold and respiratory symptoms not fulfilling NICE respiratory failure guidelines do not meet Stage 4 criteria

3. Fasciculation without wasting, weakness or reflex changes does not constitute involvement of a limb. It is acceptable as indicating involvement in the tongue

8.12   Management of Progression of ALS

Evidence based guidelines for clinical management have been published by the European Federation of Neurological Sciences and by the American Academy of Neurology. (See Suggested Reading at the end of this chapter.) Both sets of guidelines emphasize the importance of multidisciplinary care, which provides the cornerstone of ALS management. The multidisciplinary team should include a neurologist, a respiratory physician, a palliative care physician and allied professions including physiotherapy, occupational therapy, speech and language therapy, nutrition medical social services and genetic counselling (Table 8.11). Those who received care at a multidisciplinary clinic have a better prognosis than those attending a general neurology clinic, and because symptoms are addressed and treated early, management in a specialized setting is also more cost effective.

Despite a large number of clinical trials of various agents, the anti-glutamate agent Riluzole remains the one evidence based disease modifying drug for ALS. Patients with ALS should be offered Riluzole at the time of diagnosis, as clinical trials have repeatedly demonstrated that early treatment with Riluzole can increase survival by a mean of approximately 3 months.

8.12.1   Symptomatic Therapies

The aim of symptomatic therapy is to improve the quality of life of the patient and carer. The commonest symptoms and their management are outlined below.

8.12.1.1   Cramping and Spasticity

Cramping can be treated with massage and physiotherapy. Quinine sulphate (200 mg) is also effective, as are phenytoin, carbamazepine and benzodiazepines.

Spasticity can be treated with physiotherapy and hydrotherapy. Baclofen and tizanidine are effective pharmacologic agents.

Table 8.11   Multidisciplinary team for ALS management

Neurologist	Diagnosis, disclosure of diagnosis, treatment and symptom management, initiation of respiratory and nutritional interventions, unbiased information regarding research developments
Family doctor	Symptom control, drug monitoring, liaison with other teams
MND specialist nurse	Point of contact for patients and families, coordination of care, home visits, practical advice re accessing support services, patient advocacy
Speech & language therapist	Evaluation and monitoring of dysphagia and aspiration, speech therapy and advice re communication devices
Occupational therapist	Optimisation of the patient's environment. Advice re safety awareness, adaptive and splinting devices, activity modification, driving, energy conservation, home modification
Dietitian/nutritionist	Evaluation of nutritional status and the need for tube feeding, management of dysphagia, management of enteral feeding
Physiotherapist	Evaluation of muscle strength and function, advice re walking aids and orthoses, management of spasticity, safety awareness
Social worker	Advice and counselling re employment, change in lifestyle and financial issues, support for carers
Palliative care	Symptom control, pain management, maintenance of quality of life, preservation of dignity
Psychiatry and neuropsychology	Evaluation and management of cognitive impairment/dementia, adjustment disorders, anxiety and depression
Respiratory physician	Assessment of respiratory dysfunction, initiation of non-invasive ventilation, monitoring of non-invasive ventilation
Genetic counsellor	Advice regarding symptomatic testing and support for families. Discussion & counselling regarding pre-symptomatic testing

8.12.1.2 Sialorrhoea and Bronchial Secretions

Sialorrhoea (drooling or excessive salivation) is distressing to patients, and increases the risk of oral infections. It is associated with dysphagia, and a failure to effectively handle salivary secretions.

Sialorrhoea can be difficult to manage, although patients and carers can be trained to use a portable suction machine. Treatments include amitriptyline (25–50 mg), oral or transdermal hyoscine, atropine drops or glycopyrrolate. For more severe sialorrhoea, botulinum toxin can be effective, as can salivary gland irradiation.

Bronchial secretions can be treated with mucolytics and nebulized beta adrenergic antagonists and/or anticholinergics. Use of techniques such as breath stacking and mechanical cough-assisting devices (insufflator-exsufflator) are beneficial and should be introduced in the clinic.

8.12.1.3 Pseudobulbar Affect

Pathological weeping or laughing occurs in up to 50 % of patients. A combination of dextrometorphan and quinidine may be beneficial, although treatment may be limited by side effects. Fluvoxamine, amitriptyline and citalopram can also be of benefit.

8.12.1.4 Anxiety and Depression

Counseling for patients and carers is useful in managing the reactive depression associated with recent diagnosis. For more protracted depression, SSRIs can be helpful. Anxiety can be treated with benzodiazepines or buprorion.

8.12.1.5 Pain

Pain is not uncommon in ALS. Treatment should begin with simple analgesics such as paracetamol, followed by weak opioids such as tramadol, followed by strong opioids such as morphine or ketobemidon.

8.12.1.6 Communication

Dysarthria progressing to mutism occurs in bulbar ALS. As dysarthria develops, patients should be reviewed by an experienced speech and language therapist. The goal should be to optimize the communication both for the patient and the carer. Prosthetic treatments (palatal lift and/or palatal augmentation prosthesis) can be helpful to improve articulation. Augmentive and alternative communication (AAC) devices can be used in those with intact cognition. Useful technological advances include brain-computer-interfaces and thought translation devices, though these are not yet widely available.

8.12.1.7 Respiratory Insufficiency

The majority of ALS patients die of respiratory failure, and the presence of respiratory muscle weakness is an independent predictor of quality of life. Symptoms of respiratory insufficiency may be subtle. Patients should be asked directly about dyspnea, orthopnea, disturbed sleep (sleep fragmentation due to hypoventilation), nightmares, morning headaches, daytime somnolence and fatigue, poor concentration/memory and nocturia. Assessment of respiratory insufficiency includes history and examination, pulmonary function tests, and overnight pulse oximetry and early morning arterial blood gases.

Forced vital capacity is most widely used in the assessment to respiratory insufficiency in ALS but limitations include insensitivity to significant changes in respiratory function partly because of the shape of the lung pressure-volume curve, and difficulties in performing the test due to muscle weakness or apraxia. Sniff nasal inspiratory nasal pressure (SNIP) is an additional measure of declining respiratory function, although its use is also limited by apraxia. SNIP is particularly useful in patients with bulbar involvement since a face mask is not required. The SNIP correlates well with diaphragm strength and nocturnal hypoxemia and is sensitive to changes in respiratory muscle strength. A SNIP of <40 cm H_2O had a higher sensitivity for predicting 6-month mortality compared with a FVC of <50 %.

Transcutaneous carbon dioxide/oxygen sensor can be useful during home visits as it avoids the need for regular arterial blood gases. While not used as a primary tool in the assessment of the need for non-invasive ventilation, it can be a useful adjunct (Table 8.12).

Table 8.12 Indications for initiation of non-invasive ventilation

European consensus criteria for NIV (European ALS/MND Consortium and European Neuromuscular Centre workshop on non-invasive ventilation in MND, May 2002)	
Suggested criteria for non-invasive ventilation	
Symptoms related to respiratory muscle weakness. At least one of	Dyspnoea, orthopnoea, disturbed sleep (not caused by pain), morning headache, poor concentration, anorexia, excessive daytime sleepiness (ESS >9)
And	
	FVC $\leq$80 % or SNIP $\leq$40 cm H_2O
Evidence of muscle weakness	
And	
Evidence of either	Significant nocturnal desaturation on overnight oximetry OR Morning ear lobe gas pCO_2 $\geq$6.5 kPa

Non-invasive positive pressure ventilation (NIPPV) should be introduced early. Current recommendations are that NIPPV should be offered to any patient with respiratory symptoms and vital capacity less than 50 % of predicted, a SNIP of less than 40 cm H_2O, or where symptoms of respiratory insufficiency are associated with nocturnal hypoxemia. An elevated early morning blood CO_2 level is an absolute indication. Oxygen therapy is not recommended in the absence of NIPPV as there is a risk of reduction of the hypoxic drive, leading to hypercapnia. NIPPV extends survival, particularly in those who are compliant with 5 h of NIPPV each day and those without severe bulbar dysfunction. Treatment with NIPPV also improve quality of life (QOL) in patients without increasing caregiver burden or stress. Some patients have difficulty tolerating NIPPV. Factors that adversely affect the ability of patients to tolerate NIPPV including the presence of bulbar symptoms, the ability to manually adjust the mask and the presence of cognitive impairment. Pulse oximetry should be performed following commencement on NIPPV, and patients should be

reviewed at regular intervals by a respiratory physician to ensure that the pressure settings are optimized.

8.12.1.8 Weight Loss and Nutritional Support

Weight loss and malnutrition are common features of ALS. Nutritional decline can occur in the context of evolving dysphagia. In those without significant bulbar features, weight loss can result from difficulties in finishing meals because of upper extremity weakness. Weight loss may also be due to hypermetabolism, particularly in those with respiratory compromise. Dysphagia increases the risk for insufficient calorie intake, aspiration and choking. Dysphagia can be evaluated using bedside clinical scales and with videofluoroscopy and fibreoptic examination. Management includes modification of food and fluid consistency, postural advice (e.g. chin tuck: flexing the neck forward on swallowing to protect the airway), and parenteral feeding by gastrostomy.

Gastrostomy placement is indicated for those who have symptomatic dysphagia or significant weight loss. Advantages include improved nutrition, although the survival effect is likely to be marginal. Radiologically inserted gastrostomy (RIG) is preferred over endoscopic gastrostomy in patients with pronounced bulbar symptoms and/or respiratory compromise. If there is evidence of respiratory insufficiency, non-invasive ventilation should be introduced before gastrostomy (Fig. 8.2).

8.12.1.9 Management of Cognitive Impairment in ALS

Recognition of cognitive and behavioural impairment, and of deficits in social cognition is important for prognostic reasons, and in management of carer burden. Increased behavioural impairment and reduced social cognition can lead to significant increases in carer burden, and recognition that these features are symptoms of the disease can assist in the development of coping strategies for carers. Most studies of pharmacological treatment of FTD are relatively small and uncontrolled., and the

Fig. 8.2 Algorithm for
management of nutritional
decline in ALS (*FVC* forced
vital capacity, *SNIP* sniff
nasal inspiratory pressure,
PEG percutaneous
endoscopic gastrostomy, *RIG*
radiologically inserted
gastrostomy)

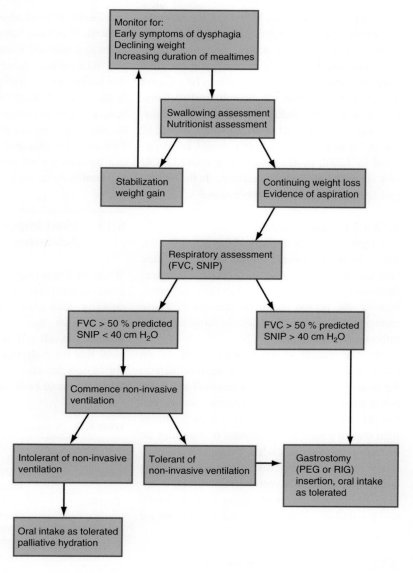

management of cognitive decline in ALS is accordingly difficult. Off-label use of medications more commonly include donepezil, rivastigmne galantamine and memantine. SSRIs are commonly used for aggression, agitation, disinhibition and depression in FTD. Treatment with SSRI is well tolerated, and they are currently the drugs of choice for behavioral control in FTD. Nocturnal agitation can be treated with low dose olanzapine, rispiridone or quetiapine. Co-management with neuro-psychiatry is recommended.

8.12.1.10 Quality of Life

Quality of life (QOL) is determined by the pleasure and satisfaction an individual draws from living. Health related QOL is determined by the impact of an individual's health on their experience of living. In ALS, health related QOL declines commensurately with physical decline, and high levels of psychological distress can occur. However, self-assessed QOL, as measured by scales in which the individual selects what is most important to them (e.g. the Schedule for Evaluation of Individual Quality of Life (SEIQoL)), does not generally decline in ALS. Moreover, the majority of patients with ALS do not exhibit high scores on depression and anxiety scales. This is because most individuals perform a psychological shift towards domains that can continue to be enjoyed despite the evolution of neurological deficits. Recognition of the ability of patients to undertake this psychological shift is an important aspect of caring for those with ALS and should be recognized by health professionals, as perceived QOL may impact on decision-making, both by the patient and the health care professional.

8.12.1.11 Carer Burden

A diagnosis of ALS impacts of the entire family. The role of the patient within the family may change—the breadwinner may become a dependent and the primary carer within the family may become the person requiring most care. These changes can have a major destabilizing effect on intimate relationships.

As the condition progresses, there is an increasing and often unacknowledged burden on the primary carer, both from a physical and emotional perspective. Many studies have shown that the self-reported QOL of carers may be lower than that of patients. The burden of care may be increased considerably when the patient is cognitively impaired. Supportive strategies including counseling for family members should be available. In the later stages of illness, regular respite and psychological support should be available for the primary carer.

8.12.1.12 Palliative Care and End of Life Decisions

ALS is an inexorably progressive condition that significantly reduces life expectancy. A palliative care approach should be taken from the time of diagnosis. The aim of palliative care is to maximize QOL of patients and families by relieving symptoms, providing emotional, psychological and spiritual support as needed, removing obstacles to a peaceful death, and supporting the family in bereavement. From the time of diagnosis, patients should be provided with a realistic projection of the trajectory of their disease. As the condition progresses, they should be encouraged to consider an advance directive regarding their end of life.

Candid discussions about the relative merits and demerits of full mechanical ventilation should take place in a planned manner, and in a comfortable and quiet setting. Assurances should be provided that palliative care strategies can control symptoms in the terminal phase of the illness. Opioids and benzodiazepines (where necessary for anxiety) can be used for symptomatic treatment of dyspnoea. Pain should be managed with opioids. Neuroleptics can be used for tor treating terminal restlessness and confusion due to hypercapnia.

8.13 Most Important Recent Advances

While ALS was originally considered to a homogeneous and pure motor system degeneration, ongoing deep phenotyping and genetic studies suggest that the condition is heterogenous. Research in cell and molecular biology also suggests that the pathophysiology of ALS and FTD are closely intertwined. A number of genes are known to cause both ALS and FTD (Table 8.13).

Table 8.13 Genes causing ALS and FTD

Chromosome 17q 21–22; MAPT gene	Disinhibiton-dementia-Parkinson-amyotrophy complex (DDPAC). Semantic language abnormalities
C9orf72	Motor symptoms followed by personality and behavioural abnormalities between fourth and seventh decades
Chromosome 9q21–q22	Five with ALS & mild cognitive impairment, nine pure FTD, ALS and/or ALS/FT
9p13.3–12, valosin-containing protein	Autosomal dominant inclusion body myopathy, Paget's disease of bone, FTD
3p12, CHMP2B	FTD and later motor syndrome (not typical ALS)
Point mutation (R1101K) in the DCTN1 gene	FTD and ALS segregate as separate traits
TDP-43	ALS-FTD
FUS	ALS-FTD
SOD1	ALS-FTD (rarely)
ANG	ALS-FTD (rarely)
Progranulin	Mostly FTD, polymorphisms associated with phenotype in ALS

Advances in neuroimaging and neuropathology have demonstrated involvement of regions of the brain outside the motor system in ALS. Detailed neuropsychological assessment of ALS patients has also identified corresponding changes in up to 50 % of patients, with evidence of fronto-temporal dementia in up to 15 %. These advances have radically changed the perspective of clinicians and researchers, and has opened new and exciting frontiers in research.

Although effective disease modifying drugs for ALS remain elusive, much progress has been made in understanding and managing the disease. From a clinical perspective, sub categorization based on phenotype and genetics will assist in appropriate stratification for future clinical trials. From a laboratory perspective, there has been a veritable explosion of new genes that are implicated in ALS and ALS/FTD. This has led to the important observation that disruptions in RNA processing may contribute to disease pathogenesis. SOD1 mouse models have identified the pivotal importance of glial tissue in the pathogenesis and progression of the disease. However, the limitations of the murine SOD1 model of ALS have also become apparent. Moreover, the identification of new genes has provided a timely opportunity to generate new animal models.

Although clinical trials have been disappointing, there have significant developments in clinical trial design and an improved recognition of the pitfalls in attempting to translate positive findings from laboratory animals into humans. It is now acknowledged that the failure of some of the more promising compounds in Phase II and III trials may have reflected a relative the paucity of pre-clinical data regarding the biological activity of the therapy. This has been coupled in some instances with a failure to identify the appropriate dose range for testing.

Notwithstanding the disappointing outcome of recent trials, clinical management has significantly improved in the recent past. There is now robust evidence to indicate that survival is enhanced by attendance at a multidisciplinary clinic. Close attention to respiratory status has led to improved secretion management and increasing use of non-invasive ventilation, with attending survival benefits of up to 9 months.

The pace of research in ALS has increased considerably in the past decade; the coming decade is likely to yield exciting results both in clinical management and in helping to understand underlying disease pathophysiology.

8.14 Most Important Developments in the Coming Years

ALS research is poised on the brink of some major and exciting advances both in clinical and basic science research. ALS researchers throughout the world are coalescing to form a variety of consortia that will pool and maximize both resources and expertise. The close biological relationship between ALS and FTD will continue to provide insights into disease pathogenesis. The recent recognition of the likely importance of RNA regulation in both diseases will have wide ranging implications in research in molecular and cell biology.

Cell-replacement therapies have become an active area of research in ALS. A major challenge relates to the diffuse nature of the disease and the important role non-neuronal cells exert in the pathological process. Neuronal stem cells, located within the adult CNS, may be genetically programmed to develop into neurons or glial cells. Efficacy of spinal mesenchymal stem cell transplantation has also been reported in the SOD-1 mouse model, with the transplanted mesenchymal stem cells evolving into astrocytes. Two recent Phase I studies have established the safety mesenchymal stem cell transplantation approaches in humans. In addition to cell-based approaches, strategies aimed at modulating gene expression are emerging as potential novel therapeutic options, particularly in light of significant advances in the understanding of the genetic causes of ALS. One such approach involves the use of an antisense oligonucleotides which, when delivered intrathecally, reduces mRNA and SOD-1 protein concentrations in brain and spinal cord in the SOD-1 transgenic mouse and prolongs survival. Strategies aimed at enhancing axonal growth, through inhibition of factors such as Nogo, may also prove therapeutically useful in

ALS. Nogo belongs to a family of proteins called Reticulon-4, which function to inhibit the outgrowth of neurites in the CNS. Three isoforms, Nogo-A, Nogo-B and Nogo-C, have been identified, with major Nogo-A isoform predominating. In ALS studies, anti-Nogo-A antibodies enhanced axonal regeneration and improved functional recovery in animal models of acute CNS injury. A randomized controlled Phase I study of the anti-Nogo-A agent ozanezumab demonstrated good safety and tolerability with a trend to efficacy, with a larger international trial currently underway.

Translation of potential therapeutic agents from animal to human models of disease will benefit from the lessons learned over the past decade. New clinical trials in ALS will be underpinned by a detailed knowledge of drug activity, bioavailability and efficacy in both the pre-clinical and clinical setting, coupled with robust proof of biological activity in the target tissue.

The new fields of transcriptomics and metabolomics are likely to be harnessed in the quest for biomarkers. Advances in high resolution neuroimaging is also likely to be helpful in tracking disease progression, as will advances in neurophysiology and neurophysics. And finally, brain computer interfaces will help to provide improved aids by using EEG signals recorded from the scalp to enable patients to both to communicate, and to interact with their environment using modern robotics.

Suggested Reading

Abrahams S, Newton J, Niven E, Foley J, Bak TH. Screening for cognition and behaviour changes in ALS. Amyotroph Lateral Scler Frontotemporal Degener. 2014;15(1–2):9–14. doi:10.3109/21678421. 2013.805784. Epub 2013 Jun 19. PubMed.

Agosta F, Al-Chalabi A, Filippi M, Hardiman O, Kaji R, Meininger V, Nakano I, Shaw P, Shefner J, van den Berg LH, Ludolph A, The WFN Research Group on ALS/MND. The El escorial criteria: strengths and weaknesses. Amyotroph Lateral Scler Frontotemporal Degener. 2014;16:1–7.

Al-Chalabi A, Calvo A, Chio A, Colville S, Ellis CM, Hardiman O, Heverin M, Howard RS, Huisman MH, Keren N, Leigh PN, Mazzini L, Mora G, Orrell RW, Rooney J, Scott KM, Scotton WJ, Seelen M, Shaw CE, Sidle KS, Swingler R, Tsuda M, Veldink JH,

Visser AE, van den Berg LH, Pearce N. Analysis of amyotrophic lateral sclerosis as a multistep process: a population-based modelling study. Lancet Neurol. 2014;13(11):1108–13. PMC4197338.

Al-Chalabi A, Hardiman O. The epidemiology of ALS: a conspiracy of genes, environment and time. Nat Rev Neurol. 2013;9(11):617–28. doi:10.1038/nrneurol.2013.203. Epub 2013 Oct 15. Review. PubMed.

Andersen PM, Abrahams S, Borasio GD, de Carvalho M, Chio A, Van Damme P, Hardiman O, Kollewe K, Morrison KE, Petri S, Pradat PF, Silani V, Tomik B, Wasner M, Weber M. EFNS Task Force on Diagnosis and Management of Amyotrophic Lateral Sclerosis EFNS guidelines on the clinical management of amyotrophic lateral sclerosis(MALS)--revised report of an EFNS task force. Eur J Neurol. 2012;19(3): 360–75.

Beghi E, Balzarini C, Bogliun G, Logroscino G, Manfredi L, Mazzini L, Micheli A, Millul A, Poloni M, Riva R, Salmoiraghi F, Tonini C, Vitelli E, Italian ALS Study Group. Reliability of the El Escorial diagnostic criteria for amyotrophic lateral sclerosis. Neuroepidemiology. 2002;21(6):265–70.

Beghi E, Millul A, Logroscino G, Vitelli E, Micheli A, SLALOM GROUP. Outcome measures and prognostic indicators in patients with amyotrophic lateral sclerosis. Amyotroph Lateral Scler. 2008;9(3):163–7.

Brooks BR, World Federation of Neurology Sub-Committee on Motor Neuron Diseases. El Escorial WFN criteria for the diagnosis of amyotrophic lateral sclerosis. J Neurol Sci. 1994;124 Suppl 1:96–107.

Brooks BR, Miller RG, Swash M, Munsat TL, The World Federation of Neurology Research Committee on Motor Neuron Diseases. El Escorial revisited: revised criteria for the diagnosis of amyotrophic lateral sclerosis. Amyotroph Lateral Scler. 2000;1:293–300.

Byrne S, Heverin M, Elamin M, Bede P, Lynch C, Kenna K, MacLaughlin R, Walsh C, Al Chalabi A, Hardiman O. Aggregation of neurologic and neuropsychiatric disease in amyotrophic lateral sclerosis kindreds: a population-based case–control cohort study of familial and sporadic amyotrophic lateral sclerosis. Ann Neurol. 2013;74(5):699–708. doi:10.1002/ana.23969. Epub 2013 Sep 10.

Byrne S, Elamin M, Bede P, Shatunov A, Walsh C, Corr B, Heverin M, Jordan N, Kenna K, Lynch C, McLaughlin RL, Iyer PM, O'Brien C, Phukan J, Wynne B, Bokde AL, Bradley DG, Pender N, Al-Chalabi A, Hardiman O. Cognitive and clinical characteristics of patients with amyotrophic lateral sclerosis carrying a C9orf72repeat expansion: a population-based cohort study. Lancet Neurol. 2012;11(3):232–40. doi:10.1016/S1474-4422(12)70014-5.

Chiò A, Hammond ER, Mora G, Bonito V, Filippini G. Development and evaluation of a clinical staging system for amyotrophic lateral sclerosis. J Neurol Neurosurg Psychiatry. 2015;86(1):38–44. doi:10.1136/jnnp-2013-306589. Epub 2013 Dec 13. PubMed.

Cronin S, Hardiman O, Traynor BJ. Ethnic variation in the incidence of ALS: a systematic review. Neurology. 2007;68(13):1002–7.

De Carvalho M, Dengler R, Eisen A, England JD, Kaji R, Kimura J, et al. Electrodiagnostic criteria for the diagnosis of ALS. Clin Neurophys. 2008;119:497–503.

DeJesus-Hernandez M, Mackenzie IR, Boeve BF, Boxer AL, Baker M, Rutherford NJ, Nicholson AM, Finch NA, Flynn H, Adamson J, Kouri N, Wojtas A, Sengdy P, Hsiung GY, Karydas A, Seeley WW, Josephs KA, Coppola G, Geschwind DH, Wszolek ZK, Feldman H, Knopman DS, Petersen RC, Miller BL, Dickson DW, Boylan KB, Graff-Radford NR, Rademakers R. Expanded GGGGCC hexanucleotide repeat innoncoding region of C9ORF72causes chromosome 9p-linked FTD and ALS. Neuron. 2011;72(2):245–56.

Elamin M, Bede P, Byrne S, Jordan N, Gallagher L, Wynne B, O'Brien C, Phukan J, Lynch C, Pender N, Hardiman O. Cognitive changes predict functional decline inALS: a population-based longitudinal study. Neurology. 2013;80(17):1590–7. doi:10.1212/WNL.0b013e31828f18ac. Epub 2013 Apr 3. PubMed.

Hardiman O, van den Berg LH, Kiernan MC. Clinical diagnosis and management of amyotrophic lateral sclerosis. Nat Rev Neurol. 2011;7(11):639–49. doi:10.1038/nrneurol.2011.153.

Logroscino G, Traynor BJ, Hardiman O, Chio A, Couratier P, Mitchell JD, Swingler RJ, Beghi E, EURALS. Descriptive epidemiology of amyotrophic lateral sclerosis: new evidence and unsolved issues. J Neurol Neurosurg Psychiatry. 2008;79(1):6–11.

Miller RG, Jackson CE, Kasarskis EJ, England JD, Forshew D, Johnston W, Kalra S, Katz JS, Mitsumoto H, Rosenfeld J, Shoesmith C, Strong MJ, Woolley SC, Quality Standards Subcommittee of the American Academy of Neurology. Practice parameter update: the care of the patient with amyotrophic lateral sclerosis: multidisciplinary care, symptom management, and cognitive/behavioral impairment (an evidence-based review): report of the Quality Standards Subcommittee of the American Academy of Neurology. Neurology. 2009a;73(15):1227–33.

Miller RG, Jackson CE, Kasarskis EJ, England JD, Forshew D, Johnston W, Kalra S, Katz JS, Mitsumoto H, Rosenfeld J, Shoesmith C, Strong MJ, Woolley SC, Quality Standards Subcommittee of the American Academy of Neurology. Practice parameter update: the care of the patient with amyotrophic lateral sclerosis: drug, nutritional, and respiratory therapies (an evidence-based review): report of the Quality Standards Subcommittee of the American Academy of Neurology. Neurology. 2009b;73(15):1218–26. Review. Erratum in: neurology. 2009;73(24):2134.

Shatunov A, Mok K, Newhouse S, Weale ME, Smith B, Vance C, Johnson L, Veldink JH, van Es MA, van den Berg LH, Robberecht W, Van Damme P, Hardiman O, Farmer AE, Lewis CM, Butler AW, Abel O, Andersen PM, Fogh I, Silani V, Chiò A, Traynor BJ, Melki J, Meininger V, Landers JE, McGuffin P, Glass JD, Pall H, Leigh PN, Hardy J, Brown Jr RH, Powell JF, Orrell RW, Morrison KE, Shaw PJ, Shaw CE, Al-Chalabi A. Chromosome 9p21 in sporadic amyotrophic lateral sclerosis in the UK and seven other countries: a genome-wide association study. Lancet Neurol. 2010;9(10):986–94. doi:10.1016/S1474-4422(10)70197-6.

Turner MR, Hardiman O, Benatar M, Brooks BR, Chio A, de Carvalho M, Ince PG, Lin C, Miller RG, Mitsumoto H, Nicholson G, Ravits J, Shaw PJ, Swash M, Talbot K, Traynor BJ, Van den Berg LH, Veldink JH, Vucic S, Kiernan MC. Controversies andpriorities in amyotrophic lateral sclerosis. Lancet Neurol. 2013;12(3):310–22. doi:10.1016/S1474-4422(13)70036-X.

Traynor BJ, Codd MB, Corr B, Forde C, Frost E, Hardiman OM. Clinical features of amyotrophic lateral sclerosis according to the El Escorial and Airlie House diagnostic criteria: a population-based study. Arch Neurol. 2000a;57(8):1171–6.

Traynor BJ, Codd MB, Corr B, Forde C, Frost E, Hardiman O. Amyotrophic lateral sclerosis mimic syndromes: a population-based study. Arch Neurol. 2000b;57(1):109–13.

Turner MR, Kiernan MC, Leigh PN, Talbot K. Biomarkers in amyotrophic lateral sclerosis. Lancet Neurol. 2009;8(1):94–109.

Valendra R, Jones A, Jivraj N, Steen IN, Young CA, Shaw PJ, Turner MR, Leigh PN, Al-Chalabi A, UK-MND LiCALS Study Group, Mito Target alS Study Group. Use of clinical staging in amyotrophic lateral sclerosis for phase 3 clinical trials. J Neurol Neurosurg Psychiatry. 2015;86(1):45–9. doi:10.1136/jnnp-2013-306865. Epub 2014 Jan 24. PubMed PMID: 24463480.

Huntington's Disease

9

Tom Burke, Colin P. Doherty, Walter Koroshetz, and Niall Pender

9.1 Introduction

HD results from an expansion of the trinucleotide repeat (Cytosine Adenine Guanine; CAG) causing an expanded polyglutamine chain in the *huntingtin* gene located on chromosome 4p16.3. While there is no unique set of symptoms which indicate the onset in HD, many patients present initially with symptoms that reflect early neurological impairment, such as brief random irregular muscle jerks (chorea), writhing movements (athetosis), difficulty walking and a tendency to fall or clumsiness. Many also present with a range of psychiatric problems including depression and anxiety. The rate of suicide in patients with HD is higher than normal base rates and accounts for 7 % of deaths in non-hospitalised HD patients. According to recent literature, the rate of suicidality between motor-symptomatic, and pre-motor symptomatic gene carriers is equal, with suicidal ideation occurring in an equal number of patients. There are also reports of self-injury, alcohol abuse, criminal offences and marital difficulties. Cognitive impairments such as poor short-term memory, poor concentration, deterioration in work performance and poor judgement have been noted in the early stages. Recent research has identified that HD patients have emerging difficulty with aspects of social cognition before movements become apparent which results in poor inter-personal relationships. As a result of degeneration in the fronto-striatal regions leading to behavioural disinhibition, patients can become aggressive or violent as the disease progresses. It has been recognised that the initial site of deterioration in HD lies within the basal ganglia and that as the disease progresses the damage extends to encompass the cortical structures.

T. Burke
Academic Unit of Neurology, Trinity Biomedical Sciences Institute, Dublin, Ireland
e-mail: burket2@tcd.ie

C.P. Doherty
Department of Neurology, St. James's Hospital, Dublin, Ireland

Academic Unit of Neurology,
Trinity Biomedical Sciences Institute,
Dublin, Ireland
e-mail: colinpdoherty@gmail.com

W. Koroschetz
Neurological Disorders and Stroke Institute,
National Institutes of Health,
Bethesda, MD, USA
e-mail: koroshetzw@ninds.nih.gov

N. Pender (✉)
Department of Neuropsychology, Beaumont Hospital,
and Academic Unit of Neurology,
Trinity College Dubln, Dublin, Ireland
e-mail: niallpender@gmail.com

© Springer International Publishing Switzerland 2016
O. Hardiman, C.P. Doherty (eds.), *Neurodegenerative Disorders: A Clinical Guide*,
DOI 10.1007/978-3-319-23309-3_9

Table 9.1 Common measures of functional disability and disease progression

Title	Authors	Scale description
Functional Capacity Rating Scale	Shoulsan and Fahn (1979)	Measures functional capacity across 5 domains on a scale of 1–5
Unified Huntington's Disease Rating Scale (UHDRS)	Kieburtz (& Huntington's disease study group; 1996)	A multi-domain measure of disease progression across 6 domains of function. Includes a Functional Assessment and Total Functional Capacity Scale
Core Assessment Program for Intracerebral Transplantation in Huntington's disease (CAPIT-HD)	Quinn et al. (1996)	A multi-domain assessment protocol originally developed for the transplantation program

9.2   Clinical Course

HD is rare but typically develops in patients between ages 40–50, although the variance of age differs greatly, ranging from 2 years-mid 80s. It has been estimated that over 25 % of cases begin after the age of 50 years whereas 7 % begin before 20 years of age.

As an autosomal dominant condition, the disease has almost equal prevalence in males and females but a marked variability in the age of onset both within and between families has been noted. As the CAG repeat is unstable in spermatogenesis, greater increases in severity, more apparently sporadic cases (although, studies have found that larger increases were most often reported in sufferers with large expansions) and earlier age of onset is often associated with inheritance through the male line of a family.

Since the genetic test became available, it has been observed that only between 40–79 % of individuals at risk for the condition reported an intention to take the test. Although many at-risk people report an intention to undertake predictive testing, the number that actually undergo testing is much lower at 12.3–14.6 % of people at risk. However, careful genetic counselling and pre-test screening is essential to manage the numerous ethical and psychological consequences of preparing to take such a test.

As the mutation is present from birth and the condition is slowly progressive, the precise onset of disease may be difficult to identify. By convention the disorder is usually diagnosed when chorea manifests. However, most patients have changes that predate chorea, which are frequently detected by close family members, some of whom have witnessed similar changes in the parent or siblings. The early changes may be in behaviour, memory, mood, speech pattern, facial expression, or gait and posture. Reduced job performance and marital discord can lead to major upheaval in those who have inherited the mutation but do not yet have chorea.

Table 9.1 lists the most common measures of disease progression and functional capacity for the clinic.

The course of Huntington's disease can nevertheless be variable. The average age of motor onset is around 42 years but HD can begin in childhood (Juvenile HD or Westphal variant) or even in the elderly. The extremes of onset age are determined in large part by the inherited CAG repeat length. Juvenile onset (onset before 20 years of age) occurs in about 5–15 % of HD cases worldwide, and presents with a bradykinetic form of the disease, which appear Parkinsonian and they may have seizures. Generally, the first signs are related to a drop in school performance. In rare pedigrees, parents of affected individuals may not have clinical evidence of disease despite living to an advanced age.

CAG repeat lengths lower than 26 are considered stable and result in no clinical symptoms or known increased risk to future generations. Repeats of 27–35 CAG repeats are considered intermediate, and symptoms are not expected to manifest in these individuals but CAG repeats of this length are 'unstable' and can lead to greater expansions with morbidity in future generations.

Repeat lengths of 36–39 CAG repeats have reduced penetrance, with most individuals becoming symptomatic, but often with a milder expression in midlife. In adults, the length of the CAG repeat expansion accounts for up to 70 % of the variability relative to age of onset. Childhood onset of HD is usually caused by an especially large CAG repeat (i.e., >50). By contrast, length of the CAG repeat appears to contribute less to the rate of disease progression.

The individual with early signs of HD has grown up in a family in which one of the parents likely became affected in adulthood and may have passed through the course of the disease and died. The newly affected individual's family life may have been severely disrupted during their childhood by the parent's change in behaviour. The psychological stress in such individuals is easy to underestimate. They may be living with a sense of dread about the insidious onset; with even minor neurologic complaints being interpreted as disease expression for instance benign myokymia is often misinterpreted as the onset of chorea. A simple mechanical fall or stumble can develop an elaborate significance it does not warrant. In the disease's prodromal phase, depression can develop years before the onset of motor symptoms, and the highest prevalence has been reported within 1 year of clinical diagnosis.

9.3 Prevalence

In the general population of the western hemisphere, the prevalence rate of HD is estimated to be 4–10 per 100,000. There is large variance in prevalence ratings, though a 20-year retrospective analysis of records in the UK recently revealed the prevalence rate has risen from 5.4 per 100,000 in 1990 to 12.3 per 100,000 in 2010. A higher prevalence has been reported in South Wales and Venezuela as compared to a lower rate found in Finland, Japan and African-American populations. This variability is due, predominantly, to the relative mobility of carriers of the gene and the existence of isolated "pockets" of families living in close proximity.

9.4 Pathology

Huntington's disease causes neuronal loss starting in the striatum but eventually leading to progressive whole brain atrophy. Early in the disease there may be little or no signs of the disease in the gross brain. However, inevitably neuronal loss develops with atrophy of the cortical surface in most and of the striatum in nearly all cases where the neuronal loss is accompanied by astrocytosis. There is a particularly severe degeneration of the caudate nucleus that begins in the tail of the caudate and then advances in predictable way to the dorsal medial aspect then to the ventrolateral side. Eventually the caudate atrophies to a thin tissue paper-like gliotic structure that is devoid of usually predominating medium spiny neurons. This gives a boxcar appearance of enlarged lateral ventricles on CT scan. The putamen is also affected in a predicable caudal to rostral vector whereas the nucleus accumbens is generally spared. Vonsattel described the standard approach to brain assessment in HD and used 1–4 grading system to standardize the pathological description from mild to severe involvement. In grades 3–4 there is much more widespread brain degeneration with cortical loss, white matter loss and extensive gliosis (see Fig. 9.1). Like many neurodegenerative disorders, Huntington's disease is associated with abnormal accumulation and misfolding of the proteins. A role of non neuronal cells is also gaining support, in Huntington's disease as well as in ALS genetic animals with the mutation in microglia or glial cells but not neurons is also associated with pathologic changes.

9.5 Symptomatology

Huntington's disease is associated with a triad of difficulties including the movement disorder as well as cognitive and neuropsychiatric conditions. Each of these is associated with a complex set of psycho-social problems. Patients with Huntington's disease face a range of difficulties from diagnosis to death and these difficulties are not confined to the patient themselves but also to

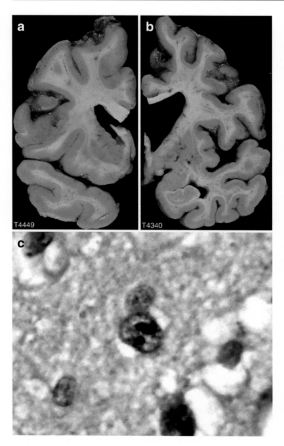

Fig. 9.1 Neuropathology of Huntington's disease. (**a**) The caudate nucleus bulges into the ventricle in normal individuals but is flattened in this 55 year old person dying with Huntington's disease as seen in this coronal section through one brain hemisphere. Characteristically the atrophy is more severe in the dorsal aspects of the caudate. (**b**) The caudate is barely visible in this 75 y.o. with severe degeneration of the caudate and globus pallidus. (**c**) The centre neuron contains a classic intranuclear inclusion composed of aggregates of the mutant huntingtin protein (Figures courtesy of Dr. Jean Paul Vonsattel of Columbia University)

the family. As an autosomal dominant disorder the disease has a particular resonance with families of sufferers.

9.5.1 Movement Disorder

By the time that chorea manifests, Huntington's disease generally includes some alteration in voluntary motor control. The ability to make rapid, repetitive, sequential movements is often abnormal.

Tests such as alternately tapping the thumb against the tips of the fingers, repetitively tapping the tip of the tongue against the top lip, alternately tapping the top, then the palm of one hand against the palm of the other hand all show slowing and irregularities in timing. There is generally great difficulty keeping the tongue protruded over a short, i.e., 10 s period.

Eye movement abnormalities are common. These include inability to make smooth pursuits due to intrusive saccades and delays in initiation of saccades. There is also dramatic slowing of saccadic velocity in some patients.

The gait of the person with early Huntington's disease demonstrates increased variability in step length and distance from the intended path. Inability to maintain position after gently pulling the patient backwards, and trouble performing tandem walking is common. Though the cerebellum is generally spared, the finger to nose test and heel to shin test generally shows dysmetria.

Chorea, from the Greek for dance, often starts as a quick flick at multiple joints in the fingers or fingers and wrist while walking. It commonly worsens to twisting turns of the limbs, involuntary neck and facial movements, with blinks, and writhing tongue movements. The progressive involvement of lingual and bulbar control leads to dysarthria and dysphagia. Food with a soft moist consistency such as pudding is easiest to swallow. Maintaining adequate nutrition can be challenging and motor symptoms tend to worsen as patients lose weight. Most become almost mute in the later stages of the illness and are completely unable to swallow without aspirating. Chorea, which can be of large amplitude and forceful enough to cause self injury, tends to slow over years and the involuntary movements evolve to dystonia in the later stages of the illness. Walking becomes more and more associated with falls and eventually the person is wheelchair or bed bound. Tone increases with disease progression. There is commonly a dramatic, reflexive increase in tone when the limb is activated. Reflexes are hyperactive. The Babinski reflex often becomes positive.

In contrast to the major motor findings, sensory abnormalities are minimal or absent. Some believe that patients with advanced HD have decreased pain sensation.

9.6   Cognition

Many of the early studies reported general intellectual and cognitive decline in HD, which is worse than in other neurodegenerative conditions. However, intellectual ability generally remains stable over time, with the most pronounced deficits seen in executive domains in parallel with pathological changes. A recent meta-analysis of the literature, which incorporated the results from 760 patients, showed maximum differences between controls and HD patients, using the effect size statistic, were found on tests of construction, and memory.

In a more recent population based cross-sectional study of motor manifest HD gene-expansion carriers, 51.8 % presented with the full symptom triad i.e., cognitive, neuropsychiatric, and motor involvement, 25 % were defined as cognitively impaired in addition to motor symptoms, and 14.3 % had neuropsychiatric symptoms along with motor symptoms. Only 8.9 % had isolated motor symptoms. Among the HD participants without motor symptoms, 39.2 % had neuropsychiatric symptoms, were cognitively impaired, or had a combination of both. Cognitive decline precedes motor signs in many gene-positive HD patients, and may be an important target in clinical trials and early intervention. Cognitive test scores may also improve the ability to predict disease onset among gene mutation carriers and help families to better plan for potential personal and economic strain.

In a recent observational report over a 36-month period of 366 participants with HD, the symbol digit modality test proved to be especially sensitive to cognitive change. Among psychiatric indicators, apathy ratings specifically showed significant increases compared to controls. Several baseline imaging, quantitative motor, and cognitive measures had prognostic value, independent of age and CAG repeat length, for predicting subsequent clinical diagnosis in pre-HD.

Cognitive reserve has been shown to have positive prognostic value in HD, comprised of composite scores derived from estimated premorbid intellectual level, occupational status, and years of education, relative to disease progression in HD. Higher cognitive reserve was significantly associated with a slower rate of change and slower rate of volumetric loss in two brain structures (caudate, putamen) for those estimated to be closest to motor disease onset. These findings demonstrate a relationship between cognitive reserve and both a measure of executive functioning and integrity of certain brain structures in pre-motor HD individuals.

Diagnostic algorithms have gained more attention in recent years in HD, where CAG-expansions are computed to obtain an estimated "years to clinical diagnosis". Stratifying groups as: *near*, estimated to be 9 years from diagnosis; *mid*, between 9 and 15 years; and *far*, >15 years, researchers conducted neurocognitive assessments on each cohort. Nineteen cognitive tasks were used to assess attention, working memory, psychomotor functions, episodic memory, language, emotional recognition, sensory and perceptual functions, and executive process. The *near* group showed significantly poorer performance on nearly all of the cognitive tests, and the *mid* group on about half of the cognitive tests. Overall, the cognitive battery accounted for 34 % of the variance. This further highlights how neurocognitive tests are robust clinical indicators of the disease process prior to reaching criteria for motor diagnosis of HD. Six main cognitive factors have to be considered when monitoring markers of disease progress, and cognitive indices should be used when monitoring cognitive function in pre-motor HD, rather than results from individual measurements or screening tools. These factors include: (1) speed/inhibition, (2) verbal working memory, (3) motor planning/speed, (4) attention-information integration, (5) sensory-perceptual processing, and (6) verbal learning/memory. Overall, motor planning/speed and sensory-perceptual processing appear to be the most important markers of disease prognosis.

Thus many studies of cognitive functioning in HD report generalised decline in cognitive functioning over the course of the condition. However, the specific nature of this decline varies between studies. It is likely that this reflects an inherent variation in the presentation of the disease within and between families as well as poor study design and differing measures. In particular, because of the relative rarity of the disease, many studies are insufficiently powered with respect to patient numbers.

9.6.1 Language Ability

Traditionally, HD patients do not present with clear cortical aphasia. However, as more sophisticated testing has emerged it has become clear that many patients presented with a range of language based functions, some of which are masked by the severity of dysarthria. Comprehension is generally thought to be intact. However, HD patients have been shown to be impaired in the comprehension of affective and propositional (command or question) prosody.

9.6.2 Executive Functions

Recently, there has been increased interest in the executive deficits experienced by patients with HD. This not only results from the earlier application of more sophisticated diagnostic testing that enables patients to complete tests sooner in the course of the disease, but also reflects the improved resolution of current neuroimaging techniques. Such techniques have facilitated a greater description of the nature of the lesions in HD and identified degeneration in the frontal lobes via fronto-striatal connections. That is, the nature of the reciprocal connections between the basal ganglia and the oculomotor region, dorsolateral prefrontal cortex and lateral orbitofrontal areas resulting in significant degeneration in fronto-striatal mediated cognitive and behavioural functions.

HD patients have been shown to be impaired on tests of planning, self-order working memory and tests of response set, all indicators of executive dysfunction. Although HD patients have been shown to perform poorly on measures of categorical fluency, more deficits are prevalent on phonological fluency (letter) rather than semantic fluency (category). Consistent with many studies, patients with a more rapidly progressive prognosis (determined using mutation size and current age) perform more slowly and with less accuracy on tests of executive function. Performance accuracy tends to be negatively related to striatal volume while both accuracy and working memory are negatively related to frontal white matter volume. Interestingly, pathological disturbances in cortico-striatal circuits in HD present similarly to other pathologies such as excessive gambling. Although similar disinhibition related symptoms are present i.e., changed sensitivity to punishments and rewards, impulsivity, and inability to consider long-term advantages over short-term rewards, both HD patients and pathological gamblers also show similar performance deficits on risky decision-making tasks and measures of executive function.

In summary, patients with HD show deficits on a range of tests of executive function. These take the form of planning, executing and inhibiting behaviour. In the context of the neuropathological data it is not surprising that HD patients should present with such difficulties. Loss of frontal white matter and neuronal cell loss have been reported in many studies and metabolic deficits in the frontal lobes have been associated with the degree of cell loss in the basal ganglia.

9.6.3 Attentional and Perceptual Functions in HD

In many studies, HD patients were found to be impaired on tests of alertness, divided attention and response flexibility. While clear disorders of perception are rare, there has been increasing interest and controversy surrounding the issue of patient's ability to perceive emotional cues. HD patients were impaired at interpreting facial and vocal expressions of emotion, and similarly, those relating to fear and disgust were disproportionately impaired. HD patients have also been shown to be impaired at comprehending emotional prosody in speech, matching facial affect, facial recognition and discriminating faces.

9.6.4 Memory

There has been a great deal of debate concerning the nature of the memory impairment in HD and the pattern of impaired and preserved skills in this patient group. It has been clear for many years that patients present with a form of memory impairment that, while severe, is distinct from other dementias such as Alzheimer's disease.

Global memory deficits are common in HD and this is unsurprising given the links between the striatum and limbic system, the reported deficits in temporal lobe function and the deficits in frontal function in this population. Unlike Alzheimer's patients where episodic memory is better for older memories, HD patients show no advantage for older memories over more recent ones. This is known as a flat temporal gradient. Procedural learning is also impaired. In particular, procedural motor tasks are more impaired than lexical tasks. It has been suggested that recognition memory is disproportionately preserved until later stages and therefore retrieval or encoding deficit are favoured by many authors. That is, the memory impairment in HD, which begins early in the course of the disease, is related to the more extensive and global deterioration in frontostriatal functions.

9.6.5 Social Cognitive Processes

Multiple reports suggest that HD patients (in both manifest and preclinical stages) have multimodal deficits in emotional processing that extend to decoding facial expressions, prosody, body language and rating of emotional scenes, with some but not all studies suggesting that negative emotions such as disgust and anger are disproportionately affected.

The term "Social Cognition" encompasses several sub-domains including emotion recognition from facial expressions, prosody or body posture, as well as, the ability to infer other people's mental states in terms of beliefs, desires, feelings, intentions, or knowledge states.

Patients with HD have been reported to make significantly more errors on measures of social cognition than controls, exhibiting difficulties in judging the social appropriateness of character's behaviour in stories, and problems inferring complex mental states through commonly used measures (the use of photographs of people's eyes).

HD patients have further evidenced lower everyday perspective taking scores relative to a matched sample. Social cognitive deficits have been shown to appear independent of executive dysfunction, however, executive deficits are linked to poor understanding of socially inappropriate remarks and errors in mental state attribution.

HD patients have notable deficits in their ability to identify fear, disgust, and anger. These results are the most consistently reported, on non-demanding tasks, and across modalities (i.e., visual and auditory). Declines in emotional recognition exist regardless of whether the emotions are being communicated by others' facial expressions or vocal intonation, although patients' emotional recognition deficits are not necessarily evident in, or associated with, increased functional problems with social interactions. This finding points to a differential impairment in emotion recognition and emotional experience in HD.

9.7 Neuropsychiatric and Behavioural Features

Depression is very common in HD. Emotional dyscontrol with outbursts of anger with a physical component can be a major source of upset in the family or in the long-term care facility. Obsessive compulsive behaviours are also common. Some have paranoid delusions but hallucinations are rare. These behaviours can lead to antisocial acts that run afoul of the law. Over time persons with HD become more and more restricted mentally. In early stages of illness they perform cognitive tests more slowly. By history they are less active mentally and can display prominent apathy. In general, patients with Huntington's disease don't completely lose one specific cognitive domain but rather lose the ability to engage these domains for goal directed behaviour. Communication can be especially difficult in the later stages. This can also be a source of tremendous frustration when the patient's primal needs are not met and communication is not possible to resolve these needs. As an example, it is not unusual for patients in the later stages to become anxious and upset when hungry but not able to transmit the fact that they are hungry to their caretakers.

9.7.1 Behavioural Difficulties

The behavioural features of HD can be conceptualised as frontal disconnection syndromes. The earliest changes can be seen as irritability with a low tolerance of frustration. These features gradually deteriorate and the episodes can become increasingly explosive and disproportionate. These features resemble the personality conditions often associated with frontal lobe impairment such as the pseudopsychopathic and the pseudodepressive states of apathy and self-neglect. Agitation and aggression can often occur in the latter stages of the disease and are often difficult to ameliorate. Up to 40 % of patients suffer from affective disorders with hypomania and mania seen in 5–10 %. These may occur before any signs of the disease are apparent. These underlying organic symptoms do also co-exist with the psychological reaction to living with such a devastating condition. The risk of suicide is increased in.

Behavioural data obtained from the European Huntington's Disease Network 'REGISTRY' study conducted using the UHDRS Behavioural Rating Scale (N = 1690) confirmed previous reports of distinct behavioural patterns within Huntington's disease comprising mainly of a depressive factor, a dysexecutive factor, an irritability factor and a psychosis factor.

Further longitudinal analysis of 91 patients with HD, without a formal psychiatric disorder at baseline, revealed that 15 % had a psychiatric disorder after 2 years, with 64 % having a major depressive disorder. The baseline characteristics of lower education, having no children, a lower level of global daily functioning were predictive of incident psychiatric disorders after 2 years. Of the 15 patients with a psychiatric diagnosis at baseline, 53 % no longer had a psychiatric disorder at follow-up. All seven patients with a persistent psychiatric disorder (47 %) were female and their most prevalent diagnosis was generalized anxiety disorder (European Huntington's Disease Network. www.euro-hd.net/html/network; EURO-HD European Huntington's Disease Network: www.euro-hd.net).

Using the Problem Behaviors Assessment for Huntington's Disease (PBA-HD), longitudinal prevalence of neuropsychiatric symptoms was notably higher than baseline prevalence. This suggests that previous studies may have underestimated the extent of this clinical problem. Apathy, irritability, and depression were each associated with distinct longitudinal profiles. Apathy progressed over time and across disease stages. Irritability also increased significantly, but only in early stages of HD. Depression did not increase significantly at any stage of disease. The neuropsychiatric syndrome of apathy appears to be intrinsic to the evolution and progression of HD.

Managing psychiatric symptoms is difficult and is exacerbated by the cognitive and physical disabilities. A marked loss of insight early in the disease might appear protective at times but can also hamper attempts to manage symptomatology. Pharmacological treatment has been widely discussed and is usually symptomatic management.

9.8 Family and Psycho-Social

There are, understandably, significant family stressors and there are marked difficulties for both affected and unaffected siblings. The suicidal rates are higher in unaffected siblings, so called survivor guilt than the general population. Similarly, unaffected parents suffer the difficulties of caring for spouses and affected children with economic and psychological difficulties.

A recent investigation by into caregiver burden found that motor impairment and symptoms of depression were the most important factors predicting caregiver burden. Significant support is needed for HD families from the multidisciplinary team, with specifically tailored psychological interventions available.

9.9 Care and Disability Management of the Person with the Huntington's Mutation

The offspring of persons with Huntington's disease have a 50 % chance of inheriting the disease. The penetrance is high. Though there can be variability most develop signs at about the same age as their parent did. The genetic test for the hun-tingtin mutation is clinically available from anal-ysis of blood DNA. The decision to be tested is a very personal one and needs to be supported with appropriate genetic counselling. The first reac-tion of many at risk persons is to jump at the chance of being tested to "get rid" of the fear of whether they have inherited the "bad gene". However those that do not have the mutation do not face the tragedy of the illness, and those that have inherited it can have their fears substantially enhanced by a "positive" test. Key to the counsel-ling process is to ensure that the at-risk individual has a sense of how it will be helpful for them to know that they will get the disease in the future. Decisions surrounding whether to have children generally predominate in presymptomatic testing but as might be expected many choose not to be tested. Most agree that children should not be tested.

As symptoms of HD develop in a person at risk, the diagnosis is made when the physician is convinced by the chorea or some other neurologi-cal sign. Gene testing may be helpful if there is a need for the diagnosis and the signs are equivo-cal. It may be helpful in cases in which there is no family history, though the implications of genetic testing need to be planned for including the dis-covery of non-paternity, or the establishment of risk within a larger family. Other diagnostic tests are not necessary in the clear-cut case of HD though the MRI shows progressive atrophy of the caudate throughout the course of the disease.

In the early stage of Huntington's disease, as well as in the later stages, the psychiatric mani-festations require management. Depression in HD can respond to anti-depressant medication but the response is often partial. Obsessive-compulsive behaviours can be very difficult to control but may respond to serotonin-uptake-inhibitors that are effective in the treatment of OCD. Sleep disorders are common and sleep studies show that awakenings from sleep are often associated with an involuntary movement. Some develop completely reversed sleep-wake cycles, remaining awake at night and sleeping much of the day. Longer acting benzodiazepines such as clonazapam at bedtime can improve sleep.

Mood disorders with frequent episodes of emotional upset can respond to mood stabilizers such as valproic acid, carbamazepine and serotonin-uptake- inhibitors. Anti-psychotics are sometimes necessary in persons with delusions and are often tried in persons with disruptive, self injurious or violent behaviours. Atypical anti-psychotics such as quetiapine may be more effec-tive than standard neuroleptics and they also do not contribute to the dystonia and motor dyscon-trol to the same extent. Some seem to respond to high doses of beta-blockers. Because these medications are generally not as beneficial as one might hope and they are fraught with side effects it is important to attempt to determine if there are environmental contributors to the disruptive behaviours.

Changes in mealtimes, discomfort in the wheel chair, misinterpretation of the caregiver, nicotine withdrawal, interruption when drowsy, etc. can be the source of behavioural disturbance.

There is no treatment for the motor dyscontrol though a novel "dopamine stabilizer", ACR16, has shown promise in an initial clinical trial. Replication studies are underway by the com-pany, NeuroSearch. Speech and swallowing ther-apy may help teach safe swallowing. Physical activity to maintain muscle tone may be helpful. Chorea will respond to low doses of neuroleptics or to tetrabenazine though it is important to check whether the drugs are associated with better over-all motor function due to the bradykinesia and dystonic side effects. Its important to also con-sider that tetrabenazine is itself associated with depression in up to 20 % of users. Often the envi-ronment simply needs to be modified; adding wheel chairs and bed rails to avoid trauma from the chorea may be critically important. Abnormal movements may be so severe that the patient is not safe in a bed and better cared for on a large mattress that rests on the floor. Use of restraints is especially problematic as combined with the choric movements the restraint ties can lead to significant harm, even strangulation.

Feeding the person with advanced HD is also challenging. Oral feedings need to be changed over time to a softer but thick consistency. Early on thin liquids like water and dry crumbly foods cause cough and aspiration. Then solid foods are too difficult to chew and swallow. One characteristic of persons with HD is that they tend to over stuff the mouth as their swallowing efficiency decreases and swallowing takes more and more time. Caregivers may continue oral feeding into the late stages with pureed foods but feeding is done very slowly over long time periods. Weight management is important as patients with HD tend to deteriorate with weight loss and in some cases have improved with weight gain. The decision to insert a feeding tube is especially difficult and needs to be discussed with the patient or family years before the decision is anticipated. Otherwise the patient may be unable to communicate when the feeding crisis occurs. In general patients with HD die of aspiration pneumonia so a feeding tube can prolong life for those who are very severely disabled.

9.10   Pathogenesis of HD

The discovery of the Huntington's disease mutation raised the expectations that a treatment to slow progression of disease might come from research. At phenotypic level research continues to investigate the manifestation of cognitive and behavioural impairments in HD. In particular, it is important to examine variations in the phenotype with age and CAG repeat length as well as investigations of the influence of frontostriatal executive dysfunction on other cognitive domains.

Genetic animal models of the disease in flies, rodents, sheep and non-human primates are now available or are soon to be available for therapeutic research. The normal huntingtin protein is found throughout the cytoplasm of all cells in the body. The mutated huntingtin protein forms abnormal aggregates in neurons. A number of other CAG repeat neurodegenerative disorders have been discovered in which the abnormally long glutamine repeat is found in different proteins. All are characterized by aggregation of the abnormal protein in neurons. In patients with Huntington's disease (except the very rare person who is homozygous for the mutation) there is one normal copy of the gene and one mutated

copy. It is now known that one normal copy is sufficient for normal brain function so the disease is caused by some abnormal toxic effect(s) of the protein due to the elongated glutamine repeat. A variety of theories of pathogenesis are supported by variable levels of evidence and some therapeutic agents are now being tested in patients. The hungtingtin protein has been implicated in a host of important cellular functions and the exact mechanism by which the mutation causes cell death is not clear. Mutant huntingtin affect the transcription of different classes of other genes and plays a role in protein trafficking, vesicle transport, postsynaptic signaling, transcriptional regulation, and apoptosis. Thus, a loss of function of the normal protein and a toxic gain of function of mutant HTT contribute to disruption of multiple intracellular pathways. Experiments have also shown that expression of the mutant protein, even if confined to glia, is still toxic to neurons.

9.11   Development of Neuro-Protective Therapies

At present, there is no medical treatment that is known to affect the rate of progression of HD. The one possible exception is the maintenance of caloric requirements, as weight loss has been associated with more rapid deterioration. The goal of scientists is to develop a neuroprotective therapy that can be used safely in persons who are gene positive to prevent the onset of disability. The National Institute of Neurological Disorders and Stroke is currently funding a large trial of coenzyme Q10 to slow progression of HD in symptomatic patients. A prior trial of Coenzyme Q10 failed to demonstrate a large effect but there was a trend toward benefit that warranted a second study of higher dose. Among its putative actions Coenzyme Q10 is important in mitochondrial function and there is some evidence of mitochondrial dysfunction in HD. In another attempt to improve energy metabolism, creatine supplementation is also being studied in an NIH funded trial. Phospho-creatine is a major source of stored energy in the brain.

A major focus of research is on how best to "turn off" the mutant huntingtin gene. Recent research has shown that complete loss of the huntingtin protein is embryonically lethal suggesting that complete "turn off" of both alleles would be dangerous. The discovery that short strands of RNA can attach to messenger RNA and prevent transcription of protein raises the possibility that such interference RNA (iRNA) can be engineered to stop the production of the mutant protein. Whether iRNA treatment would be beneficial if it "turns down" the expression of both the mutant and the normal allele is not clear. If not, then an allele-specific iRNA may be custom engineered for individual families so that it interacts with only the mutant gene may be required. Anti-sense RNA therapy is also being pursued with similar aims. The challenge facing human use of these exciting therapies is how to deliver to the brain without adverse effects.

A variety of efforts are now ongoing to understand how to clear the protein aggregates from neurons which seem to be the signature feature of most neurodegenerative diseases. To that end techniques are being developed to introduce key components of antibodies into cells, called intrabodies. These are designed to attach to and promote clearance of abnormally deposited proteins like mutant huntingtin. Drugs which promote the metabolism of protein deposits may also prove beneficial. There are now attempts to use high throughput screening techniques to find drugs that prevent the aggregation or decrease production of the huntingtin protein. The mutant huntingtin protein also has been shown to alter the transcription of a variety of other genes. The down regulation of brain derived neurotrophic factor (BDNF) is one example of an important consequence of the effect of huntingtin on gene transcription. Drugs which modify gene transcription, particularly histone deacetylase (HDAC) inhibitors are under study as potential therapeutic agents.

Conclusions

Huntington's disease is a progressive neurodegenerative disease for which there is currently no cure. However, despite this, there is a wealth of information available to provide evidence based efficacious treatments for the management of the patient's condition. Patients present with a triad of cognitive, movement and psychiatric difficulties which progress slowly over a 15–20 year period. Each of these domains requires careful assessment and management in order to maintain the person's quality of life and functional ability. Extensive advances have been made in the understanding of the pathophysiology of the condition but further care is required if services are to avoid a nihilistic approach to HD.

Selected Bibliography

Banaszkiewicz K, Sitek EJ, Rudzińska M, Soltan W, Slawek J, et al. Huntingotn's disease from the patient, caregiver and physician's perspective: three sides of the same coin? J Neural Transm. 2012;119:1361–5.

Bates G, Harper P, Jones L. Huntington's disease. 3rd ed. Oxford: OUP; 2002.

Bonner-Jackson A, Long JD, Westervelt H, Tremont G, Aylward E, et al. Cognitive reserve and brain reserve in prodromal Huntington's disease. J Int Neuropsychol Soc. 2013;19:739–50.

Calder AJ, Keane J, Young AW, Lawrence AD, Mason S, Barker RA. The relation between anger and different forms of disgust: implications for emotion recognition impairments in Huntington's disease. Neuropsychologia. 2010;48:2719–29.

David AS, Fleminger S, Kopelman MD, Lovestone S, Mellers JDC. (eds) (2009) Index, in Lishman's Organic Psychiatry: A Textbook of Neuropsychiatry, Fourth Edition, Wiley-Blackwell, Oxford, UK.

Douglas I, Evans S, Rawlins MD, Smeeth L, Tabrizi SJ, Wexler NS. Juvenile Huntington's disease: a population-based study using the General Practice Research Database. BMJ Open. 2013;3:e002085. doi:10.1136/bmjopen-2012-002085.

Eddy CM, Sira-Mahalingappa S, Rickards HE. Is Huntington's disease associated with deficits in theory of mind? Acta Neurol Scand. 2012;126:376–83.

Eddy CM, Sira-Mahalingappa S, Rickards HE. Putting things into perspective: the nature and impact of theory of mind impairment in Huntington's disease. Eur Arch Psychiatry Clin Neurosci. 2014;264(8): 697–705.

Epping EA, Paulsen JS. Depression in the early stages of Huntington disease. Neurodegener Dis Manag. 2011;1(5): 407–14.

Evans SJW, Douglas I, Rawlings MD, Wexler NS, Tabrizi SJ, et al. Prevalence of adult Huntington's disease in the UK based on diagnoses recorded in general practice records. J Neurol Neurosurg Psychiatry. 2013;84:1156–60.

Harrington DL, Smith MM, Zhang Y, Carlozzi NE, Paulsen JS, et al. Cognitive domains that predict time to diagnosis in prodromal Huntington disease. J Neurol Neurosurg Psychiatry. 2012;83(6):1–7.

Hart EP, Dumas EM, Giltay EJ, Middelkoop HAM, Roos RAC. Cognition in Huntington's disease in manifest, premanifest and converting gene carriers over ten years. J Huntingtons Dis. 2013;2:137–47.

Henley SMD, Marianne NJU, Frost C, King J, Tabrizi SJ, Warren JD. Emotional recognition in Huntington's disease: a systematic review. Neurosci Biobehav Rev. 2012;36:237–53.

Hersch S, Jones R, Koroshetz W, Quaid K. The neurogenetics genie: testing for the Huntingtons disease mutation. Neurology. 1994;44:1369–73.

Hubers AA, Reedeker N, Giltay EJ, Roos RA, Van Dujin E, et al. Suicidality in Huntington's disease. J Affect Disord. 2012;136:550–7.

Huntington's Disease Collaborative Research Group. A novel gene containing a trinucleotide repeat that is expanded and unstable on Huntington's disease chromosomes. Cell. 1993;72:971–83.

Ille R, Holl AK, Kapfhammer HP, Reisinger K, et al. Emotional recognition and experience in Huntington's disease: is there a differential impairment? Psychiatry Res. 2011;118:377–82.

Johnson CD, Davidson BL. Huntington's disease: progress toward effective disease-modifying treatments and a cure. Hum Mol Gen. 2010;19(Rev issue 1): R98–102.

Kalkhoven C, Sennef C, Peeters A, Van den Bos R. Risk-taking and pathological gambling behaviour in Huntington's disease. Front Behav Neurosci. 2014;8: 1–12.

Kayson E, Darnell M, Weber J, Biglan K, Shoulsan I, et al. Depression and suicidality at baseline in the prospective Huntington's At Risk Observational Study (PHAROS). Mov Disord. 2004;19:1128.

Klöppel S, Stonnington CM, et al. Irritability in preclinical Huntington's disease. Neuropsychologia. 2010;48:549–57.

Krainc D. Clearance of mutant proteins as a therapeutic target for neurodegenerative diseases. Arch Neurol. 2010;67:388–92.

Lundin A, Dietrichs E, Haghighi S, et al. Efficacy and safety of the dopaminergic stabilizer pridopidine (ACR16) in patients with Huntington's disease. Clin Neuropharmacol. 2010;33:260–4.

Mestre T, Ferreira J, Coelho MM, Rosa M, Sampaio C. Therapeutic interventions for symptomatic treatment in Huntington's disease. Cochrane Database Syst Rev. 2009. Issue 3. Art. No.: CD006456. doi:10.1002/14651858.CD006456.pub2.

Marder K, Zhao H, Eberly S, Tanner CM, Oakes D, Shoulson I, Huntingtons Study Group. Dietary intake in adults at risk for Huntington disease: analysis of PHAROS research participants. Neurology. 2009;73:385–92.

Maroon DA, Gross AL, Brandt J. Modeling longitudinal change in motor and cognitive processing speed in presymptomatic Hungtington's disease. J Clin Exp Neuropsychol. 2011;33(8):901–9.

Mellers JDC, Pender N. Neuropsychiatry of Huntington's disease. Adv Clin Neurosci Rehabil. 2001;1(5):15–6.

Morrison PJ. Accurate prevalence and uptake of testing for Huntington's disease. Lancet Neurol. 2010; 9:1147.

Novak MJ, Tabrizi SJ. Huntington's disease. Br Med J. 2010;340:c3109. doi:10.1136/bmj.c3109.

Papp KV, Snyder PJ, Mills JA, Duff K, Westervelt HJ, et al. Measuring executive dysfunction longitudinally and in relation to genetic burden, brain volumetrics, and depression in prodromal Huntington disease. Arch Clin Neuropsychol. 2014;28:156–68.

Paulsen J. Cognitive changes in Huntington's disease. Adv Neurol. 2005;96:209–25.

Paulsen S, Langbehn DR, Stout JC, et al. Detection of Huntington's disease decades before diagnosis: the Predict-HD study. J Neurol Neurosurg Psychiatry. 2008;79:874–80.

Potter NT, Spector EB, Prior TW. Technical standards and guidelines for Huntington disease testing. Genet Med. 2004;6(1):61–5.

Quinn N, Brown R, Craufurd D, Goldman S, Hodges J, et al. Core Assessment Program for Intracerebral Transplantation in Huntington's Disease (CAPIT-HD). Mov Disord. 1996;11(2):143–50.

Reedeker W, van der Mast RC, Giltay EJ, Kooistra TAD, et al. Psychiatric disorders in Huntington's disease: a 2-year follow-up study. Psychosomatics. 2012;53:220–9.

Rickards H, DeSouza J, van Walsem M, van Duijn E, Simpson SA, et al. Factor analysis of behavioural symptoms in Huntington's disease. J Neurol Neurosurg Psychiatry. 2011;82:411–2.

Ross CA, Tabrizi SJ. Huntington's disease: from molecular pathogenesis to clinical treatment. Lancet Neurol. 2011;10:83–98.

Rosas HD, Feigin AS, Hersch SM. Using advances in neuroimaging to detect, understand, and monitor disease progression in Huntington's disease. NeruoRx. 2004;1:263–73.

Shoulson I, Fahn S. Huntington disease: clinical care and evaluation. Neurology 1979;29:1–3.

Snowden JS, Austin NA, Sembi S, Thompson JC, Craufurd D, Neary D. Emotional recognition in Huntington's disease and frontotemporal dementia. Neuropsychologia. 2008;46:2638–49.

Snowden J, Crauford D, Griffiths HL, Neary D. Longitudinal evaluation of cognitive disorder in Huntington's disease. J Int Neuropsychol Soc. 2001;7: 33–44.

Snowden JS, Gibbons ZC, Blackshaw A, Doubleday E, Thompson J, Craufurd D, Foster J, Happe F, Neary D. Social cognition in frontotemporal dementia and Huntington's disease. Neuropsychologia. 2003;41: 688–701.

Stout JC, Paulsen JS, Queller S, Solomon AC, Whitlock KB, et al. Neurocognitive signs in prodromal Huntington disease. Neuropsychology. 2010;25(1):1–14.

Sutherland GR, Richards RI. Dynamic mutations on the move. J Med Genet. 1993;30:978–81.

Tabrizi SJ, Langbehn DR, Leavitt BR, et al. Biological and clinical manifestations of Huntington's disease in the longitudinal TRACK-HD study: cross-sectional analysis of baseline data. Lancet Neurol. 2009;8: 791–801.

Tabrizi SJ, Scahill RI, Owen G, Durr A, Leavitt BR, et al. Predictors of phenotypic progression and disease onset in premanifest and early-stage Huntington's disease in the TRACK-HD study: analysis of 36-month observational data. Lancet Neurol. 2013;12:637–49.

Testa JA, Brumback RA, et al. Neuropathology and memory dysfunction in neurodegenerative diseases. In A. Troster (Ed.), Memory in neurodegenerative disease: Biological, Cognitive and Clinical Perspectives 1988. Cambridge University Press, UK.

Thompson JC, Harris J, Sollom AC, Stopford CL, Howard E, et al. Longitudinal evaluation of neuropsychiatric symptoms in Huntington's disease. J Neuropsychiatry Clin Neurosci. 2012;24(1):53–60.

Vinther-Jensen T, Larsen IU, Hjermind LE, Budtz-Jørgensen E, et al. A clinical classification acknowledging neuropsychiatric and cognitive impairment in Huntington's disease. Orphanet J Rare Dis. 2014;9:114–23.

Vittori A, Breda C, Repici M, Orth M, Roos RA, et al. Copy-number variation of the neuronal glucose transporter gene SLC2A3 and age of onset in Huntington's disease. Hum Mol Genet. 2014;23(12):3129–37.

Vonsattel JP, DiFiglia M. Huntington disease. J Neuropathol Exp Neurol. 1998;57(5):369–84.

Wetzel HH, Gehl CR, Dellefave-Castillo L, Schiffman JF, Shannon KM, et al. Suicidal ideation in Huntington disease: the role of comorbidity. Psychiatry Res. 2011;188(3):372–6.

Zakzanis KK. The subcortical dementia of Huntington's disease. J Clin Exp Neuropsychol. 1998;20(4): 565–78.

Parkinsonism-Plus Syndromes

10

Seán O'Dowd, Daniel Healy, and David Bradley

10.1 Introduction

Parkinsonism is a clinical syndrome encompassing some or all of four cardinal features: bradykinesia, rigidity, tremor and postural instability. Idiopathic Parkinson's disease is the pathological substrate in approximately 80 % of cases. The remaining 20 % of cases are largely attributable to other primary neurodegenerative disorders, termed "parkinsonism-plus" or atypical parkinsonian disorders, whilst a smaller number are considered to represent "secondary parkinsonism", wherein non-neurodegenerative processes such as vascular, iatrogenic or parainfectious mechanisms are at play. Parkinsonism can also be seen as a feature of some rare heredo-degenerative disorders. The latter, and secondary parkinsonism, are considered outside the scope of this chapter, but are listed in Table 10.1.

The four main parkinsonism-plus disorders are the synucleinopathies multiple system atrophy (MSA) and dementia with Lewy bodies (DLB), and the taupoathies progressive supranuclear palsy (PSP) and corticobasal degeneration (CBD). These are neurodegenerative disorders that are frequently confused with idiopathic Parkinson's disease (PD). In fact, about 30 % of pathologically proven parkinsonism plus syndromes are initially misdiagnosed as PD. It is important to concede however that even where strict clinical criteria are retrospectively applied there is incomplete, even poor, clinicopathological correlation in this group of disorders. Whilst PSP, MSA and CBD have clear pathological diagnostic features, the distinction of DLB from Parkinson's disease dementia (PDD) is clinical, and the concept of a spectrum of "Lewy body disease", rather than splitting the two disorders, is advocated by some authorities.

Accurate differentiation between parkinsonism plus syndromes and PD is important for several reasons, the two most significant being (i) life expectancy is much lower in parkinsonism plus, and (ii) treatments such as levodopa and deep brain stimulation are generally ineffective in parkinsonism plus.

A complete history and neurological examination is critical in establishing a correct diagnosis. General features of an atypical syndrome are symmetric clinical features at onset (with the exception of corticobasal degeneration), and poor L-Dopa response. Features that do occur in Parkinson's Disease later on in the disease should

S. O'Dowd • D. Bradley (✉)
Department of Neurology, St. James's Hospital,
Dublin, Ireland
e-mail: DBradley@STJAMES.IE

D. Healy
Royal College of Surgeons in Ireland, Dublin, Ireland

Department of Neurology, St. James's Hospital,
Dublin, Ireland

© Springer International Publishing Switzerland 2016
O. Hardiman, C.P. Doherty (eds.), *Neurodegenerative Disorders: A Clinical Guide*,
DOI 10.1007/978-3-319-23309-3_10

Table 10.1 Classification of parkinsonism

Idiopathic Parkinson's disease	Parkinson's disease Genetic forms of Parkinson's disease
Parkinsonism plus syndromes	Progressive supranuclear palsy Multiple system atrophy Cortico-basal ganglionic degeneration Dementia with lewy Bodies
Hereditary neurodegenerative Parkinsonism	Huntington's disease Wilson' disease Autosomal dominant spinocerebellar ataxias Lubag (X-linked dystonia-parkinsonism) Neuroacanthocytosis Familial basal ganglia calcification Fronto-Temporal dementia with parkinsonism Brain Iron accumulation disorders Pallidopyramidal syndromes (usually genetic)
Secondary (acquired, symptomatic) Parkinsonism	Infectious: postencephalitic, AIDS, SSPE, Creuzfeldt-Jakob disease Drugs: dopamine receptor blocking drugs; reserpine, lithium, flunarizine, valproate Toxins: MPTP, CO, Mn, Hg, cyanide, methanol, ethanol Vascular: multi-infarct Trauma: pugilistic encephalopathy Other: parathyroid abnormalities hypothyroidism, hepatocerebral degeneration, brain tumour, paraneoplastic, normal pressure hydrocephalus

Table 10.2 'Red flag' features in parkinsonism

Clinical feature	Likely cause of parkinsonism
Young onset	Juvenile PD, MSA
Axial rigidity	PSP
Pill rolling rest tremor	
Myoclonus	MSA, CBD
Vertical gaze palsy	PSP
Early falls backwards (1st year)	PSP
Asymmetric onset	PD, CBD
Alien limb/apraxia	CBD
Poor response to levodopa	PSP, CBD, MSA
Dysautonomia	MSA
Early cognitive impairment	PSP, CBD
Laryngeal stridor	MSA
Palilalia	PD, PSP
Cerebellar signs	MSA
Pyramidal signs	MSA

arouse suspicion if they occur <u>early</u> in the clinical course: early falls, early autonomic features and early cognitive impairment should raise suspicion of a parkinsonism plus syndrome. Some syndromes have specific features that are not seen in IPD, for example square wave jerks or the supranuclear gaze palsy of PSP. Table 10.2 provides a guide to some clinical red flags that should make the examiner consider an alternative diagnosis to PD. Importantly, patients with suspected Parkinson's disease may declare specific features of a parkinsonism-plus syndrome after their initial presentation, so the physician must keep an open mind and keen observation during follow-up visits.

10.2 Multiple System Atrophy

10.2.1 Clinical Features

Like PSP and CBD, MSA is a progressive, sporadic, adult- onset neurodegenerative disorder. The first cases were described over a hundred years ago by Dejerine and Thomas who referred to olivopontocerebellar atrophy. The term MSA was introduced in 1969 by Graham and Oppenheimer indicating that multiple brain systems are involved (extrapyramidal, pyramidal, cerebellar and autonomic (in any combination)). Patients are clinically classified according to the predominant motor presentation i.e. cerebellar (MSA-C) and parkinsonian (MSA-P) subtype. When autonomic failure predominates or there is primary autonomic failure, MSA is sometimes termed Shy-Drager syndrome, although this term is rarely used nowadays.

Autonomic dysfunction is usually the earliest feature in both MSA-P and MSA-C, with 97 % ultimately developing symptoms. Genitourinary dysfunction is the most frequent initial complaint in women, and early erectile dysfunction is almost

Fig. 10.1 This figure provides an illustration of the major clinical features of Multiple System atrophy (MSA)

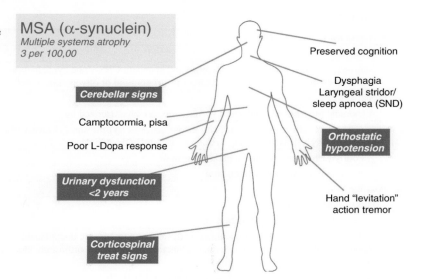

invariable in men by 2 years. Orthostatic hypotension is common and is present in at least 68 % of patients. Symptoms associated with orthostatic hypotension include presyncope (lightheadedness, dizziness, blurred vision), fatigue, yawning, "coathanger pain" across the neck and shoulders, and syncope. Akinesia and rigidity are prominent in MSA-P but are usually also evident in the later stages of MSA-C. Cerebellar dysfunction is predominant in MSA-C with gait and limb ataxia the prominent features, but also is seen in a significant proportion of MSA-P cases over time. Notable features supporting a diagnosis of MSA include rapid progression (wheelchair bound <10 years from onset), orofacial dystonia (spontaneous or levodopa-induced), camptocormia (forward trunk flexion resolving in certain postures, typically lying down), Pisa syndrome (lateral trunk flexion), disproportionate antecollis (severe neck flexion or 'dropped head syndrome'), dysphonia (hoarse/harsh/ high pitched), dysarthria, dysphagia, inspiratory stridor, cold hands and feet, emotional incontinence, pyramidal signs (Babinski and hyper-reflexia), and a jerky myoclonic postural/action tremor of the digits and/or hands (poliminimyoclonus). Only one third of patients with MSA-P respond to levodopa and about 90 % are unresponsive to long-term therapy.

MSA progresses rapidly and most patients develop motor impairment within 1 year of onset. Motor impairment can be caused by cerebellar dysfunction and/or extrapyramidal involvement; corticospinal tract dysfunction can also occur but is not a major symptomatic feature of the condition. At least 50 % of all patients with probable MSA are disabled or wheelchair- bound within 5 years after onset and the median survival is 9.8 years.

Figure 10.1 provides an illustration of the major clinical features of MSA. Table 10.3 shows an international bedside classification system for MSA according to differing levels of diagnostic certainty- possible, probable or definite.

10.2.2 Epidemiology

There is an estimated incidence of 1.2–4.1 cases per 100,000 population per year, with an estimated prevalence of 0.9–8.4 cases per 100,000. However, as with the other atypical parkinsonian disorders, ascertainment (due to frequent misdiagnosis) poses a significant problem, so this is probably under-estimated. About 30 % of patients with late-onset sporadic cerebellar ataxia have MSA. MSA has been reported in Caucasian, African and Asian populations. MSA-P predominates in western countries (68–82 %) whilst in Eastern countries, MSA-C is more common, constituting 67–83 % of patients. Most studies indicate a slight male predominance and the mean patient age at onset is 54.3 years with a range of 33–78 years.

Table 10.3 Criteria for MSA

A. **Criteria for diagnosis of MSA**
Definite MSA
Neuropathological findings of widespread and abundant CNS alpha-synuclein-positive glial cytoplasmic inclusions with neurodegenerative changes in striatonigral or olivopontocerebellar structures.
Probable MSA
A sporadic progressive, adult (>30 y)- onset disease characterized by
Autonomic failure involving urinary incontinence or an orthostatic decrease of blood pressure within 3 min of standing by at least 30 mmHg systolic or 15 mmHg diastolic and
Poorly Levodopa-responsive parkinsonism or
A cerebellar syndrome/dysfunction
Possible MSA
Parkinsonism or
A cerebellar syndrome/dysfunction and
At least one feature suggesting autonomic dysfunction (otherwise unexplained urinary urgency, frequency or incomplete bladder emptying, erectile dysfunction or significant orthostatic blood pressure that does not meet the level required in probable MSA) and
At least one of the additional features shown in Table 10.1b
B. **Additional features of possible MSA**
Possible MSA-P or MSA-C
Pyramidal signs – Babinski sign with increased tendon reflexes
Stridor
Possible MSA-P
Rapidly progressive parkinsonism
Poor response to Levodopa
Postural instability within 3 years of motor onset
Gait ataxia, cerebellar dysarthria, limb ataxia, or cerebellar oculomotor dysfunction
Dysphagia within 5 years of motor onset
Atrophy on MRI of putamen, middle cerebellar peduncle, pons or cerebellum
Hypometabolism on FDG-PET in putamen, brainstem or cerebellum
Possible MSA-C
Parkinsonism
Atrophy on MRI of putamen, middle cerebellar peduncle, or pons
Hypometabolism on FDG-PET in putamen
Presynaptic nigrostriatal dopaminergic denervation on SPECT or PET

Reproduced and modified with permission of Wolters Kluwer Health from Gilman et al. (2008), from the second consensus statement on the diagnosis of multiple system atrophy

MSA multiple system atrophy, *MSP-P* MSA with predominant parkinsonism, *MSA-C* MSA with predominant cerebellar ataxia, *FDG* (18) fluorodeoxyglucose

10.2.3 Neuropathology and Molecular Pathology

The neuropathological substrate of MSA-C is olivopontocerebellar degeneration (inferior olivary nucleus, pons, and cerebellum) whilst that of MSA-P is striatonigral degeneration (substantia nigra, putamen, caudate nucleus and globus pallidus). Even though they can be clinically very different, MSA-C and MSA-P share oligodendroglial cytoplasmic inclusions (GCIs) as a unifying pathological feature. Both subtypes display neural loss and gliosis in their respective regional brain distributions and both are frequently accompanied by neurodegeneration of the autonomic nervous system; the severe clinical correlate of this is Shy-Drager syndrome.

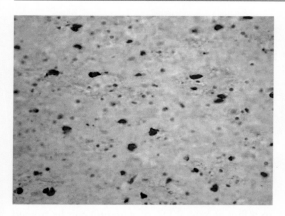

Fig. 10.2 Alpha-synuclein immunostaining to show cytoplasmic immunopositivity in glial cells (glial cytoplasmic inclusions (GCI)) within subcortical white matter (magnified ×40 before photo enlargement). The authors acknowledge Professor Michael Farrell for this image

Table 10.4 Selected synucleinopathies and tauopathies

Synucleinopathies	Tauopathies
Progressive supranuclear palsy	Parkinson's disease
Fronto-temporal dementia	Multiple system atrophy
Corticobasal disease	Lewy body dementia
Pick's disease	
Argyrophilic brain disease	
PD – dementia complex – Guam	
Post-encephalitic PD	

Approximately 30 % of Caucasian patients have principally striatonigral pathology, 20 % olivopontocerebellar pathology and the remaining 50 % have equal amounts of both. Pathological degeneration of the putamen appears to correlate with the poor levodopa response in MSA.

Oligodendroglial cytoplasmic inclusions, which define MSA neuropathology, are formed by fibrillized (aggregated, insoluble) alpha-synuclein protein (see Fig. 10.2). Genome-wide screening in MSA has identified an association between certain SNPs in the alpha synuclein gene and MSA risk, and transgenic mice over-expressing alpha synuclein under the control of specific oligodendroglial promoters develop GCI-like inclusions. These findings confirm MSA as a 'synucleinopathy' similar to PD and dementia with Lewy Bodies (see Table 10.4)

but it appears that oligodendrogliopathy precedes neuronal degeneration in MSA.

Aberrant myelin basic protein may also be pathogenic in MSA raising the possibility that this is a primary disorder of myelin-producing oligodendroglial cells. However, no studies to date have linked these two plausible hypotheses.

10.3 Laboratory Tests

Investigations of autonomic function include the table-tilt test or active stand to measure orthostatic blood pressure and sphincter electromyography. The latter detects denervation in the external urethral sphincter secondary to degeneration of Onuf's nucleus in the spinal cord. Cardiac scintigraphy demonstrates reduced sympathetic MIBG uptake in the heart in PD but not MSA. Clinically, this test is more commonly used in Eastern countries than in the West. Video-polysomnography can be helpful in identifying the sleep disturbances associated with MSA (sleep apnoea, nocturnal stridor, REM sleep behaviour disorder (REMBD)).

10.3.1 Radiological Findings

MRI findings in MSA-P often show decreased signal intensity in the posterolateral putamen bilaterally on T2 weighted images. In addition to putaminal hypointensity on T2, a characteristic finding in MSA is the slit-hyperintensity in the lateral margin of the putamen, related to putaminal atrophy. The MRI abnormalities of MSA-C consist of atrophy of the pons, middle cerebellar peduncles, and cerebellum. A characteristic "hot cross bun sign" is described, produced by selective loss of myelinated transverse pontocerebellar fibers and neurons in the pontine raphe with relative preservation of the pontine tegmentum and corticospinal tracts (Fig. 10.3).

10.3.2 Management

There is no effective disease-modifying therapy and a multidisciplinary approach is recommended,

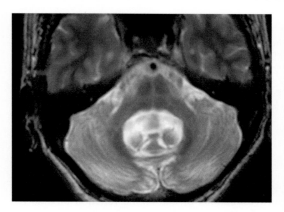

Fig. 10.3 Axial T2-MRI showing a cross of signal hyperintensity within the body of the pons originally described by Quinn as a hot cross bun

It is worth considering Levodopa replacement but the results are usually poor, with only a minority of patients witnessing benefit, which is typically short-lived. A trial of L-Dopa is considered negative if a dose of 1,000 mg per day is reached with no clinical benefit. Caution must be exercised given the risk of exacerbating non-motor features, in particular orthostatic hypotension.

RBD can be treated symptomatically with clonazepam or melatonin; sleep apnoea may be ameliorated by continuous positive airway pressure (CPAP). Concomitant depression (estimated to affect at least 40 % of patients) can be treated effectively with selective serotonin reuptake inhibitors (SSRIs) or SNRIs.

with supportive care from the allied health professional team. A number of symptomatic therapies are can be deployed to good effect. Orthostatic hypotension is often the earliest and most debilitating symptom. Along with simple explanation and advice regarding care when standing, the addition of liberal salt, increasing fluid intake, head elevation when sleeping and elastic stockings may improve standing blood pressures. Several drugs are used for the management of orthostatic hypotension including fludrocortisone (mineralocorticoid), midodrine (alpha1-adrenoreceptor agonist), droxidopa (synthetic precursor of norepinephrine), and less commonly NSAIDs (possible inhibition of vasodilator prostaglandins) and pyridostigmine (putative vasoconstrictive effect). Therapy can be limited by supine hypertension which affects up to 60 % of patients. Bladder symptoms including urinary retention and incontinence are relatively common and troublesome problems. Formal urodynamics with measurement of post micturition volumes are important, particularly with co-existing prostatism. Overactive bladder symptoms may improve with anti-muscarinics such as oxybutynin or tolterodine while some patients require intermittent self catherisation. Medication may also be considered for constipation and erectile dysfunction, although silenafil and other phosphodiesterase inhibitors should be used with caution as they frequently exacerbate orthostatic hypotension.

10.4 Progressive Supranuclear Palsy: Clinical Features

Steele, Richardson and Olszewski presented the first clinicopathological descriptions of PSP in 1963 and 1965. Unsteadiness of gait, with falls within the first year, frequently backwards, represents the presenting feature in more than 60 % of cases. Bradykinesia and rigidity may be associated, often resulting in a misdiagnosis of PD, but these features have an axial predominance in PSP, unlike PD which tends to have asymmetric lateralised features in the early stages. In a minority of cases gaze difficulties, dysarthria, dysphagia or cognitive impairment may be the prominent early symptoms (see Fig. 10.4). The illness progresses to an immobile state over less than 10 years in the majority of cases. Recent years have witnessed a considerable expansion in the volume of clinic-pathological series describing PSP and there is now widespread recognition that there can be considerable phenotypic heterogeneity, particularly in the early years of the disease. This has given rise to the proposed clinical subdivision of PSP into a number of sub-entities, and there is some pathological data to corroborate this. Such clinical subtypes include the classic phenotype as described by Steele et al. (PSP-RS); PSP-parkinsonism (PSP-P) which can mimic IPD with asymmetric features, tremor and partial levodopa responsivity for a number of years, as

Fig. 10.4 This figure provides an illustration of the major clinical features of Progressive Supranuclear Palsy

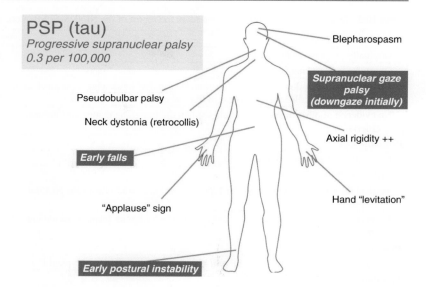

PSP (tau)
Progressive supranuclear palsy
0.3 per 100,000

Blepharospasm

Pseudobulbar palsy

Neck dystonia (retrocollis)

Supranuclear gaze palsy (downgaze initially)

Axial rigidity ++

Early falls

Hand "levitation"

"Applause" sign

Early postural instability

well as a corticobasal syndrome (PSP-CBS), a primary progressive aphasia phenotype (PSP-PNFA), and rarely, gait initiation failure and freezing of gait, speech or writing in the absence of other parkinsonian signs (PSP-PAGF). Ultimately, however, the disease evolves in the vast majority of patients into the classical picture of axial rigidity, postural instability, oculomotor palsies, bulbar dysfunction and cognitive (particularly frontal lobe) impairment.

In contrast to the short and shuffling gait, stooped posture, narrow base, and flexed knees typically seen in PD, PSP patients tend to be erect with a stiff and broad-based gait, often with poor safety awareness and impulsivity ("motor recklessness"). They tend to pivot when turning, which further compromises balance. Although the PSP gait can appear ataxic, cerebellar signs are not a feature.

Oculomotor abnormalities are common in PSP. Symptomatic eye movement difficulty is typically present within 4 years after the onset. Prior to this, most patients have slowing of vertical saccades, saccadic pursuit, breakdown of opticokinetic nystagmus in the vertical plane, poor convergence and square-wave jerks (SWJs). The latter occurs in nearly all patients with PSP and rarely in PD. Vertical supranuclear ophthalmoparesis is a prominent feature of PSP. The patient loses range of vertical gaze, with

downgaze usually worse than upgaze, and will describe difficulty walking down stairs. This voluntary gaze restriction is supranuclear; it therefore can be overcome by using the vestibulo-ocular reflex ("Doll's eye" manoeuvre) achieved by passive flexion/extension of the neck. Involuntary orbicularis oculi contractions producing blepharospasm and 'apraxia' of eyelid opening and eyelid closure affect up to one third of PSP patients.

Pseudobulbar symptoms in PSP patients are characterised by dysarthria, dysphagia and emotional lability. The classic speech is a low pitched "growling" dysarthria. Some patients have severe stuttering and palilalia.

Cognitive impairment is a prominent feature of PSP, often presenting as cognitive slowing, impairment of executive function, and occasionally with non-fluent aphasia. Apathy and hypoactive behaviours have been attributed to a dysfunction in the frontal cortex and associated circuits. Sleep problems are common, particularly confusional awakenings, and often correlate with worsening dementia. REMBD is however very rarely seen in PSP, as it is almost exclusively associated with the synucleinopathies.

Similarly, relative sparing of olfaction helps to differentiate PSP from PD and MSA.

Inexorable decline characterises the clinical course of PSP with death, often by aspiration, usually occurring within 10 years of onset with a

Table 10.5 Diagnostic criteria for PSP – based on the report of the NINDS-SPSP international workshop

Possible PSP
Gradually progressive disorder
Onset age ≥40 or later
Vertical (upward or downward gaze) supranuclear palsy[a] *or* slowing of vertical saccades[a] and prominent postural instability with falls in the first year of disease onset[a]
No evidence of other disease that could explain the foregoing features, as indicated by mandatory exclusion criteria
Probable PSP
Gradually progressive disorder
Onset age ≥40 or later
Vertical (upward or downward gaze) supranuclear palsy[a] *and* prominent postural instability with falls in the first year of disease onset
No evidence of other disease that could explain the foregoing features, as indicated by mandatory exclusion criteria
Definite PSP
Clinically probable or possible PSP *and* histopathologic evidence of typical PSP[b]
Mandatory exclusion criteria
Recent history of encephalitis
Alien limb syndrome, cortical sensory deficits, focal frontal or temporoparietal atrophy
Hallucinations or delusions unrelated to dopaminergic therapy
Cortical dementia of Alzheimer's type.
Prominent, early cerebellar symptoms or prominent, early unexplained dysautonomia (marked hypotension and urinary disturbances)[a]
Severe, asymmetric parkinsonian signs
Neuroradiologic evidence of a relevant structural abnormality (i.e. basal ganglia or brainstem infarct, lobar atrophy)
Whipple's disease, confirmed by polymerase chain reaction, if clinically indicated
Supportive criteria
Symmetric akinesia or rigidity, proximal more than distal
Abnormal, neck posture, especially retrocollis
Poor or absent response of parkinsonism to levodopa therapy
Early dysphagia and dysarthria
Early onset of cognitive impairment including at least two of the following: apathy, impairment in abstract thought, decreased verbal fluency, imitation behaviour and frontal release signs

Reproduced and modified with permission of Wolters Kluwer Health from Litvan et al. (1996)
[a]Upward gaze is considered abnormal when pursuit or voluntary gaze, or both, have a restriction of at least 50 % of the normal range
[b]Definite PSP is a clinicopathologic diagnosis

mean survival of about 6 years. Table 10.5 provides a summary of the current diagnostic criteria for PSP.

10.5 Epidemiology

There is an estimated incidence of 0.3–1.1 cases per 100,000 population per year, with an estimated prevalence of 6.2–7.4 cases per 100,000, but cognisance must be taken of a clinical misdi-

agnosis rate of approximately 25 % confounding these data. No racial predilection is known. Men are more commonly affected and the mean age of onset is 63 years.

10.5.1 Neuropathology and Molecular Pathology

PSP shares histological and molecular similarities with other 'tauopathies' such as Alzheimer's

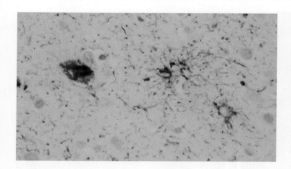

Fig. 10.5 Tau immunostaining to show a neuronal cytoplasmic tau positive neurofibrillary tangle (on the left as you look at the image) and tau positive tufted astrocyte (on the right as you look at the image) (magnified ×40 before photo enlargement). The authors acknowledge Professor Michael Farrell for this image

disease, frontotemporal dementia and argyrophilic grain disease (Table 10.4). Tau is a microtubule-associated protein meaning that it regulates the structure and stability of a major axon protein trafficking system. When tau protein is hyperphosphorylated it tends to form aggregates/ inclusions. These are termed neurofibrillary tangles when occurring in glial cells, coiled bodies in oligodendrocytes and 'tufted' inclusions in astrocytes (see Fig. 10.5). The neurofibrillary tangles in PSP are single straight filaments and are common in subcortical regions whereas in Alzheimer's disease they are paired helical filaments and cortical.

Alternative exon splicing of the tau gene (*MAPT*) produces six isoforms in human brain. Isoforms containing exon 10 have four microtubule binding domains (4R tau) and those that splice out exon 10 have three (3R tau). In the normal brain 3R and 4R tau isoforms have similar ratios; in PSP and CBD there is a 4R preponderance and in Pick's disease a 3R preponderance. Certain tau gene mutations, including some that disrupt the stem loop structure that splices exon 10, cause an autosomal dominant frontotemporal dementia with parkinsonism (FTDP-17), supporting the key role of the tau gene in tauopathy-associated neurodegeneration (Chap. 6). Mitochondrial dysfunction has also been implicated in the aetiopathogenesis of PSP and certain compounds known to inhibit complex I have been shown to increase 4R tau levels in neuronal cell culture.

Certain tau mutation carriers with FTDP-17 have a phenotype similar to PSP but tau mutations do not cause PSP and in clinical practice familial clustering of PSP is very rare. However, one of the most compelling and robust associations between gene and phenotype across all known human disorders is the association between sporadic PSP and a specific H1 haplotype formed by a balanced inversion of the region surrounding the tau gene about three million years ago. A number of polymorphisms on the H1 haplotype that influence gene expression have been implicated. Genetic testing of the tau gene is unnecessary in PSP unless one is considering an alternative differential diagnosis such as autosomal dominant FTDP-17.

10.6 Radiological Findings

Generalised brain atrophy is common in PSP, especially in the frontal lobes, but the characteristic finding of dorsal midbrain atrophy is best seen on a dedicated sagittal MRI where it produces a picture sometimes similar to a humming bird and on axial views to "Mickey Mouse" (Fig. 10.6).

10.7 Laboratory Tests

There are no diagnostic tests currently available for PSP; the diagnosis remains a clinical one (Table 10.4).

10.8 Management

There is no effective disease-modifying treatment for PSP and therapy is symptomatic or supportive in nature. A multidisciplinary team approach is recommended; physiotherapists may improve mobility, reduce falls, prevent contractures and provide hip protectors and walking aids; occupational therapists and social workers can assist with adapting patients' homes. Speech and language therapists may provide communication devices if required.

Fig. 10.6 (**a**) Sagittal T1-MRI through the brainstem showing volume loss in the midbrain with relative preservation of the pons. The upper convexity of the midbrain is lost giving a hummingbird appearance. (**b**) Axial MRI of midbrain shows severe volume loss giving a "Mickey Mouse" appearance

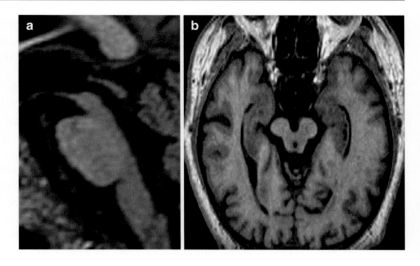

If parkinsonism is a prominent feature a trial of levodopa is recommended, increasing the dose to at least 1 g per day before deciding it is of no benefit. Forty to fifty percent of patients show some improvement although this is often short lived. Adverse effects include visual hallucinations and rarely dystonia, dyskinesias and apraxia of eye-lid opening. Amantadine may benefit 15 % of patients but the response is usually modest. Dopamine agonists, monoamine oxidase inhibitors and catechol-O-methyl transferase inhibitors are of no proven benefit. Anticholinergics should be avoided as there is an unusual sensitivity to cholinergic blockade in these patients. Lorazepam and low-dose quetiapine could be considered for management of psychiatric and behavioural symptoms.

Blepharospasm, with or without eyelid freezing, can be effectively treated with botulinum toxin. Dysphagia is progressive and some patients choose PEG insertion. Sialorrhoea can be treated with sublingual atropine drops, or targeted botulinum toxin or radiotherapy to the salivary glands.

10.9   Corticobasal Degeneration

10.9.1 Clinical Features

CBD was first described by Rebeiz et al. in 1968 in three patients of Irish descent with parkinsonism, myoclonus, supranuclear palsy and apraxia who were found at autopsy to have 'cortico-dentato-nigral degeneration with neuronal achromasia.' This disorder has an insidious onset, typically with progressive asymmetric levodopa-unresponsive rigidity and apraxia. Severe disability and death typically occurs within 6–7 years. Definite diagnosis requires histological examination.

CBD is an exception to the rule that atypical parkinsonian syndromes are symmetric (unlike IPD). Cortical dysfunction may manifest as asymmetric ideomotor apraxia (disorder of skilled, learned, purposeful movement) and/or an alien limb ('my hand has a mind of its own'). A typical description by the patient may be that they have a 'useless' hand or arm that is stiff, wayward and clumsy. The motor alien hand must be differentiated from a sensory syndrome associated with a lesion in the thalamus or temporal-occipital lobe. Eye movement abnormalities with slow initiation of horizontal movements as well as upgaze are common. However restricted downgaze is more suggestive of PSP. Limb dystonia is common and asymmetrical limb contractures are more prevalent in this condition than in the other parkinsonism- plus syndromes. Figure 10.7 provides a summary of the main clinical features of CBD.

Clinicopathological series have delineated the frequency of certain motor and other features, all of which increase over time from initial presentation as the disease evolves. The rates of occurrence of motor features over the entire disease course are as follows: limb rigidity 85 %, bradykinetic/

Fig. 10.7 This figure provides an illustration of the major clinical features of Corticobasal degeneration (CBD)

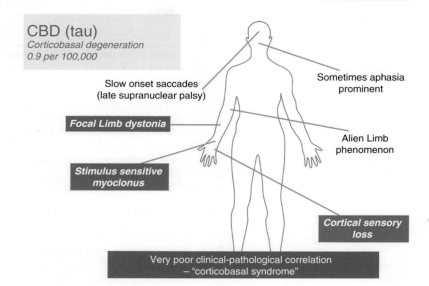

CBD (tau)
Corticobasal degeneration
0.9 per 100,000

Slow onset saccades (late supranuclear palsy)

Sometimes aphasia prominent

Focal Limb dystonia

Alien Limb phenomenon

Stimulus sensitive myoclonus

Cortical sensory loss

Very poor clinical-pathological correlation – "corticobasal syndrome"

clumsy limb 76 %, postural instability 78 %, falls 75 %, abnormal gait 73 %, axial rigidity 69 %, tremor 39 %, limb dystonia 38 %, myoclonus 27 %. Abnormal eye movements were seen in 60 % and speech abnormalities in 53 %. Higher cortical deficits include cognitive impairment in 70 %, limb apraxia in 57 %, aphasia in 52 %, cortical sensory loss in 27 % and alien limb phenomena in 30 %. Behavioural changes were seen in 55 % of patients. These data underscore the wide phenotypic variability seen in this condition and hence the significant challenges posed in devising robust clinical diagnostic criteria. Furthermore, numerous clinicopathological studies have demonstrated that many patients who present with a corticobasal syndrome ultimately do not have CBD pathology, but instead another neurodegenerative process, such as Alzheimer's disease or frontotemporal dementia. Unfortunately, even the most rigorously devised clinical diagnostic criteria (see Tables 10.6 and 10.7) have been unable to distinguish CBD from other causes of CBS antemortem, underlining the need to identify robust paraclinical biomarkers for this condition.

10.9.2 Epidemiology

There is a dearth of reliable data on the incidence and prevalence of CBD, largely attributable to the high misdiagnosis rate. Clinicopathological series indicate however that it is rare, with an estimated incidence of less than 1 cases per 100,000 population per year, with an estimated prevalence of 4.9–7.3 per 100,000. No racial predilection is known. The condition tends to occur in older age groups (60–80 years), with a mean age of onset of 63 years. CBD may be more common in women.

10.10 Radiological Findings

MRI brain findings are non-specific but often show asymmetric posterior parietal and frontal cortical atrophy with "knife-like" gyri. Atrophy of the corpus callosum has also been described.

10.10.1 Neuropathology and Molecular Pathology

CBD is another tauopathy with similar molecular characteristics to PSP, differing mainly in regional brain pathology. Rebeiz described CBD in 1968 as "corticodentatonigral degeneration with neuronal achromasia'; patients with prominent frontoparietal degeneration get limb apraxia and dementia and those with prominent

Table 10.6 Proposed clinical diagnostic criteria for corticobasal degeneration

Syndrome	Features
Probable Cortico-Basal Syndrome (CBS)	An *asymmetric* presentation including **2 or more** of the following: (a) Limb rigidity/akinesia, (b) Dystonia, or (c) Myoclonus, as well as **2 or more** of the following features: (d) Apraxia (Orobuccofacial or Limb) (e) Alien limb phenomena (more than levitation) (f) Cortical sensory deficit,
Possible Cortico-Basal Syndrome (CBS)	**At least 1** of the following (can be symmetrical) : (a) Limb rigidity/akinesia, (b) Dystonia, or (c) Myoclonus, as well as **1 or more** of the following features: (d) Apraxia (Orobuccofacial or Limb) (e) Cortical sensory deficit, (f) Alien limb phenomena (more than levitation)
Frontal Behavioural Spatial (FBS) Syndrome	**2** of: the following (a) Executive dysfunction, (b) Behavioral or personality changes, (c) Visuospatial deficits
Non-fluent/Agrammatic variant of primary progressive apahasia (NAV)	Effortful, agrammatic speech plus at **least 1** of: (a) Impaired grammar/sentence comprehension with relatively preserved single word comprehension, or (b) Groping, distorted speech production (apraxia of speech),
Progressive Supranuclear Palsy (PSP) Syndrome	**3** of following (a) Axial or symmetric limb rigidity or akinesia, (b) Postural instability or falls, (c) Urinary incontinence, (d) Behavioural changes, (e) Supranuclear vertical gaze palsy or decreased velocity of vertical saccades

Reproduced and modified with permission of Wolters Kluwer Health from Armstrong et al. (2013)

Table 10.7 Proposed clinical diagnostic criteria for corticobasal degeneration

	Clinical research criteria for probable sporadic CBD	Clinical criteria for possible CBD
Presentation	Insidious onset and gradual progression	Insidious onset and gradual progression
Median duration of symptoms	1	1
Age at onset (years)	>50	No minimum
Family History (2 or more relatives)	Exclusion	Permitted
Permitted phenotypes	(1) Probable CBS or (2) FBS or NAV plus at least one CBS feature (a–f)	(1) Probable CBS or (2) FBS or NAV plus at least one CBS feature (a–f)
Genetic mutations (e.g. *MAPT* gene)	Exclusion	Permitted

Reproduced and modified with permission of Wolters Kluwer Health from Armstrong et al. (2013)

frontotemporal atrophy get progressive primary aphasia. Severe substantia nigra depigmentation is invariable and most patients have some extrapyramidal features/ parkinsonism.

CBD and PSP are both 4R tauopathies and the tau H1 haplotype is a shared risk factor. However CBD and PSP cannot be considered different manifestations of the same disorder since their classical clinical presentations can be strikingly different and the neuropathological diagnostic criteria of CBD and PSP are validated with high sensitivity and specificity. Both share neuronal tau accumulation but astrocytic plaques are the hallmark of CBD and tufted astrocytes the hallmark PSP. Prominent cortical and subcortical neuronal loss, often highly asymmetric, also separates CBD from PSP. Ballooned swollen neurons with loss of cytoplasmic staining (achromasia), is supportive when present in the cortex and basal ganglia.

10.10.2 Management

To date no effective treatment has been found. Occasionally the extrapyramidal symptoms including rigidity, bradykinesia and tremor may respond to levodopa, but this is usually short-lived. Clonazepam and levetiracetam can be tried for myoclonus, with valproate usually avoided. Painful rigidity and dystonia may improve with botulinum toxin injections; occasionally gabapentin can be helpful. Physiotherapy, speech and language therapy and occupational therapy are important components of multidisciplinary management.

10.11 Dementia with Lewy Bodies

Dementia with Lewy bodies (DLB) occupies a somewhat unusual place within the rubric of parkinsonism plus syndromes as it shares many characteristics (clinical, radiological and pathological) with Parkinson's disease dementia. As such, unlike the other three disorders discussed in this chapter, it is not a pathologically distinct entity. DLB is a diagnosis made on clinical 'operational criteria' grounds, based on the appearance of cognitive symptoms prior to, or within 1 year of, the development of spontaneous parkinsonism. The evolution of cognitive symptoms after 1 year in a picture otherwise supportive of a diagnosis of IPD, is then considered to represent Parkinson's Disease Dementia (PDD). This arbitrary "one-year" rule was established by consensus in 2005 in order to facilitate phenotyping for research, but is now widely used standard clinical practice.

10.11.1 Clinical Features

DLB is characterised by a slowly progressive dementing process, which classically commences with impairment in cognitive domains other than memory (particularly visuospatial, attentional and frontal-executive function). Core diagnostic features (Table 10.8) include clear fluctuations in cognition, with variations in alertness and attention, which has considerable differentiating value from Alzheimer's disease; spontaneous features of parkinsonism which can be indistinguishable from that of IPD but frequently is more symmetrical; and recurrent visual hallucinations. The latter are typically well formed and detailed and patients generally retain insight. These hallucinations tend to take human form (often a familiar person such as a deceased relative), and are not distressing to the patient, but this is not invariably

Table 10.8 Clinical diagnostic criteria for dementia with Lewy bodies

Central features (essential for a diagnoses of dementia with Lewy bodies (DLB)
Dementia defined as a progressive cognitive decline of sufficient magnitude to interfere with normal social or occupational function
Prominent or persistent memory impairment may not necessarily occur in the early stages but is usually evident with progression
Deficits on tests of attention, executive function, and visuo-spatial ability may be especially prominent
Core features (two or more are sufficient for a diagnoses of parobable DLB, one for possible DLB)
Fluctuating cognition with pronounced variations in attention and alertness
Recurrent visual hallucinations that are typically well formed and detailed
Spontaneous features of parkinsonism
Suggestive features (if one or more are present in the presence of one or more core features, a diagnoses of DLB can be made. In the absence of any core features, one or more suggestive features are sufficient for possible DLB but probable DLB should not be diagnosed on the basis of suggestive features only)
REM sleep behavior disorder
Severe neuroleptic sensitivity
Low dopamine uptake in basal ganglia demonstrated by SPECT or PET imaging

Reproduced and modified with permission of Wolters Kluwer Health from McKeith et al. (2005)

Fig. 10.8 This figure provides an illustration of the major clinical features of dementia with Lewy bodies (DLB)

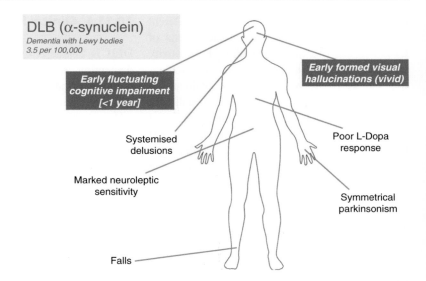

DLB (α-synuclein)
Dementia with Lewy bodies
3.5 per 100,000

Early fluctuating cognitive impairment [<1 year]

Early formed visual hallucinations (vivid)

Systemised delusions

Poor L-Dopa response

Marked neuroleptic sensitivity

Symmetrical parkinsonism

Falls

the case. Hallucinations in other modalities are rarer, but well described. Patients will often acknowledge retrospectively that formed visual hallucinations were preceded by visual misperceptions, and occasionally by "extracampine" hallucinations which are characterised by a sense of an invisible human presence. These symptoms are often undetected unless specifically sought by the clinician.

As in PD, premotor symptoms of REM sleep behaviour disorder and depression are frequently present; the former is quite specific for synucleinopathy and hence helpful in distinguishing from AD. Alpha-synuclein is frequently found in the autonomic nervous system in DLB and hence autonomic symptoms including orthostatic hypotension, constipation and urogenital symptoms are often harbingers of the condition. Systematized delusions are not infrequent and also constitute a suggestive feature in the validated diagnostic criteria. Antipsychotics must be used with great caution however: patients with DLB are exquisitely sensitive to typical neuroleptics, with consequences ranging from drowsiness and mild encephalopathy through to a catastrophic neuroleptic malignant syndrome which can be fatal. Figure 10.8 provides an illustration of the major clinical features of DLB.

10.11.2 Epidemiology

DLB is widely regarded to be the second most common cause of neurodegenerative dementia after AD. Precise prevalence data are lacking, but it is estimated to be responsible for between 7.5 and 30 % of all dementias. Incidence is estimated at 3.5 cases per 100,000 person years, which increases sharply with age. There is a male predilection, possibly up to 2:1.

10.11.3 Neuropathology and Molecular Pathology

The characteristic pathological hallmark of DLB is the synonymous Lewy body, an intracellular insoluble aggregate of alpha-synuclein protein. It is postulated that Lewy body pathology spreads sequentially from medullary structures rostrally through the pons, midbrain and subcortex, before ultimately affecting the neocortex itself (as described in the Braak staging process). DLB patients tend to have a higher neocortical burden of disease than PDD patients, but this is not invariable. Interestingly, some DLB cases with cortical involvement have limited involvement of subcortical and brainstem structures; the precise mechanistic reasons for this are unclear. A considerable proportion of DLB patients have concomitant Alzheimer's pathology- this is greater than that seen in PDD and may go some way towards explaining the more aggressive phenotype of DLB. As in other neurodegenerative proteinopathies, debate continues as to what constitutes the neurotoxic entity in DLB. Increasing evidence implicates earlier alpha-synuclein oligomeric aggregates as the noxious species, which form a nidus promoting further misfolding and aggregation, with the Lewy body merely representing the end stage of this process rather than being neurotoxic *per se*. There is some evidence that such soluble early aggregates may be able to propagate cell-to-cell in a prion like manner, which makes these species an attractive potential target for neuroprotective strategies.

10.11.4 Radiology

There are no pathognomonic features of DLB on standard structural imaging. The role of functional imaging modalities (both FDG-PET and [123] I-FP-CIT SPECT) is discussed elsewhere in this chapter; in early disease occipital PET hypometabolism differentiates from AD.

10.11.5 Management

As for any dementing process, supportive care and early involvement of the multidisciplinary team are key tenets in the management of DLB.

In general, the cognitive and neuropsychiatric symptoms of DLB exceed the motor symptomatology, and as such the movement disorder only requires treatment if truly responsible for functional impairment. The parkinsonism of DLB is somewhat less levodopa-responsive that PD but if required, levodopa should be initiated at the lowest dose possible and titrated very cautiously, as patients are sensitive to both the neuropsychiatric and cardiovascular adverse effects. Dopamine agonists and other antiparkinsonian medications are poorly tolerated in this cohort and should be avoided. From a cognitive perspective, the acetylcholinesterase inhibitors (AChEis) such as donepezil, rivastigmine and galantamine have a proven, albeit modest stabilising effect. The role of the NMDA antagonist memantine is less clear. Psychosis can be problematic in DLB, and the choice of neuroleptic is inherently limited by the pronounced sensitivity of patients to these agents. Based on tolerability and efficacy data, clozapine is the agent of choice but its use is complicated by the need for rigorous surveillance for potential agranulocytosis. In practice, low dose quetiapine is generally used; well tolerated with variable efficacy, although its use has not been definitively validated by well designed studies. Orthostatic hypotension can be managed as suggested for MSA.

10.12 Other Environmental Tauopathies

Clusters of PSP-like disorders exist in a number of remote parts of the world. In Guadeloupe, a PSP-like presentation of parkinsonism is as common as idiopathic PD. The consumption of soursop which contains high concentrations of annonacin has been implicated, as annonacin can cause direct inhibition of mitochondrial complex −1, and has been shown to cause excess accumulation of 4R tau *in vitro*. Interestingly, association between Guadeloupian parkinsonism and the H1 tau haplotype has been reported, as has 4R tau pathology at post mortem.

A parkinsonism-dementia complex sometimes with features of motor neuron disease is another tauopathy described amongst the Chamorro population of Guam and isolated villages on the Kii peninsula of Japan. The incidence of this disorder has declined since the original 1945 description by Zimmerman. Flour made from the false sago palm (Cycas Micronesica) has been implicated as it contains high levels of an excitatory amino acid BMAA, but this theory remains completely unproven. Familial clustering is described as is weak genetic association with the tau gene.

Encephalitis lethargica (EL) is characterised by somnolence, sleep inversion, oculogyric crises, and behavioural disorders. Most cases of EL occurred during the 1918/19 influenza pandemic and an aetiological association has been suggested but not proven. Many patients who recovered from the somnolent phase developed partial dopa responsive parkinsonism sometimes years after the acute disease. Sporadic cases still occur rarely. Pathologically EL shows subcortical and brainstem neurofibrillary pathology comprised of both 3R and 4R tau.

10.13 Hereditary Mimics

A number of single gene disorders can occasionally mimic the atypical parkinsonisms. We have already described how tau (*MAPT*) mutation carriers (FTDP-17) can clinically mimic PSP, or even CBD. Progranulin (*GRN*) mutation carriers, typically present with a frontal lobe behaviour and language disturbance which can partly resemble PSP and CBD. The neuropathological substrate is accumulation of TAR DNA-binding (TDP)-43 protein; tau pathology is lacking. LRRK2 mutation carriers typically display PD and Lewy body neuropathology, but in some kindreds, primary tau pathology resembling PSP occurs for unknown reasons. A potential association between the *c9orf72* repeat expansion and atypical parkinsonian syndromes is contentious; whilst reported in a handful of patients with clinical features of PSP or CBD, these patients also had features of ALS. The *c9orf72* mutation has not yet been associated with any autopsy-proven case of PSP, CBD or MSA despite a number of rigourous retrospective pathological studies. The fragile X tremor-ataxia syndrome (FXTAS) and a number of the autosomal dominant spinocerebellar ataxias (SCA) clinically mimic MSA-C. SNCA mutations and multiplication are implicated in familial PD; rarely these mutations can manifest as DLB, with prominent early cognitive decline.

10.14 Biomarkers in PSP, MSA, CBD and DLB

Presently there are no completely reliable markers for PSP, MSA, CBD or DLB. Whilst many studies are confounded by a lack of neuropathological corroboration of clinical diagnosis, a number of rigorous prospective studies have robustly interrogated radiological and biochemical markers in confirmed cases. It appears likely that a combination of clinical phenotyping, radiological and biochemical markers deployed together will give the greatest yield.

CSF presents an attractive and accessible window to the CNS but the search for a reliable biochemical biomarker in the atypical parkinsonian disorders has been disappointing thus far. It was postulated that phosphorylated-tau and total-tau protein levels might distinguish PD from the parkinsonism plus spectrum but results have been inconsistent and further confounded by elevated tau levels in overlapping neurodegenerative disorders like Alzheimer's disease. Total alpha-synuclein levels appear to be lower (although not consistently in all studies) in PD cohorts versus normal controls; this also appears to hold true for the other synucleinopathies, MSA and DLB, but does not discriminate between the three entities. It may be helpful in distinguishing DLB from AD however. Neurofilament light chain (NF-L) levels appear to reflect the greater burden of neurodegeneration in the atypical disorders and hence may prove to be the most promising CSF discriminator of PD from the parkinsonism plus syndromes.

As discussed, standard MRI may show suggestive (but not specific) features in PSP (mid brain atrophy (hummingbird sign)), MSA (pontocerebellar atrophy (hot cross bun) and lateral putaminal sclerosis (putaminal slit sign)), and CBD (frequent asymmetrical parietal lobe atrophy). Functional evaluation of the presynaptic dopaminergic system using dopamine transporter SPECT scanning is widely available in clinical practice but does not reliably differentiate PD, PSP or MSA and therefore is of little discriminatory value. Evidence of dopaminergic dysfunction can however be helpful however in distinguishing DLB from AD. The role of MIBG cardiac scintigraphy in distinguishing MSA from PD has already been discussed.

A more promising modality is fluorodeooxy-glucose (FDG)-PEt although this is not widely available. Recent computer programmes for FDG-PET analysis that recognise disease specific patterns show remarkable accuracy in differentiating parkinsonisms even before examination by a clinician. In PD the pattern is increased pallido-thalamic and pontocerebellar metabolic activity and reduced activity in premotor cortex, supplementary motor area, and parietal association regions. MSA is characterised by bilateral metabolic reductions in putaminal and cerebellar activity and PSP by reductions in the upper brainstem, medial frontal cortex, and medial thalamus. Prominent occipital hypometabolism suggests a diagnosis of DLB; in the presence of sparing of the posterior cingulate this has good discriminatory value versus AD.

FDG-PET is most specific in the early phase of disease when the clinical diagnosis is hardest and accords with the time window where disease modifying treatment approaches might be more effective. Later in the course of any of these conditions, widespread PET hypometabolism often precludes any useful diagnostic interpretation. Functional imaging of the cholinergic system and of activated microglia hold promise for the future. Imaging technologies that directly indentify intraneuronal inclusions such as NFTs and Lewy bodies are in development; like the use of Pittsburgh compound B (PiB) to image senile plaques in AD (see Chaps. 2 and 3), these developments may add considerably to the diagnostic arsenal.

REM sleep behaviour disturbance (RBD) is common to synucleinopathies (PD, MSA, DLB) and rare in tauopathies (PSP, CBD) and often invariably precedes the movement disorder. A significant Majority of patients diagnosed with RBD go on to develop PD , DLB or MSA making RBD a clinically useful biomarker and identifying a target patient group for future disease modifying therapies. Neuropsychological tests (e.g. Frontal Assessment Battery) may show disproportionately early frontal pathology, apathy and/or executive dysfunction and hence aid in the differentiation of PSP from PD and other atypical parkinsonisms. The simple 3-clap applause test is a very sensitive bedside test with perseveration pointing to PSP. Similarly, early disproportionate visuospatial dysfunction may support a diagnosis of DLB in the correct clinical context.

10.15 Future Advances

The identification of robust biomarkers of the atypical parkinsonian disorders remains something of a "holy grail" in neurodegenerative research and continues apace. This is important as the earlier these conditions are identified, the sooner potential neuroprotective or disease modifying strategies can be investigated and evaluated in randomised trials. At this time, no neuroprotective therapies exist, but a shift in emphasis towards targeting molecules implicated "upstream", in the early stages of the neurodegenerative cascade has recently led to the identification or development of a number of pharmacotherapies. Drugs that inhibit alpha-synuclein aggregation have been an area of active investigation in PD, DLB and MSA. The antibiotic rifampicin inhibits alpha-synuclein aggregation in transgenic mouse models of MSA. Unfortunately a recent randomised clinical trial in patients was discontinued for futility at an early stage.

Rodent studies have shown that embryonic striatal graft transplantation can partially restore L dopa responsiveness which if applied to humans might be analogous to turning the parkinsonism of MSA into that of PD; however this has to yet to be trialled in human subjects. One small single-centre study demonstrated some benefit from intra-arterial infusion of mesenchymal stem cells in halting disease progression in a cohort of MSA-C patients; however there are concerns about the safety of this approach and the sustainability of the response. Most recently, monoclonal antibody-based approaches to prevent protein spread and possibly eventually aid clearance have been a focus of research and early trials.

In PSP and CBD, one of the most tractable treatment strategies is to block the aggregation of tau; the hyperphosphorylation step in particular appears to be integral to the pathological process.

Therefore one therapeutic approach is protein kinase inhibitors that inhibit tau phosphorylation. One such agent, tideglusib, failed to be clinically efficacious however; another novel compound, davunetide, which exerts its effects partly through preventing hyperphosphorylation similarly has failed to make a successful transition from bench to bedside. Like other neurodegenerative conditions, strategies that promote tau clearance through proteolytic and/or autophagosomal degradation pathways are also under consideration. Anti-tau immunisation has been attempted in transgenic mice with encouraging early data. Interfering with splicing machinery to decrease the 4R:3R ratio might be another. From the clinical experience to date however, it seems likely that early diagnosis will be essential for neuroprotective strategies to be worthwhile.

Conclusion

The parkinsonism-plus syndromes are uncommon but encountered in clinical practice with enough frequency to warrant careful clinical attention. Their diagnosis is predominantly clinical, and index of suspicion an important element, with some availability of supporting additional investigations. These disorders may declare themselves over time in a parkinsonian patient, making careful repeat assessments important. There are several important prognostic, planning and treatment implications with all of these disorders. While there is no effective disease-modifying treatment, symptomatic treatments can significantly improve quality of life and involvement of the multidisciplinary team is critical in achieving optimal management.

Suggested Reading

Armstrong MJ, et al. Criteria for the diagnosis of corticobasal degeneration. Neurology. 2013;80:496–503.

Alexander SK, et al. Validation of the new consensus criteria for the diagnosis of corticobasal degeneration. J Neurol Neurosurg Psychiatry. 2014;85:923–7.

Donaghy PD, McKeith IG. The clinical characteristics of dementia with Lewy bodies and a consideration of prodromal diagnosis. Alzheimers Res Ther. 2014; 6(4):46.

Gilman S, et al. Second consensus statement on the diagnosis of multiple system atrophy. Neurology. 2008; 71(9):670–6.

Golbe LI. Progressive supranuclear palsy. In: Watts RL, Koller WC, editors. Movement disorders neurological principles and practice. Pa: McGraw-Hill; 1997. p. 279–97.

Lang AE, Riley DE, Bergeron C. Cortical-basal ganglionic degeneration. In: Calne DB, editor. Neurodegenerative diseases. Philadelphia: WB Saunders; 1994. p. 877–94.

Litvan I, et al. Clinical research criteria for the diagnosis of progressive supranuclear palsy (Steele-Richardson-Olszewski syndrome): report of the NINDS-SPSP international workshop. Neurology. 1996;47(1):1–9.

McKeith IG, et al. Diagnosis and management of dementia with Lewy bodies: third report of the DLB consortium. Neurology. 2005;65:1863–72.

Rebeiz JJ, Kolodny EH, Richardson Jr EP. Corticodentatonigral degeneration with neuronal achromasia. Arch Neurol. 1968;18(1):20–33.

Respondek G, et al. The phenotypic spectrum of progressive supranuclear palsy: a retrospective multicenter study of 100 definite cases. Mov Disord. 2014;29(14): 1758–66.

Wenning GK, et al. The natural history of multiple system atrophy: a prospective European cohort study. Lancet Neurol. 2013;12(3):264–74.

Wenning GK, Litvan I, Tolosa E. Milestones in atypical and secondary parkinsonisms. Mov Disord. 2011; 26(6):1083–95.

Williams DR, Lees AJ. What features improve the accuracy of the clinical diagnosis of progressive supranuclear palsy-parkinsonism (PSP-P). Mov Disord. 2010; 25(3):357–62.

Medical Mimics of Neurodegenerative Diseases

Lewis P. Rowland, Peter Bede, Marwa Elamin, and Orla Hardiman

11.1 Introduction

In this chapter, we consider syndromes that resemble neurodegenerative disorders but differ in some essential way. It is important to recognize these mimic syndromes, which may differ from a neurodegenerative condition not only in natural history with periods of stability or even spontaneous improvement, but also because the mimic may be treatable. Clinical examination and judicious use of ancillary studies, as described in each chapter of this book, usually exclude the mimic syndrome, as described in the pages that follow.

11.2 Mimics of Amyotrophic Lateral Sclerosis (ALS)

11.2.1 Benign Fasciculation

Blexrud et al. introduced this term in 1993, identifying the benign clinical course of 121 people

L.P. Rowland
Department of Neurology, The Neurological Institute of New York, Columbia University Medical Center, New York, USA

P. Bede • M. Elamin • O. Hardiman (✉)
Academic Unit of Neurology,
Trinity Biomedical Sciences Institute,
Dublin, Ireland
e-mail: Orla@hardiman.net

with fasciculation with no other abnormality on examination or in electrodiagnostic studies. On follow-up by telephone 2–32 years after this diagnosis, not one of the 121 patients had developed symptomatic ALS. As indicated by Eisen and Stewart in 1994, in response to that report, however, fasciculation may the first manifestation of ALS. Blexrud et al. responded that those patients usually have "weakness or incoordination" in addition to the visible twitching and, additionally, other EMG abnormalities are usually present by that time. Others, including de Carvalho and Swash, reported similar cases in 2004. Bruyn et al. described a patient who had PLS for 27 years before lower motor neuron signs appeared.

11.2.2 Multifocal Motor Neuropathy with Conduction Block

Another important consideration in the differential diagnosis of ALS is multifocal motor Neuropathy with conduction block (MMNCB).

ALS almost always progresses inexorably to death, regardless of therapy. Neither ALS nor MMNCB responds to corticosteroid therapy or plasmapheresis. In contrast, however, MMNCB improves with intravenous immunoglobulin therapy (IvIG) in doses of 400 mg/kg body weight over 5 days. Efficacy has been proven in four randomized controlled trials but there is no consensus about dosage or frequency of treatments

© Springer International Publishing Switzerland 2016
O. Hardiman, C.P. Doherty (eds.), *Neurodegenerative Disorders: A Clinical Guide*,
DOI 10.1007/978-3-319-23309-3_11

to maintain the original improvement. Benefit may be seen within a week of the first series of treatments, and lasting for a variable number of weeks before symptoms may recur. Disability may be severe, but the disease is only rarely fatal.

Demonstration of conduction block in nerve conduction studies is the sine qua non for the diagnosis. Antibodies against GM1 are found in up to 80 % of cases. Clinical clues to the presence of MMNCB include onset before age 50; men affected three times more often than women; hands affected more than legs and bulbar innervated muscles spared; stuttering course and distribution of weakness suggesting mononeuropathy multiplex; more weakness than atrophy; visible fasciculations in about half the patients; and no cutaneous sensory loss. Tendon reflexes are usually absent but may be active in some cases. Hoffmann and Babinski signs are rarely seen. The CSF protein content is usually normal or only slightly elevated up to 80 mg/dl (in contrast to the values near or above 100 mg/dl seen in chronic inflammatory demyelinating polyneuropathy).

Table 11.1 Spinal MRI features of Hirayama disease in Neutral and flexion position

Cervical spine MRI in Hirayama-disease
In neutral neck position
Inferior cervical cord segmental atrophy
Segmental cord flattening
High signal in the anterior aspect of the lower cervical cord
Loss of cervical lordosis
Loss of attachment (LOA) between the posterior dural sac and subjacent lamina
In neck flexion
Anterior shifting of the posterior wall of the dural canal
Enlarged posterior epidural component
Thoracic extension of the inferior cervical posterior epidural component
Prominent posterior epidural flow voids
Asymmetrical cord flattening on axial imaging
Post contrast enhancement of epidural component (Sonwalkar et al. 2008)

11.2.3 Multifocal Acquired Motor Axonopathy

Conduction block is not present in all patients who have the clinical features of motor neuropathy. These patients also respond well to IVIG therapy. In other words, this disorder is a clinical look-alike for MMNCB but lacks the defining physiological characteristics in nerve conduction studies. Moreover, an axonal motor neuropathy is difficult to differentiate from a disease of the cell body itself, i.e., the progressive muscular atrophy (PMA) form of motor neuron disease, although mltifocal acquired motor axonopathy (MAMA) is more likely to be subacute than PMA, which is slowly progressive.

11.3   Hirayama Disease

Hirayama disease (HD), or Juvenile muscular atrophy of the distal upper extremity (JMADUE), is a relatively benign lower motor neuron syndrome. HD is a segmental inferior cervical myelopathy which typically presents with unilateral or asymmetrical upper limb weakness and atrophy in young male patients of Asian descent. The aetiology of the condition is unclear, but the disproportionate growth of the spinal column during growth spurt, anterior horn trauma due to repetitive neck flexion, and posterior epidural venous engorgement were implicated. A background of strenuous physical activity, competitive sport, and repetitive neck flexion is frequently noted. Pathological characterisation of Hirayama's disease was not available until 1982, when histological examination revealed anterior horn degeneration at C7 and C8 with neuronal loss, lipofuscin accumulation, chromatolysis and mild astrogliosis. Spinal imaging in neutral neck position often contain diagnostic clues for Hirayama disease which warrant further imaging in neck flexion to capture disease specific features (Table 11.1). The disease is self-limiting but spinal fusion is occasionally considered to prevent progression. Alternatively, patients are advised to wear a protective collar to prevent excessive neck movements.

11.3.1 Brachial Amyotrophic Diplegia (BAD)

The term brachial amyotrophic diplegia (BAD) has been used to describe a slowly progressive lower motor neuron disorder affecting proximal arm muscles. The wasted arms hang limply at the sides giving the person the appearance of "a man in a barrel." Another moniker is the "flail arm syndrome". In most cases there is no obvious cause but reports have implicated HIV or HTLV-1 infection. In one case an axial view of the cervical spinal cord showed high signal in the anterior horns of the gray matter. Sjögren syndrome was held responsible for one patient with BAD who improved with combination therapy that included prednisone, plasmapheresis, and IVIG.

11.3.2 Cervical Spondylotic Myelopathy

The clinical manifestations of cervical spondylotic myelopathy can rarely mimic ALS. Observations from the Irish and Scottish ALS Registers suggest that cervical spondylotic myelopathy is more likely to show slowly progressive wasting of the arms and hands plus spastic paraplegia. However, there have been few documented reports of visible fasciculation. Also, the rate of progression is slower than in ALS, and the condition may be more symmetric than in ALS. Key clinical features identified by the Irish and Scottish Registers that raised the possibility of cervical myelopathy included the presence of upper motor signs caudal to lower motor signs, early bladder involvement, the absence of bulbar involvement, presence of sensory symptoms and the relatively slow progression. Neuroimaging is helpful in making the diagnosis. However, some people over the age of 40 have spondylosis with cord compression and may even show high signal within the cord—but they are asymptomatic. Also, 5–10 % of people with documented ALS have had cervical decompressive operations without benefit.

Misdiagnosing ALS as cervical myelopathy is more common than the converse.

11.3.3 HIV-Associated ALS

Brachial diplegia has been reported in HIV-positive patients. In 2006, Verma and Berger raised doubts about possibility that HIV might cause ALS because HIV is not a neurotropic virus and because, in comparison with HIV-negative ALS patients, the reported HIV-infected patients were younger, the course of ALS was more rapid, had atypical features and, perhaps most important, the ALS improved in some of those treated with highly active antiretroviral therapy (HAART) for the HIV-infection. On the other hand, about half of the treated HIV-infected patients succumbed to ALS. They concluded that "the causal relationship remains uncertain." Primary lateral sclerosis may also appear with HIV-infections, but is rare.

11.3.4 Other Causes of Reversible Motor Neuron Disease

Motor neuron diseases usually progress inexorably to death. However, cases of complete resolution of sporadic motor neuron diseases with upper and lower motor neuron signs have been reported. The underlying pathology is unclear and such cases are extremely rare: no spontaneous resolutions of ALS have been noted among over 1400 population-based cases collected by the Irish ALS Register over 16 years. West Nile virus infections can cause a reversible poliomyelitis that differs from the others in having a much more acute course. Electrical injury, HTLV-1 infection, and lead intoxication can also cause reversible motor neuron syndromes.

11.4 Reversible Causes of Cognitive Decline

11.4.1 Delirium

This term implies an "acute impairment of cognition with a fluctuating course," including a change in the level of consciousness. Impaired cognition, the acute and transient course, and also the many evident causes of delirium including metabolic, infectious and toxic, differentiate this cerebral dysfunction from both neurodegeneration and from dementia.

However, patients with an underlying dementia are more susceptible to delirium in the context of infection, metabolic changes, or drugs (see also Chaps. 3, 4, 5, and 12).

11.4.2 Mild Cognitive Impairment

Alzheimer disease (AD) classically presents with both subjective and caregiver reports of memory dysfunction which is sub-acute in onset but progressive. The condition tends to evolve with the pathological recruitment of other networks including dorsolateral prefrontal cortex causing executive dysfunction and language networks causing word finding problems. In clinical practice, most physicians deal regularly with patients with subjective complaints in any or all these domains, the majority of whom do not have a neurodegenerative disorder. In many cases, depression, anxiety or psychosocial stress can play a significant role. The lack of objective concern in family and caregivers, and the performance on standardized delayed word recall testing are usually enough to reassure. Nevertheless, there are some patients with mild subjective symptoms, without any negative effective on work or social performance who score poorly on testing and may have what we call "mild cognitive impairment" (MCI). This condition is believed to be in excess of what might be expected with normal aging and is a risk factor for the development of clinical dementia. The exact risk is unclear but about 80 % of MCI patients progress eventually to AD (see also Chap. 4). The remaining 20 % either remain stable or may even improve, two features that point towards a mimic syndrome rather than a neurodegenerative one. The mechanisms underpinning stable or improving MCI are unclear.

11.4.3 Drug Induced Encephalopathy

Medications are listed as the most common cause of reversible "dementia" but some drug effects must also include obtundation in addition to cognitive decline. That would be defined as delirium rather than dementia. Common causal drugs include anticholinergics, tricyclic antidepressants, opiate analgesia, antipsychotics, bismuth (in the form of bismuth subsalicylate, available as an over-the-counter medication), bromides, digoxin, antihistamines, antiepileptics, dopamine antagonist antiemetics, and lithium (See Table 11.2).

The evaluation of a patient with cognitive impairment should therefore include a careful medication history, including a complete review of all over-the-counter medications.

11.4.4 Epilepsy

Non-convulsive status epilepticus or clusters of non-convulsive seizures may be focal onset or be part of a generalized epileptic syndrome. Occasionally, the only clinical manifestation may be altered mental status that appears more like delirium than dementia. Some patients, however, especially the elderly, may maintain such vigilance that the patient merely appears cognitively impaired. This has been called 'epileptic pseudodementia' a rare disorder that can be diagnosed only in the presence of unequivocal prolonged epileptiform discharges on the electroencephalogram (EEG) of the cognitively impaired patient. Treatment is that for other forms of non-convulsive status but as the term 'epileptic pseudodementia' implies a prolonged course, the prognosis for eventual recovery is poor.

11.4.5 Subdural Hematoma

Chronic subdural hematoma is the most frequent type of intracranial hemorrhage and may occur in the elderly following minor trauma. Patients may

Table 11.2 Common drugs that can cause cognitive impairment

Drug	Effect
Amitriptyline	Anticholinergic properties: Sedation, confusion, delirium, or hallucinations
Anticholinergics	Sedation, confusion, delirium, or hallucinations
Anticonvulsants valproate, levetiracetam	Confusion, sedation, elevated ammonia Confusion, hallucinations
Antihistamines	Anticholinergic properties: sedation, confusion, delirium, or hallucinations
Antipsychotics	Confusion, sedation
Antispasmodics (GI)	Anticholinergic properties : Confusion, delirium, or hallucinations
Baclofen	Hallucinations, impaired memory, catatonia, mania
Barbiturates	Drowsiness, lethargy, depression, severe CNS depression
Long-acting benzodiazepines	Sedation, drowsiness, ataxia, fatigue, confusion, weakness, dizziness, vertigo, syncope, psychological changes
Bismuth subsalicylate	Encephalopathy resembling dementia. Encephalopathy resembling CJD
Chlorpropamide	Hypoglycemia, which can result in altered mental state (confusion, amnesia, coma)
Digitalis	Headache, fatigue, malaise, drowsiness, and depression
H2 Receptor Antagonists	Confusion, hallucinations, agitation
Indomethacin	Headache, dizziness, vertigo, somnolence, depression, fatigue
Lithium	Confusion, sedation, movement disorder
Methyldopa	May exacerbate depression
Muscle Relaxants	Anticholinergic properties, weakness, confusion, delirium, or hallucinations
Pentazocine	Confusion, hallucinations, dizziness, lightheadedness, euphoria, and sedation
Reserpine	Depression, sedation

show a slow decline in cognitive function with confusion, impaired memory, headache and motor deficits or aphasia. Chronic subdural hematoma or hygroma should therefore be considered in the differential dementia of cognitive impairment. Diagnosis is by neuroimaging, and treatment is surgical evacuation.

11.4.6 Sleep Apnea

Sleep apnea can be associated with memory loss. Patients may present with symptoms suggestive on cognitive decline, and can account for up to 8 % of patients attending a young onset dementia clinic. Symptoms include daytime somnolence, snoring, and morning headache. The reversible cognitive decline is thought to relate to sleep deprivation and nocturnal hypoxemia. The diagnosis is established by overnight polysomnography with oxygen saturation monitoring. Treatment is with non invasive ventilation using a continuous positive air way pressure (CPAP) device.

11.4.7 Neuropsychiatric Conditions Associated with Reversible Cognitive Decline

11.4.7.1 Depression
Depressive pseudodementia has been defined as a reversible cognitive impairment of the type seen in dementia. It is associated with delusions and a history of affective illness.

There are few studies of the frequency of depressive pseudodementia, although rates as high as 18 % have been reported in specialist dementia referral centers.

Patients with cognitive impairment and concomitant depression should be treated aggressively with antidepressants and psychotherapy. However, clinically depressed patients with signs of pseudodementia are at higher risk of developing irreversible dementia in 2 or more years. This suggests that depression with reversible cognitive

Table 11.3 Abnormal signs in catatonia

Motor	Speech & language	Behavioral	Autonomic	Laboratory
Akinesia	Mutism	Agitation	Hypertension	Leukocytosis
Bradykinesia	Aphasia	Impaired	Pyrexia	Elevated creatine
Parkinsonism	Palilalia	judgment	Diaphoresis	kinase (CPK)
Tremor		Impaired insight	Insomnia	Abnormal EEG
Stupor			Tachycardia	
Primitive Reflexes				
Upgoing Plantars				
Oculomotor signs				
Tics				

impairment could be a prodromal phase for dementia rather than a risk factor, and that patients with depressive pseudodementia should be followed closely.

The prevalence of depression in people with Parkinson disease varies in different reports from 20 to 80 % and often starts before the motor signs appear (See also Chap. 5). This problem of diagnosis is compounded because some syndromes are common in both conditions: bradykinesia, bradyphrenia, sleep and autonomic disorders, anorexia and weight loss, apathy, and loss of libido. However, the fundamental signs of parkinsonism (include tremor, cogwheel rigidity, loss of dexterity, deterioration of handwriting, frequent falls or loss of postural control) are not seen in patients with depression.

Severe depression may also mimic a predominantly apathetic presentation of FTD; cognitive testing should help distinguish the two with dysexecutive features much more prominent in the dementia (see also Chap. 7).

11.4.7.2 Catatonia

This complex neuropsychiatric syndrome may be seen with either a primary psychiatric disorder or with a general medical condition. Catatonia may mimic other neurodegenerative conditions including, FTD and Parkinson disease (Table 11.3). The acute onset of catatonia, with alternating agitation, stupor, and dysautonomia may respond to high-dose lorazepam or electroconvulsive therapy.

11.4.7.3 Conversion Disorder

Conversion disorder is characterized by loss or alteration of physical function that suggests a physical disorder, but that has a psychological

Table 11.4 DSM IV criteria for conversion disorder

Patient has one or more symptom affecting voluntary, motor or sensory function that suggests a neurological or medical condition.
Psychological factors are associated with the symptom or deficit.
Symptom or deficit is not intentionally produced, but is maintained by secondary gain.
Symptom or deficit cannot be fully explained by a general medical condition, by direct effects of a substance, or as a culturally sanctioned behavior or experience.
Symptom or deficit causes clinically significant distress or impairment in social, occupational or other important areas of functioning, or warrants medical explanation.
Symptom or deficit is not limited to pain or sexual dysfunction, and is not better accounted for by another mental disorder.

basis. Although conversion disorder are more likely to occur in younger patients—onset is unusual after 35 years of age, symptoms can mimic neurodegenerative disease. Common psychogenic mimic symptoms include limb paralysis, diverse movement disorders, gait disturbances, blindness and deafness. The patient's behavior seems inappropriately accepting of or indifferent to the serious physical symptoms.

The Diagnostic and Statistical Manual of Mental Disorders (DSM IV) lists six criteria that must be filled for the diagnosis of conversion disorder (Table 11.4). All neurological and medical causes must be excluded.

11.4.7.4 Late Onset Psychiatric Disease

Late onset psychiatric disease may mimic frontotemporal dementia.

Of the three main clinical syndromes of FTD (See Chap. 7), the behavioral variant FTD (bv-FTD), is the one most likely to be confused with a mimic disorder, the others having a more characteristic language dysfunction (semantic dementia or progressive aphasia). Detailed neuropsychological testing is helpful in distinguishing organic disease from a late onset psychiatric disorder.

11.4.8 Nutritional Causes of Reversible Cognitive Decline

Nutritional causes of cognitive decline may be detected by clues in different systems.

11.4.8.1 Wernicke Encephalopathy
This is the result of thiamine deficiency, usually with other nutritional deprivations with alcohol abuse. In addition to the cognitive disorder, the full syndrome includes ophthalmoparesis and ataxia. It is also seen with dialysis, after bariatric surgery or intravenous administration of glucose. Subacute forms have been reported in a range gastrointestinal conditions such as Crohn's disease, celiac disease, pancreatitis and other malabsorption syndromes.

11.4.8.2 Pellagra
Vitamin B3 deficiency (niacin deficiency) may manifest by dementia, dermatitis, and diarrhea. Vestibular symptoms, ataxia, nystagmus and peripheral neuropathy often precede dementia. Carcinoid syndrome may lead to relative niacin deficiency because neuroendocrine tumors synthetize serotonin instead of niacin from the essential amino acid tryptophan. Isoniazid and chloramphenicol also reduce niacin synthesis. If unrecognized and untreated, it may be fatal.

Both Wernicke syndrome and pellagra differ from neurodegeneration syndromes in younger age at onset, more acute onset, more rapid progression, and reversibility with replacement therapy.

11.4.8.3 B12 Deficiency
Whether B12 deficiency causes a dementia-like disorder has been controversial, but it seems to be standard practice to test blood levels routinely and, if values are low, to administer the missing cobalamin. The neurological syndrome ("combined system disease") that accompanies pernicious anemia results from both myelopathy and sensorimotor polyneuropathy. Severity of the disorder is related to duration of symptoms before treatment. Symptoms may include ataxia of gait, distal paresthesias, dementia, psychosis, or visual loss. Many individuals with B12 deficiency are asymptomatic these days but some have one or more co-morbid autoimmune diseases. Tendon reflexes may be increased or decreased and upper motor neuron signs may be evident. Distal sensory loss and impaired perception of limb position may be found.

Almost all patients improve with treatment and, in about half, recovery is complete. Dementia has been reversed by treatment even when B12 levels are still in the low normal range.

11.4.8.4 Refeeding Syndrome
Refeeding syndrome is a complex metabolic and hormonal disturbance which may lead to delerium, convulsions and coma if not considered in severely malnourished patients. During refeeding, insulin levels increase and glucose, potassium and magnesium are shifted intracellularly. This rapidly leads to significant serum hypophosphataemia, hypomagnesaemia and hypokalaemia hich are responsible for refeeding syndrome. Careful monitoring and replacement of these electrolytes in malnourished patients along with B12 vitamin supplementation makes this a preventable syndrome.

11.4.9 Toxic Exposures

Many heavy metals, pesticides, solvents and gasses can lead to neurological deficits that can mimic a neurodegenerative process. For example, manganese toxicity can induce a parkinsonian syndrome, lead and arsenic toxicity can induce an encephalopathy, and chronic inhalation of low dose elemental mercury is associated with ataxia and cognitive impairment.

11.4.9.1 Alcohol

The most common toxic exposure is to ethanol. Alcohol abuse is associated with a wide range of neurological and neuropsychiatric syndromes including cerebellar degeneration, alcoholic polyneuropathy, Wernicke-Korsakoff syndrome, and alcohol-related dementia. Although the concept of a dementia that is directly related to alcohol abuse remains controversial, in the United States, it is estimated that alcohol-related dementia accounts for up to 20 % of admissions to state psychiatric facilities. The mechanism of alcohol-associated cognitive decline is poorly understood, and there are no established treatment protocols other than abstinence with psychosocial supports.

11.4.9.2 Carbon Monoxide

Acute exposure to carbon monoxide is one of the most common causes of poisoning requiring admission to hospital. In the United States the incidence of suspected carbon monoxide poisoning is approximately 1/10,000 per annum. Acute intoxication can lead to encephalopathy and coma. Up to 50 % of individuals with carbon monoxide poisoning subsequently develop neurologic, neurobehavioral, or cognitive sequelae. Some patients experience a progressive course, with development of a persistent akinetic-mute state. Other patients experience a delayed relapse after an initial recovery period of approximately 3 weeks. Those with the delayed relapsing course can develop a parkinsonian state with behavioral and cognitive impairment. Brain MRI reveals multiple lesions in the subcortical white matter and basal ganglia, mostly in the globus pallidus, and to a lesser extent in putamen, and caudate.

Diagnosis should be suspected if the partial pressure of blood oxygen is low, in the presence of apparently normal oxygen saturation. Carboxyhemoglobin to hemoglobin ration can either be measured directly or estimated using Pulse CO-oximeters. Treatment is with hyperbaric oxygen.

11.4.10 Endocrine Causes of Reversible Cognitive Decline

11.4.10.1 Thyroid Disease

Clinical hypothyroidism may cause cognitive impairment, which can be reversed if treated early. There are no long term cognitive sequelae in treated hypothyroidism.

Hyperthyroidism can cause tremulousness, chorea and encephalopathy. Symptoms resolve with treatment.

11.4.10.2 Hashimoto Encephalopathy

Encephalopathy in people with high levels of antibodies to thyroid antigens (thyroperoxidase and thyroid microsomal proteins) has long been considered a specific syndrome, one likely to respond to prednisone therapy, and called "Hashimoto encephalopathy". Most of the cases with this neurologic syndrome have had Hashimoto thyroiditis. Other autoimmune thyroid diseases have also been described, mainly Graves disease. The pathogenesis of this encephalopathy is still unknown and largely debated. Cerebral symptoms include stroke-like episodes, coma, seizures, subacute cognitive decline, and hallucinations. However, high serum levels of the same thyroid antibodies may be found in many asymptomatic people. Moreover, it has not been proven that the antibodies cause the symptoms (or how they might do so) and steroid therapy may fail in 50 % of otherwise typical cases. Some authors have advocated brain biopsy as an important diagnostic test, primarily to exclude Creutzfeldt-Jakob disease.

In 1999, Caselli et al. proposed a more formal name, but the simpler eponym, honoring Hashimoto, has not disappeared. The syndrome is subacute in onset and course, another difference from the chronic features of neurodegeneration.

11.4.11 Posterior Reversible Encephalopathy Syndrome

Posterior reversible encephalopathy syndrome (PRES) or reversible posterior leukoencephalopathy syndrome (RPLS) has been first described in

Table 11.5 Paraneoplastic neurological syndromes

Antibody	Tumor	CNS syndrome
Hu	Small cell lung carcinoma	Encephalomyelitis, paraneoplastic cerebellar degeneration, limbic encephalitis
CV2 (CRMP 5)	Small cell lung carcinoma, Thymoma	Encephalomyelitis, Chorea, Cerebellar degeneration Limbic encephalitis
Amphiphysin	Breast, small cell lung carcinoma	Stiff person syndrome, encephalomyelitis
Ri	Breast, small cell lung carcinoma	Brainstem encephalitis, cerebellar degeneration, opsoclonus myoclonus
Yo	Breast, ovary	Paraneoplastic cerebellar degeneration
Ma2	Testicular	Limbic encephalitis, brainstem encephalitis
Voltage gated potassium channel	Small cell lung cancer, thymoma	Limbic encephalitis, Morvan syndrome, Creutzfeldt Jacob-like syndrome
NMDA Receptor	Ovarian teratoma	Encephalitis with catatonia, dystonia, psychiatric symptoms
AMPA Receptor	Small cell lung carcinoma, Thymoma	Limbic encephalitis, psychosis
Gaba B Receptor	Small cell lung carcinoma	Limbic encephalitis
Glycine Receptor	Lung carcinoma	Encephalomyelitis, stiff person syndrome

1996 by Hinchey et al. It may manifest as delirium, seizures, visual disturbance, nausea and vomiting with poorly localizing but alarming constellation of neurological signs. PRES is diagnosed clinically, but supported by bilateral occipital, parietal and pontine signal intensities on T2-weighted or FLAIR MR imaging. The thalami and basal ganglia may also be involved. Typically, no gadolinium enhancement is observed, but mild sulcal effacement and mass effect with oedema is frequently noted. PRES is associated by a number of systemic conditions such as eclampsia, sustained hypertension, renal failure, post-partum, or following cytotoxic or immunosuppressive therapy, such as cyclophosphamide administration. The mainstay of management is the treatment of the underlying condition which typically leads to radiological and clinical resolution within 1–2 weeks,

11.4.12 Paraneoplastic Causes of Cognitive Decline

Cognitive impairment is sometimes seen in patients with malignant tumors, especially small cell lung cancer, lymphoma, thymoma or testicular cancer (Table 11.5). The complex paraneoplastic syndromes include disordered sleep patterns, hallucinations, behavioral anomalies, orthostatic hypotension and the Morvan syndrome (neuromyotonia, hypersalivation, hyperhidrosis, and insomnia). The clinical picture is that of limbic encephalitis with manifestations that evolve in days or weeks.

Other features that distinguish these syndromes are imaging abnormalities in the temporal lobes, non-infective CSF pleocytosis, and presence of serum antibodies to the Hu antigen, anti-Ma, and (in the Morvan syndrome) anti-voltage-gated potassium channels (VGKC) as well as other antigens.

11.4.13 Non-Paraneoplastic Autoimmune Syndromes

Antibodies to VGKC have been found in several reversible conditions without an underlying neoplasm, but the critical antigen and target of the antibodies is the synaptic protein leucine-rich glioma-inactivated 1 (LGI1). The ensuing condition is an autoimmune synaptic encephalopathy. The clinical features of the associated limbic encephalitis may be the subacute onset of episodic memory impairment, disorientation and agitation. Movement disorders may also occur, and some patients have hyponatremia.

Treatment with prednisone, intravenous immunoglobulins, or plasmapheresis leads to improvement of about 80 % of patients with VGKC antibodies. Although these findings suggest autoimmunity, it is not clear how these or other antibodies damage the brain.

11.5   Superficial Siderosis

Superficial siderosis is a relatively uncommon condition caused by hemosiderin deposition in anatomical structures exposed to the cerebrospinal fluid in the subarachnoid space. It typically results from chronic subarachnoid haemorrhage from arteriovenous malformations, ependymoma, neurosurgery or prior CNS trauma. Frequently no underlying aetiology is identified despite extensive neuroimaging. The manifestations of superficial siderosis are diverse ranging from cognitive impairment, ataxia, sensorineural hearing loss, anosmia and it may manifest in upper motor neuron dysfunction. A hypointense rim may be visible on axial T2-weighted MR imaging around the spinal cord, medulla, pons and cerebellum. The identification of the source of the bleeding can be challenging and if not identified treatment with iron chelators such as deferiprone is often attempted.

11.6   Mimics of Parkinson Disease

11.6.1   Tauopathies, Dementia, and Parkinsonism

Neurodegeneration may cause parkinsonian disorders that can be divided into two major categories based on postmortem histological findings. First, are the synucleinopathies, which include Parkinson disease dementia (PDD), dementia with Lewy bodies, and multiple system atrophy. Disorders in the second group are "tauopathies", including progressive supranuclear palsy and corticobasal degeneration, as well as AD and FTLD. Both categories are multisystem syndromes and both include clinical manifestations of parkinsonism in combination with dementia, oculomotor abnormalities and other basal ganglia signs (Table 11.6). Therefore, parkinsonism can result from other mimic conditions. (See also Chaps. 4, 6, 7, and 10).

11.6.2   Drug-Induced Parkinsonism

Fifty years ago, reserpine was found to cause parkinsonian symptoms and signs, an observation leading to the discovery that dopamine content in the brain is depleted in Parkinson disease. Tetrabenazine administration also depletes dopamine and can also cause parkinsonism. Later came the antipsychotic neuroleptics, which act by a different mechanism, blocking receptors for dopamine and also inducing parkinsonism. Some neuroleptic drugs were first thought to cause fewer extrapyramidal disorders and were therefore called 'atypical' but that view was proven wrong with continued experience.

The neuroleptic drugs include haloperidol, chlorpromazine and metoclopramide. Other pathophysiological mechanisms seem to be involved in the parkinsonian syndromes ascribed to fluoxetine, lithium, amiodarone or valproic acid (Table 11.7). Mild parkinsonism is sometimes tolerated for the beneficial antipsychotic effects of quetiapine, olanzapine, and risperidone.

Drug-induced parkinsonism can mimic Parkinson disease in all major features including rigidity, bradykinesia, tremor and postural abnormalities. Bradykinesia is the most common symptom. The condition can be distinguished from idiopathic Parkinson disease by the history of drug exposure in the context of symptom-onset, age at onset, duration of symptoms, the nature of the tremor (pill rolling tremor is rare in drug-induced parkinsonism), the presence of symmetry (Parkinson disease tends to be asymmetric), and response to anticholinergics (Table 11.8). Neuroleptic-induced parkinsonism usually improves when the offending drug is discontinued, but recovery may take several weeks.

Table 11.6 Classification of Parkinsonian dementia syndromes

Etiology	Clinical manifestations
Degenerative	
PDD	Parkinsonism precedes dementia.
DLB	Visual hallucinations, fluctuating mental state; variable parkinsonism; REM sleep disorder; neuroleptic sensitivity; falls.
PSP	Impaired balance, bulbar signs, down-gaze limited.
CBD	Dementia with limb apraxia, myoclonus, parkinsonism
MSA Cerebellar (OPCA)	Brainstem signs; cerebellar atrophy; oculomotor disorders.
MSA Parkinsonism	Parkinsonism; autonomic disorders (urinary incontinence; orthostatic hypotension; cerebellar signs).
Prion Disorders	Rapidly progressing dementia, ataxia, PRES.
Secondary Parkinsonism	
Drug-induced	Neuroleptics; metaclopramide, promethazine, valproate.
Vascular	Subcortical infarcts, white matter lesions.
NPH	Magnetic gait, urinary incontinence, dementia.
Hereditable metabolic disorders	
Wilson disease	Abnormal copper metabolism, hepatic failure, Kayser-Fleischer rings.
Hallervorden-Spatz ("Neurodegeneration with brain iron accumulation", NBIA)	Iron deposits in basal ganglia; familial or sporadic with parkinsonism, dystonia, dementia.
Basal ganglia calcification (Fahr disease).	Familial, autosomal dominant or recessive dementia with parkinsonism.

Reproduced from Possin and Kaufer (2010)
Abbreviations: *CBD* Corticobasal degeneration, *CBS* Corticobasal syndrome, *DLB* Dementia with Lewy bodies, *PDD* Parkinson disease dementia, *MSA* Multiple system atrophy, *NPH* Normal pressure hydrocephalus, *OPCA* Olivopontocerebellar syndrome, *PRES* Posterior reversible encephalopathy syndrome, *PSP* Progressive supranuclear palsy, *REM* Rapid eye movement

Table 11.7 Drugs that can MIMIC Parkinson disease

Neuroleptics
Reserpine
Tetrabenazine
Methyldopa
Alpha methyltyrosine
Lithium
Diazoxide
Physostigmine
Metocolpramide
Trazodone
Meperidine
Cimetidine
Cinnarizine
Flunarizine

Table 11.8 Differentiation of Parkinsonian disorders

	Idiopathic Parkinson disease	Drug induced Parkinsonism
Exposure to neuroleptics	No	Yes
Age at onset	>50	<50
Natural history	Progressive	Resolves after discontinuation of neuroleptic
Tremor	4–6 Hz, supination pronation	Action/Postural
Distribution	Asymmetric	Symmetric

11.6.3 Street Drugs and Frozen Addicts

Sometimes, persistent parkinsonism after withdrawal of the offending drug proves to be the onset of true Parkinson disease.

In 1984, Langston and associates described the appearance of parkinsonism in men who were using a home-brewed version of meperidine. The contaminant that proved to be causal was

N-methyl-4-phenyl-1,2,3,6-tetrahydropyridine (MPTP). The parkinsonian features were comparable those seen in PD and were partially responsive to levodopa but seemed permanent. Animal models of PD have been created with MPTP and 5-hydroxy tryptophan. Ephedrone (methcathinone) is another intoxicant that can cause parkinsonism in opiate addicts.

11.6.4 Vascular Parkinsonism

Whether cerebrovascular disease can cause parkinsonism is a question that does not go away. Critics point out that both conditions are relatively common and affect elderly people. Even by chance, the presence of either disorder is probably a risk factor for the other. Nevertheless, vascular parkinsonism and Parkinson disease differ in clinical manifestations

Vascular parkinsonism is less likely to include the pill-rolling tremor, and is more likely to affect the lower body, with postural instability, freezing, and falling, as well as hyperactive tendon reflexes with Hoffmann and Babinski signs. These patients are more likely to have had a history of stroke, are more likely to have stroke risk factors (hypertension, smoking, diabetes, hyperlipidemia, heart disease) and are much less likely to benefit from levodopa therapy.

This debate involved two of neurology's leaders. In a multi-authored 1954 book on parkinsonism, the editor (Lewis J. Doshay) asked Houston Merritt to write the preface. He opined: "It is also possible that degeneration of the basal ganglia, as a result of arteriosclerosis, can produce the characteristic symptoms, but the pathological evidence for such a relationship is not unequivocal. In addition, there are few satisfactory criteria for the establishment of the clinical entity of arteriosclerotic parkinsonism." Merritt attributed the disorder to "unknown cause" or "so-called idiopathic parkinsonism". A few pages later, Denny-Brown wrote a section entitled "Arteriosclerotic Parkinsonism.". Neither author referred to the other.

11.6.5 Normal Pressure Hydrocephalus

Normal pressure hydrocephalus (NPH) is the main problem in differential diagnosis of vascular parkinsonism; bradykinesia is seen in almost half of NPH patients and frank parkinsonism has been reported in up to 11 % of those patients. The clinical syndrome is the triad of dementia, ataxia, and urinary incontinence. Numerous imaging tests have been advocated to improve prediction of a good response to diverting the outflow of CSF. If CSF drainage and shunting help relieve NPH, the parkinsonism may also improve.

11.6.6 Binswanger Disease (Subcortical Vascular Cognitive Impairment, Leukoaraiosis)

Vladimir Hachinski, the modern authority on this syndrome, concluded that the eponym should not be used. With John Bowler, he writes that "Binswanger" has become a popular term in the era of modern imaging to describe asymptomatic changes seen in MRI or CT. However, they prefer the word "leukoaraiosis" for that asymptomatic condition. A dictionary definition of leukoaraiosis is: "Decreased vascular density, especially in deep white matter in the brain, on MRI or CT; may be caused by demyelination, gliosis, or decreased perfusion." Bowler and Hachinski describe MRI changes of "extensive deep white matter lesions sparing subcortical U-fibers and corpus callosum." That is, the disorder is defined by the MRI appearance of diffuse high signal in the white matter. It is often seen in asymptomatic people but may be seen with dementia or parkinsonism. Cognitive impairment is seen more often than the vascular parkinsonism described above. Despite admonitions from respected authorities, the eponym honoring Binswanger is still used for the combination of dementia with imaging evidence of "subcortical vascular cognitive impairment". (See also Chap. 4.)

11.6.7 Hepatolenticular Degeneration (Wilson Disease) and Other Hereditary Movement Disorders

According to a literature review by Lorincz, parkinsonism is seen about 17 % of patients with Wilson disease, with onset of symptoms at about age 20. Liver failure is usually evident and cerebellar tremor is seen more often than parkinsonism (mean 36 %) so the correct diagnosis is usually evident. Pfeiffer, however, was skeptical about any association of parkinsonism with Wilson disease. Similarly, juvenile parkinsonism may be seen with mutations of other movement disorder genes, including Huntington disease, dentatorubro-pallidoluysian atrophy, Hallervorden-Spatz disease, and neuronal intranuclear inclusion disease as well as mutations of mitochondrial DNA.

11.6.8 Idiopathic Basal Ganglia Calcification (FAHR Syndrome)

Once again, experts disparage use of the eponym in reviewing this syndrome. Yet, once again, the eponym continues to be used. The disease is defined by the imaging abnormalities that show widespread intracranial calcification of the basal ganglia, with or without concomitant hypoparathyroidism, and clinically manifest by dementia, parkinsonism, or both. In some families, inheritance seems to be autosomal dominant. Calcific deposits are sometimes seen with other diffuse cerebral disorders.

11.6.9 Pantothenate Kinase-Associated Neurodegeneration (PKAN) (Hallervorden-Spatz Disease)

Most often this is a disease of children but symptom-onset occurs after age 10 in about 25 % of affected people. Inheritance is autosomal

recessive and caused by mutations in *PANK2*, which leads to iron deposition in the basal ganglia. Symptoms include dystonia, dysarthria, pigmentary retinopathy, and lower body parkinsonism. Orobuccolingual dystonia may cause mutilating tongue-biting. Upper motor neuron signs may be seen. MRI shows the eye-of-the-tiger sign, a central hyperintensity surrounded by hypointensity on T2 images of the globus pallidus.

Conclusion

Careful attention to history and clinical examination is required to ensure that important clues to a mimic syndrome are not overlooked. Atypical features should be assiduously assessed and pursued. Systemic signs may point to an underlying neoplasm, raising the possibility of a paraneoplastic disorder. A history of poor sleep and loud snoring may reveal a diagnosis of sleep apnea.

Routine hematological and biochemical tests should be performed in all cases, as should CSF analysis and detailed neuroimaging. Heavy metal screening may be useful in those with occupational exposures. EEG can be helpful in differentiating clinical sydromes-for example the preservation of alpha rhythm in the FTDs and its early disintegration in AD (Chaps. 4 and 7); or the presence of epileptiform changes in a patient with epilepsy associated amnesia. Nerve conduction studies can identify evidence of conduction block in patients with multifocal motor neuropathy (Chap. 8).

The course of mimic syndromes often differs from true neurodegenerative disease, and perhaps the most important diagnostic test is careful clinical evaluation over time. Patients should be reviewed regularly.

Failure to progress, or the development of new or atypical signs should trigger a full re-evaluation. And during each clinical review, the clinical should pose the question: "Could this be a mimic syndrome?"

Further Reading

Blexrud MD, Windebank AJ, Daube JR. Long-term follow-up of 121 patients with benign fasciculations. Ann Neurol. 1993;34:622–5.

Bowler JV, Hachinski V. Subcortical vascular cognitive impairment. Medlink, 16 Sep 2009, http://www.medlink.com/article/wilson_disease.

Bosco DA, Morfini G, Karabacak NM, Song Y, Gros-Louis F, Pasinelli P, Goolsby H, Fontaine BA, Lemay N, McKenna-Yasek D, Frosch MP, Agar JN, Julien JP, Brady ST, Brown Jr RH. Wild-type and mutant SOD1 share an aberrant conformation and a common pathogenic pathway in ALS. Nat Neurosci. 2010;13(11):1396–403. Epub 2010 Oct 17.

Bruyn RP, Koelman JH, Troost D, de Jong JM. Motor neuron disease (amyotrophic lateral sclerosis) arising from longstanding primary lateral sclerosis. J Neurol Neurosurg Psychiatry. 1995;58(6):742–4.

Caselli RJ, Boeve BF, Schellhauser BW, O'Duffy JD, Hunder GG. Nonvasculitic autoimmune inflammatory meningoencephalitis (NAIM): a reversible form of encephalopathy. Neurology. 1999;53:1579–81.

de Carvalho M, Swash M. Cramps, muscle pain, and fasciculations: not always benign? Neurology. 2004;63(4):721–3.

Eisen A, Stewart H. Not-so-benign fasciculation. Ann Neurol. 1994;35:375.

Graus F, Saiz A, Dalmau J. Antibodies and neuronal autoimmune disorders of the CNS. J Neurol. 2010;257:509–17.

Iqbal S, Clower JH, Boehmer TK, Yip FY, Garbe P. Carbon monoxide-related hospitalizations in the U.S.: evaluation of a web-based query system for public health surveillance. Public Health Rep. 2010;125(3):423–32.

Lorincz MT. Wilson disease. 24 Jun 2009. http://www.medlink.com/article/subcortical_vascular_cognitive_impairment.

Meuth SG, Kleinschnitz C. Multifocal motor neuropathy: update on clinical characteristics, pathophysiological concepts and therapeutic options. Eur Neurol. 2010;193:204.

Mills KR. Characteristics of fasciculations in amyotrophic lateral sclerosis and the benign fasciculation syndrome. Brain. 2010;133(11):3458–69. doi: 10.1093/brain/awq290. Epub 2010 Oct 19.

Parry GJ, Clarke S. Multifocal acquired demyelinating neuropathy masquerading as motor neuron disease. Muscle Nerve. 1988;11:103–7.

Pfeiffer RF. Wilson's disease. Semin Neurol. 2007;27:123–32.

Possin KL, Kaufer DI. Parkinsonian dementias. Continuum Minneap Minn. 2010;16(2):57–79.

Sáez-Fonseca JA, Lee L, Walker Z. Long-term outcome of depressive pseudodementia in the elderly. J Affect Disord. 2007;101(1–3):123–9.

Singh V, Gibson J, McLean B, Boggild M, Silver N, White R. Fasciculations and cramps: how benign? Report of four cases progressing to ALS. J Neurol. 2010;258(4):573–8. published online.

Toothaker TB, Rubin M. Paraneoplastic neurological syndromes: a review. Neurologist. 2009;15(1):21–33.

Traynor BJ, Codd MB, Corr B, Forde C, Frost E, Hardiman O. Amyotrophic lateral sclerosis mimic syndromes: a population-based study. Arch Neurol. 2000;57(1):109–13.

Tucker T, Layzer RB, Miller RG, Chad D. Subacute, reversible motor neuron disease. Neurology. 1991;41(10):1541–4.

Tullberg M, Ziegelitz D, Ribbelin S, Ekholm S. White matter diffusion is higher in Binswanger disease than in normal pressure hydrocephalus. Acta Neurol Scand. 2009;120:226–34.

Verma A, Berger JR. ALS syndrome in patients with HIV-1 infection. J Neurol Sci. 2006;240:59–64.

Winnikates J, Jankovic J. Clinical correlates of vascular parkinsonism. Arch Neurol. 1999;56:98–102.

Prion Diseases

12

Simon Mead and Peter Rudge

12.1 Introduction

Prion diseases are a diverse group of human and animal neurodegenerative disorders; examples include sheep scrapie, bovine spongiform encephalopathy (BSE) and human Creutzfeldt–Jakob disease (CJD). The most notable feature of these diseases is the potential for transmission between humans and animals. The pathogenesis of these conditions involves a cell surface glycoprotein termed the 'prion protein' (or PrP^C, "C" for cellular or normal isoform). Human prion diseases are most usefully classified by aetiology as inherited, acquired or unknown (sporadic). In general physicians should consider these diseases in patients presenting with rapidly progressive dementias and in those with dementia and additional neurological signs or psychiatric symptoms. As will be described below however, the group is remarkable for its heterogeneity and has mimicked virtually all other neurodegenerative syndromes in the early phases.

The infectious agent of prion disease comprises an abnormal isoform of the prion protein (termed PrP^{Sc}, "Sc" for scrapie isoform). PrP^C is found on cell surfaces throughout the body, but with enhanced expression in the nervous and immune systems. It predominantly has an alpha helix structure and its function is unknown (Fig. 12.1). The

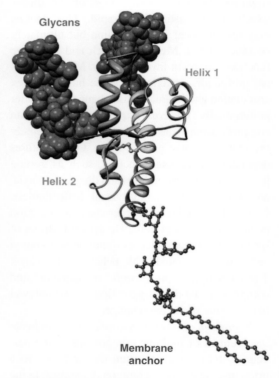

Fig. 12.1 Image of the structure of PrP^C showing three alpha helices, a single disulphide bond, up to two carbohydrate moieties and attachment to the cell surface via a glycosylinositolphosphate anchor. An N-terminal region containing octapeptide repeats appears to be unstructured and is not shown

S. Mead (✉) • P. Rudge
MRC Prion Unit, Department of Neurodegenerative Disease, UCL Institute of Neurology, Queen Square, London WC1N 3BG, UK

NHS National Prion Clinic, National Hospital for Neurology and Neurosurgery, University College London Hospitals NHS Foundation Trust, London, UK
e-mail: simon.mead@prion.ucl.ac.uk

© Springer International Publishing Switzerland 2016
O. Hardiman, C.P. Doherty (eds.), *Neurodegenerative Disorders: A Clinical Guide*,
DOI 10.1007/978-3-319-23309-3_12

disease-associated form of the protein is largely of beta-sheet structure although the precise structure of the infectious form remains uncertain. Many prion diseases are transmissible; it is hypothesized that transmission occurs because the misfolded protein acts as a template that encourages conversion of normal host prion protein into the form detected in disease.

12.2 Clinical Features of Prion Diseases

12.2.1 General Overview

Although there is considerable heterogeneity in the clinical picture of the prion diseases there are a number of core features. All are associated with *cognitive* decline at some stage of the illness which characteristically is rapid. This decline may remain focal for some time but ultimately becomes global. Memory, speech and executive functions are often involved early. Many patients are profoundly apraxic and some have complex articulation and language disturbances. The latter preferentially involves expression rather than comprehension in most cases and can be extremely prominent in some genetic types. Other features dependent on parietal function, such as getting lost in familiar surroundings and dressing apraxia, are frequent. Frightening visual hallucinations frequently occur but high order visual dysfunction is uncommon except in the Heidenhain variant of sporadic CJD. Executive dysfunction is common and often associated with behavioural change. The latter may require careful management and comprise irritability, aggression or withdrawal from normal social interchange.

Neurological symptoms and signs indicate involvement of multiple components in the nervous system, which is often the first clue to a prion disease vs. more common dementias. In the motor systems, ataxia, especially of gait, and dysarthria are early features in many types of CJD including variant CJD (vCJD), kuru, iatrogenic CJD (iCJD) and some types of sporadic CJD. Abnormal movements, especially myoclonus of cortical or subcortical type, is characteristic

of most types of prion disease, especially sporadic CJD. Chorea is found in a proportion of sporadic and variant CJD, and exceptionally alien limb phenomena and epilepsia partialis continua have been reported. Stiffness with increased tone in the limbs and neck occurs in many types of CJD. This tone increase commonly has extrapyramidal features, especially in the upper limbs, in addition to spasticity. Fasciculation rarely occurs. Power in general is relatively preserved but hemiparesis or a stroke-like onset has been described.

Sensory loss is not often detected because the patients are frequently not capable of cooperating with the examination. Hyperaesthesiae is typical of vCJD and iCJD due to growth hormone and loss of thermal sensation occurs in some inherited prion disease. Sensory loss and autonomic failure is prominent in PrP-systemic amyloidosis associated with truncating mutations of *PRNP*.

Late in the course of all these diseases incontinence develops. Ultimately most patients enter a state of akinetic mutism. Death generally follows decreasing conscious level, pneumonia and respiratory failure or sepsis.

12.3 Sporadic CJD

Sporadic CJD (sCJD) is the most frequent type of spongiform encephalopathy in man. Although a rare disease with an incidence of 1–2 per million throughout the world, ascertainment in old age, when dementia is prevalent, remains an important unknown. The most frequent phenotype is of a rapidly progressive disease characterised by cognitive decline, visual disturbance, apraxia, ataxia and myoclonus. Typically the age of onset is between 55 and 70 years but many cases occur outside this range; cases in the 70–85 years range have probably been overlooked in the past but cases under the age of less than 45 years are rare. Only three cases of sporadic CJD younger than 30 years old have been identified in the UK since 1970. The disease affects males slightly less frequently than females. Death typically occurs in 5 months from onset in the majority, with only an atypical 10 % surviving up to 2 years, or exceptionally even longer, from onset.

Table 12.1 MRI-CJD consortium criteria for sporadic Creutzfeldt–Jakob disease

I- Clinical signs (with a symptom duration of less than 2 years)
Dementia
Cerebellar or visual
Pyramidal or extrapyramidal
Akinetic mutism
II- Tests
Periodic sharp wave complexes on the EEG
14-3-3 protein detection in the CSF
High signal abnormalities in caudate nucleus and putamen or at least two cortical regions (temporal, parietal or occipital) either in diffusion-weight imaging (DWI) or fluid attenuated inversion recovery (FLAIR) MRI
Probable CJD
Two out of I and at least one out of II
Possible CJD
Two out of I and duration less than 2 years

Clinicians have long recognised different phenotypes of sCJD, that described by Jones and Nevin being the most frequent. Myoclonus is characteristic at some stage of the disease in virtually all cases but can be subtle. The Heidenhain variant is not infrequent and is characterised by visual disturbance culminating in cortical type blindness.

Other phenotypes include an ataxic variant, a thalamic variant and a panencephalitic type with extensive white matter change, these latter being mainly in the Japanese literature but may merely reflect long duration of disease where more grey matter is destroyed. It is uncertain if an amyotrophic type occurs and these cases, if they exist, have not been transmitted. Some case series describe groups with long pure cognitive and/or psychiatric phases early in the clinical course. Whether or not these different phenotypes represent distinct disease entities or extremes of a range of involvement of different neurological systems is not clear.

12.3.1 Diagnostic Criteria

The World Health Organisation have drawn up criteria for diagnosing various types of CJD and recently MRI criteria have been recommended to be added (Table 12.1). While these criteria are useful in epidemiological surveys ensuring uniformity of data, they may be restrictive in clinical trials where early diagnosis is essential.

12.4 Pathology

Macroscopically the cerebral hemispheres in sCJD are often of normal appearance although atrophy occurs in long standing cases. Cerebellar atrophy occurs in kuru, iCJD, vCJD and Gerstmann–Sträussler–Scheinker syndrome (GSS) and there is striking thalamic atrophy in familial fatal insomnia.

The characteristic microscopic features of prion diseases on haematoxylin and eosin staining are spongiform degeneration of the cerebral cortex, neuronal loss and gliosis associated with amyloid deposition in some cases (Fig. 12.2). Spongiform change begins in the dendrites, especially the presynaptic zones, and expands to form vacuoles in the neuropil. This is different to some animal prion diseases in which only the latter is usually apparent. Typically the vacuoles are 2–20 µm but can expand into much larger structures. The vacuoles have numerous membranous fragments in them on electron microscopy. In sporadic disease cortical layers four and five are most affected in the typical case with additional pathology in the basal ganglia, thalamus and cerebellum. Some of the inherited diseases have relatively little or no vacuole formation. There is substantial neuronal loss in most cases that increases with time.

The distribution of pathology is dependent on the type of CJD. In vCJD and the insomnias thalamic damage is prominent while in Gerstmann Straussler Scheinker disease (P102L) the cerebellum is most involved. Neuronal loss and gliosis occur in a similar distribution. It should be emphasised that these changes are variable between patients even in those with the same phenotype.

Understanding the microscopic pathology has been greatly enhanced by the development of specific PrP immunostains, which not only demonstrate amyloid plaques better, but also show other abnormalities not apparent on routine

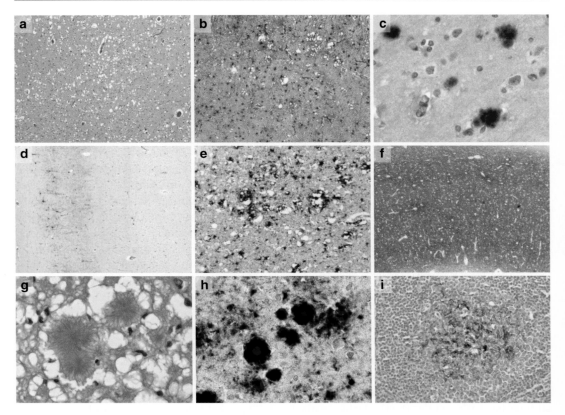

Fig. 12.2 Examples of prion pathology courtesy of Professor Sebastian Brandner, UCL Institute of Neurolgy. (**a**) spongiform change in sCJD (H&E), (**b**) gliosis and spongiform change in sCJD (GFAP), (**c**) kuru-like plaques in sCJD (ICSM35), (**d**) perineuronal PrP staining in sCJD (ICSM35), (**e**) perivacuolar PrP staining in sCJD (ICSM35), (**f**) synpatic PrP staining in sCJD (ICSM35), (**g, h**) florid plaques in vCJD (H&E, ICSM35), (**i**) PrP deposition in a tonsillar biopsy specimen in vCJD (ICSM35)

stains. Amyloid plaques, comprising aggregations of PrP^{Sc}, occur in a variety of prion diseases. In sCJD they occur in about 10 % of patients; they have a dense core with a fibrillary halo, the so called kuru plaques (Fig. 12.2). Some inherited disorders such as GSS (P102L) have numerous plaques in the cerebellum which have a multicentric appearance while those patients with the 6-OPRI mutation have a pathognomonic linear arrangement in the cerebellum perpendicular to the surface. In contrast patients with familial insomnia have no amyloid plaques. vCJD patients have numerous large florid plaques with a characteristic pattern of fibrillary structure surrounded by spongiform change (Fig. 12.2).

Non-plaque deposition occurs in all cases of sCJD. The deposits can be granular synaptic,

perineuronal decorating the neurones, or perivacuolar; the type of deposition depends on the subtype of sCJD and usually one type dominates (Fig. 12.2). In some cases there are so called mini-plaques which occur particularly in iCJD.

Tau inclusions are common in all types of CJD and are particularly prominent in vCJD in spite of the young age of the patients. Tau co-localises with prion amyloid. The morphology of Tau deposits is different to that seen in Alzheimer's disease. In the latter the deposits are thread like whereas in CJD they form minute rods.

The pathology in the spinal cord and nerve roots is less well documented. Few autopsy studies have been done in sCJD but in iCJD with P102L mutation there is loss of fibres in the corticospinal, spinocerebellar and gracile tracts.

Patients carrying the E200K mutation sometimes have a mixed axonal and demyelinating sensori-motor neuropathy.

While the pathology in sCJD, the insomnias, inherited disease and some of the iatrogenic disease (growth hormone and dural implantation) the abnormalities are confined to the CNS including the spinal cord, this is not the case with vCJD, or PrP systemic amyloidosis. These diseases have systemic pathology, notably in vCJD in the lymphoreticular system, including the spleen, and in this respect are similar to cervid chronic wasting disease (CWD), ovine and caprine scrapie, and to a lesser extent BSE. Prion staining is positive early in the course of the disease in animals and precedes the encephalopathy, a situation that almost certainly applies to man. The deposition in the lymphatic tissue is the basis of tonsil biopsy for diagnosis in vCJD where all definite cases have been positive (Fig. 12.2).

PrP systemic amyloidoses are a group inherited prion diseases, of which Y163X is the best documented, and are characterised by vascular and parenchymal PrP amyloid with a broad distribution in the CNS and systemic organs. These patients present with diarrhoea, autonomic failure, sensory neuropathy and urinary incontinence.

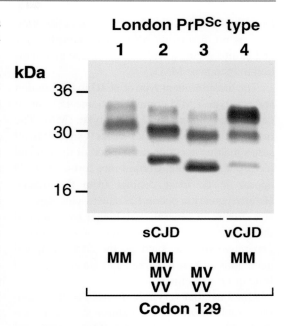

Fig. 12.3 Western blot (*left*) of four patient brain samples prepared by homogenization in phosphate buffered saline, partial protease digestion using proteinase K, and immunoblotting. Three PrP immunoreactive bands are seen related to three glycosylation states (un-, mono-, and diglycosylated). Types 1–3, distinguished by molecular weight, are seen in sCJD with restriction to certain codon 129 genotypes (below). Type 4, distinguished from sporadic types by the predominance of the diglycosylated (*top*) band, is exclusively seen in vCJD

12.4.1 Molecular Classification

Since the advent of prion protein gene (*PRNP*) analysis and prion protein analysis by Western blotting, a molecular classification of sporadic CJD has emerged. Although the subdivision of sCJD in this way is of interest from a research perspective, to date, it has little clinical relevance. Nevertheless some new facts have emerged. Firstly, a polymorphic genetic variant at *PRNP* codon 129 between methionine and valine, is one factor that is particularly important in determining the clinical phenotype and type of PrP^{Sc} observed by Western blot. Second, two classifications have been developed in which the genotype at codon 129 is combined with prion protein electrophoretic pattern on Western blot after partial digestion with protease viz that of Parchi and colleagues, and that of the London (MRC Prion Unit). The

patterns of PrP staining after Western blot (Fig. 12.3) are different because of differential protease cleavage and differing predominance of three glycosylation states. The situation is further complicated by the sensitivity of Western blot protocols to changes in the experimental conditions and the frequent coexistence of types when multiple brain areas are examined.

As a starting point in the following discussion the London classification will be used and this is compared to the Parchi typing. In general, homozygosity at codon 129 causes a more aggressive disease. Type 1 patients who are 129MM tend to have the classical CJD phenotype with a mean age of 55–60 years and survival of weeks. Type 2 patients who are 129MM differ in that the course of the disease is usually longer (a few months) and they are younger with a mean age of onset of about 50 years, although ascertainment may be an influence here. In the Parchi classification there is no distinction between London types 1 and 2, thus giving a wider range of age and duration in their type MM1.

The most frequent type of sCJD in the London series is type 2 MM comprising some 45 % of all cases while about 16 % were type 1MM. The number of homozygous VV cases is smaller in all series making accurate description of the clinical picture less reliable. Certain rare forms of sCJD appear to be most distinct from the others. Heterozygosity at codon 129 causes a less aggressive disease in general, with longer survival, and the patients can initially mimic other neurodegenerative disease such as the frontotemporal dementias or have a marked apraxia at onset, and little or no myoclonus.

One final, but very rare, form of sCJD is sporadic fatal insomnia, a condition that is associated with autonomic features. This condition is characterised by thalamic involvement. There is a wide age range with a mean of about 50 years and duration of 16 months. The cases are classified as Parchi MM2 (thalamic) type.

A new type of sporadic prion disease was described in 2008 and 2010 termed variably proteinase sensitive prionopathy. These patients have clinical courses of 6 months – 4 years, and a predominance of behavioural and cognitive signs, compared with motor or cerebellar features. The condition also differs from sporadic CJD in its histopathological and immunoblotting features, with a ladder like electrophoretic profile on Western blot.

Development of a molecular classification for human prion disease may have implications for epidemiological research into the causes of sporadic CJD, whose aetiology remains obscure. Spontaneous conversion of PrP^C to PrP^{Sc} as a rare stochastic event, or somatic mutation of *PRNP*, resulting in expression of a pathogenic PrP mutant are plausible explanations for sporadic CJD. However other causes for at least some cases including environmental exposure to human prions, or exposure to animal prions may also be important. In this regard, the number of prion strains causing sheep scrapie has yet to be established and epidemiological data cannot exclude this as a cause of a minority of cases. As future research begins to provide a more precise understanding of the origins of human prion disease, this will facilitate re-analysis of epidemiological data, and is likely to reveal important risk factors that might have been obscured by analysing sporadic CJD as a single entity.

12.5 Inherited Prion Disease (IPD)

There are at least 35 different pathological mutations causing inherited prion disease (IPD, Fig. 12.4). There are broadly three types of mutation viz: alteration of the normal number of a nonapeptide followed by four octapeptide repeats between codons 51 and 91 of *PRNP*, or point mutations in the C-terminal portion of the protein, and premature truncation of the protein by stop codon mutations.

Phenotypes can be highly variable even in patients with the same mutation and within a family. Some of these cases have been transmitted to other species but many have not, particularly those reported from a single family. Failure of transmission in experimental situations does not necessarily mean that transmission will not occur given the appropriate route of inoculation and genetic background of the recipient. A summary of the mutations so far described is shown in Table 12.2.

12.5.1 Octapeptide Repeat Insertion Mutations (OPRI)

In the UK a number of families with six extra octapeptide repeats have been described. The largest group of over 100 patients has a 144 bp insertion (6-OPRI). These patients have a mean age of onset of symptoms of 35 (20–53) years and mean age at death of 45 (30–65) years. Interestingly those with methionine homozygosity at codon 129 have an earlier onset (by about 10 years) than heterozygotes although the duration of the illness is similar between genotypes. Younger patients have a slightly longer course. Typically patients present with cortical cognitive deficits encompassing

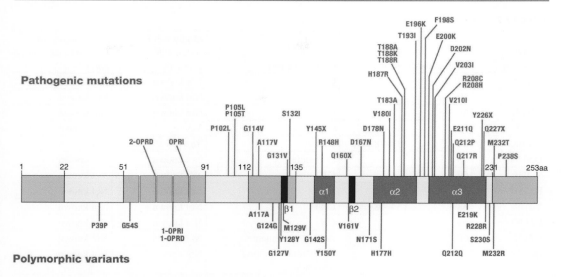

Fig. 12.4 Pathogenic mutations (*red above*) and polymorphic changes (*green below*) in the prion protein gene are shown on this schematic. The central grey bar also illustrates the secondary structural features of the prion protein

Table 12.2 In this table the mean age (years) of onset, range of ages and clinical features of IPD mutations is shown

PRNP mutation	Median onset	Range	Clinical features	Modification by codon 129 genotype	Transmission of disease to laboratory animals
P102L	50	25–70	GSS, CJD, psychiatric presentations, heterogenous	Possible	Yes
P105L	45	38–50	GSS, spastic paraparesis	Not known	Not known
G114V	22	18–27 in one family	GSS, Neuropsychiatric and extrapyramidal signs prominent	Not known	Not known
A117V	40	20–64	GSS with early cognitive, neuropsychiatric, extrapyramidal features	Yes	No
G131V	42		GSS	Not known	Not known
Y145X	38		Alzheimer-like dementia	Not known	No
R148H	72	63–82	CJD	Not known	Not known
Q160X	40	32–48	Unspecified dementia	Not known	Not known
D178N	50	20–72	FFI, CJD	Possible	Yes
V180I	74	58–81	CJD	Not known	Not known
T183A	45	37–49	Prominent behavioral abnormalities, one patient with dementia and no additional signs	Not known	Not known
Y163X	30	30–50	Early diarrhea and autonomic neuropathy Late development of CNS symptoms	Not known	No
H187R	32	20–53	Early onset with personality disorder in one family	Not known	Not known

(continued)

Table 12.2 (continued)

PRNP mutation	Median onset	Range	Clinical features	Modification by codon 129 genotype	Transmission of disease to laboratory animals
T188A	82		CJD	Not known	Not known
T188K	59		CJD	Not known	Not known
E196K	69		CJD	Not known	Not known
F198S	56	40–71	GSS	Yes	Not known
E200K	58	33–78	CJD	Yes	Yes
D202N	73		Dementia	Not known	Not known
V203I	69		CJD	Not known	Not known
R208H	59	58–60	CJD	Not known	Not known
V210I	58	54–68	CJD	Not known	Not known
E211Q	69		CJD	Not known	Not known
Q212P	60		Ataxia, no dementia	Not known	Not known
Q217R	64	62–66	CJD, frontotemporal dementia	Not known	Not known
4-OPRI	62	56–82	CJD	Not known	Not known
5-OPRI	45	26–61	GSS, CJD, Alzheimer-like, variable, some with prominent extrapyramidal signs	Yes	Not known
6-OPRI	34	20–53	GSS, CJD, variable, personality and psychiatric features and extrapyramidal signs	Yes	Yes
7-OPRI	29	23–35	GSS, CJD, variable, personality and psychiatric features	Not known	Yes
8-OPRI	38	21–55	GSS, CJD, variable, personality and psychiatric features	Not known	Yes
9-OPRI	44	34–54	GSS	Not known	Not known
2-OPRD			CJD	Not known	Not known

Modification by codon 129 and transmission to laboratory animals is also shown where known. In the table, Gerstmann-Straussler-Scheinker syndrome (GSS) is used to refer to the clinical combination of a slowly progressive ataxia, spasticity and later dementia, rather than the pathological phenotype which is not known in all cases

acalculia, language dysfunction, apraxia and memory impairment together with frontal behavioural disturbance. There is some evidence that scholastic achievement is poor before overt clinical signs are apparent. Similarly work history often shows a progressive decline before the diagnosis is established. Physical signs include ataxia, corticospinal and extrapramidal features. Myoclonus occurs but seizures are rare. The phenotype is variable within families suggesting genetic or other factors, additional to codon 129, play an important part in the clinical picture.

A number of different 5-OPRI mutations have been described including at least five families from the UK, South Africa and N. Ireland. The phenotypic variation is probably greater in this group than with any other mutation. The age of onset ranges from the third to the seventh decade and the duration from of the illness from 4 months to 15 years. Some patients are indistinguishable from sCJD but most have a slower dementing disorder mistaken for Alzheimer's disease, only later accompanied by apraxia, ataxia and sometimes myoclonus. Additional features include pyramidal signs in many and less commonly myoclonus and extrapyramidal features.

Seven, eight and nine octapeptide repeat insertions have been described all with pathological evidence of prion disease. A 7-OPRI mutation has been reported in an American family with multiple system involvement in young people (23–35 years) and the disease has a prolonged course (10–13 years). A similar clinical picture is seen in three families with 8-OPRI; the disease is of variable duration extending up to 13 years. A single case of 9-OPRI insertion in a 54 year old English woman with dementia, rigidity and myoclonus lasting about 5 years has been described; there was no convincing family history of a similar illness. The largest insertional mutation described is 12-OPRI.

Occasionally patients with a clinical phenotype typical of sCJD have other octapeptide repeat mutations, but the exact significance of these mutations in this group is unclear in many. Those involving one, two or three additional repeats may be coincidental findings, or rare risk factors as these have been found in healthy control populations. Four repeat insertions have been reported more frequently associated with a late-onset, short duration course with an absence of family history in most and so are often mistaken for sCJD.

There are only two reports of a deletion in the repeat region (2-OPRD) in patients with CJD; this has not been found in controls and is probably causal of disease. A 1-OPRD is a relatively uncommon polymporphism of the healthy population and is therefore not causal of disease.

12.5.2 Point Mutations

A large number of point mutations have been described. Some show marked ethnogeographic clustering. Some of the more prevalent mutations in Europe are described here.

12.5.3 P102L (Gerstmann Straussler Scheinkler Disease)

In the UK the most frequent point mutation is P102L which usually presents as the archetypal Gerstmann Straussler Scheinker disease. Ataxia is the commonest symptom with cognitive decline, leg weakness and lower limb pain, especially burning discomfort, occurring later. Additional features include psychiatric symptoms and pyramidal and extrapryramidal signs in a minority. Myoclonus is uncommon. A particularly striking feature is the presence, on clinical testing, of distal sensory loss especially marked in the lower limbs due to involvement of the central spino-thalamic and posterior column pathways. Occasional CJD-like atypical patients are seen. Many of the patients reside in southern or mid-England and may well have a common ancestor dating back before the seventeenth century. The age of onset is 27–66 (mean 51) years and death occurred from 33 to 69 (mean 55) years. Again those who were homozygous for methionine at codon 129 had an earlier age of onset (mean 47 years) than heterozygotes but the range of durations of the illness is wide and may be independent of codon 129.

12.5.4 P105L

Originally described in Japanese families this condition occurs more widely. Age of onset is in the fourth to fifth decade with a duration of about 5 years. All have dementia, rigidity, and some a spastic paraparesis. There are plaques in the cerebral cortex but not in the cerebellum.

12.5.5 A117V

This mutation was first described in France and subsequently has been reported from a number of countries. Parkinsonian features are frequent with dementia and there is a severe loss of ability to speak but with relative preservation of understanding. The age of onset is variable between 20 and 64 years and a duration of several years. Amyloid plaques are plentiful and there is often associated tau pathology. There is one large UK family under the care of the National Prion Clinic.

12.5.6 Y163X

We recently described a pedigree diagnosed with hereditary sensory and autonomic neuropathy which segregates for the Y163X mutation. Onset of autonomic symptoms, particularly diarrhoea is in the fourth decade. The condition is only very slowly progressive with increasing sensory loss, ataxia, incontinence, fluctuating weight loss and eventually cognitive decline.

12.5.7 D178N (Including Familial Fatal Insomnia)

Fatal familial insomnia, due to a mutation most frequently on the 129 methionine allele, was the first described in Italians but occurs extensively. Onset is between 36 and 62 (mean 51) years and duration wide varying between 1 and 6 (mean 2.5) years. Insomnia is the cardinal feature of the disease often preceded by lack of attentiveness. The insomnia may be masked by apparent excessive day time sleeping as a result of lack of nocturnal somnolence. This is soon accompanied by autonomic symptoms such hypertension, excessive sweating, evening pyrexia, salivation and impotence. Later hallucinations occur, often related to dreams, and the patients may have limb movements related to the dreaming. As the disease progresses ataxia, pyramidal signs and myoclonus occurs in many patients.

Usually, but not exclusively, 178 N on a valine 129 allele is a rare cause of a CJD type picture. These patients present with memory impairment often at a younger age than sCJD, and have a more prolonged course and have no periodic complexes on EEG.

12.5.8 E200K

This is the most frequently occurring inherited prion disease and common in localised populations e.g. in Eastern Europe, North Africa and Chile, but is less common in the UK. E200K patients are on average slightly younger than sCJD subjects but there is great variation. They are indistinguishable from the sCJD apart from some having a peripheral neuropathy of mixed axonal and demyelinating type and seizures are more common than in sCJD. There are rare reports of this mutation being on the valine allele

where the patients are reported to have a longer course and more ataxia.

12.5.9 V210I

This is the commonest form of IPD in Italy but also described in other countries. The phenotype is like sCJD but with a mean age of onset at 55 years.

12.5.10 Other Point Mutations

A number of other point mutations have been described often in a single family. These patients may present a clinical phenotype of sCJD (R148H), Alzheimer's disease (G131V, F198S), fronto-temporal dementia (T183A), early onset dementia (Q160X), rapidly progressive dementia (E196K) or psychiatric symptoms (G114V). The significance of other mutations is less certain because of lack of pathological confirmation or inconsistent occurrence of morbidity in carriers within a family (various substitutions at codon 188).

12.5.11 Genetic Counselling and Presymptomatic Testing

PRNP analysis allows unequivocal diagnosis in patients with inherited prion disease. This has also allowed pre-symptomatic testing of unaffected, but at-risk, family members, as well as antenatal testing following appropriate genetic counselling. The effect of codon 129 genotype on the age of onset of disease associated with some mutations also means it is possible to determine within a family whether a carrier of a mutation will have an early or late onset of disease. Most of the well recognised pathogenic PRNP mutations appear fully penetrant, however experience with some mutations is extremely limited. In families with the E200K mutation there are examples of elderly unaffected gene carriers who appear to have escaped the disease.

12.6 Variant CJD (vCJD)

In late 1995, two cases of sporadic CJD were reported in the UK in teenagers. Only four cases of sporadic CJD had previously been recorded in teenagers, and none of these cases occurred in the UK. In addition, both were unusual in having kuru-type plaques at autopsy. Soon afterwards a third very young sporadic CJD case occurred. These cases caused considerable concern and the possibility was raised that they were BSE-related. By March 1996, further extremely young onset cases were apparent and review of the histology of these cases showed a remarkably consistent and unique pattern. These cases were named "new variant" CJD.

Review of neuropathological archives failed to demonstrate such cases. The statistical probability of such cases occurring by chance was vanishingly small and ascertainment bias seemed unlikely as an explanation. It was clear that a new risk factor for CJD had emerged and appeared to be specific to the UK. The UK Government Spongiform Encephalopathy Advisory Committee (SEAC) concluded that, while there was no direct evidence for a link with BSE, exposure to specified bovine offal prior to the ban on its inclusion in human foodstuffs in 1989, was the most likely explanation. A case of vCJD was soon after reported in France. Direct experimental evidence that vCJD is caused by BSE was provided by molecular analysis of human prion strains and transmission studies in transgenic and wild type mice.

The striking feature of vCJD is the young age of the patients. The mean age of onset is 29 (range 16–74) years and the mean duration 14 months. Surprisingly for a disease with a point source of infection, the average age of onset has not progressively increased with time; the reason for this is unknown but may be related to lymphoid tissue mass being greatest in the young and providing a maximal permissive environment for prion protein replication. Presentation of vCJD is with behavioural and psychiatric disturbances and, in some cases, sensory disturbance. Initial referral, with depression, anxiety, withdrawal and behavioural change, is often to a psychiatrist. Suicidal ideation is, however, infrequent and

response to anti-depressants poor. Delusions, which are complex and unsustained, are common. Other features include emotional lability, aggression, insomnia and auditory and visual hallucinations. Dysaesthesiae, or pain in the limbs or face, which was persistent rather than intermittent and unrelated to anxiety levels is a frequent early feature, sometimes prompting referral to a rheumatologist. A minority of cases have early memory loss or gait ataxia but in most such overt neurological features are not apparent until some months later. Typically, a progressive cerebellar syndrome then develops with gait and limb ataxia followed with dementia and progression to akinetic mutism. Myoclonus is frequent, and may be preceded by chorea. Cortical blindness develops in a minority of patients in late disease. Upgaze paresis, an uncommon feature of classical CJD, has been noted in some patients.

Extensive human infection almost certainly resulted from widespread dietary exposure to BSE prions. Cattle BSE was subsequently reported, albeit at much lower levels than in the UK, in most member states of the EU, Switzerland, USA, Canada and Japan. Fortunately, the number of recognised cases of vCJD (177) in the UK has been relatively small and the incidence has been falling for some years; no cases have been reported since 2012 in the UK. Patients have been identified in a number of other counties notably France and including Ireland, Italy, USA, Canada and Hong Kong. However, the number of healthy but infected individuals is unknown. Human prion disease incubation periods, as evidenced by kuru, are known to span decades. While estimates based on mathematical modelling and clinically recognised vCJD, suggest the total epidemic will be small key uncertainties, notably with respect to major genetic effects on incubation period suggest the need for caution: such models cannot estimate the number of infected individuals and it is these that are most relevant to assessing risks of secondary transmission. Also, the possibility of sub-clinical carrier states of prion infection in humans, as recognised in several animal models, must also be considered. An attempt to estimate prevalence of vCJD prion infection in the UK by anonymous screen of archival appendix tissue, found an estimated prevalence of 1 in 2000.

Secondary transmission of vCJD via surgical procedures is not known to have occurred and the risk is unquantifiable at present. As discussed below, vCJD is transmissible by blood transfusion, also prions are known to be resistant to convention sterilisation and indeed iatrogenic transmission from neurosurgical instruments has long been documented. The wider tissue distribution of infectivity in vCJD, unknown prevalence of clinically silent infection, together with the recent experimental demonstration of the avid adherence to, and ease of transmission from, surgical steel surfaces highlight these concerns. Studies in transgenic mouse models of human susceptibility to BSE prion infection suggest that BSE may also induce propagation of a prion strain indistinguishable from the commonest type of sporadic CJD, in addition to that causing variant CJD. Other novel human prion disease phenotypes may be anticipated in alternative *PRNP* genotypes exposed to BSE prions.

No *PRNP* mutations are present in vCJD and gene analysis is important to exclude pathogenic mutations, as inherited prion disease presents in this age group and a family history is not always apparent. The codon 129 genotype has uniformly been homozygous for methionine at *PRNP* codon 129 to date in all definite cases with the exception of one case thought clinically to be vCJD in an MV heterozygote.

Clear ante mortem tissue based diagnosis of vCJD can be made by blood test and/or tonsil biopsy with detection of characteristic PrP immunostaining and PrP^{Sc} type. In 2011 a prototype blood test for vCJD was published in The Lancet, which relies on the binding and concentration of abnormal PrP on stainless steel surfaces, followed by immunodetection. In a blind panel of samples, sensitivity for vCJD was 70 % with no false positives.

It has long been recognised that prion replication, in experimentally infected animals, is first detectable in the lymphoreticular system, considerably earlier than the onset of neurological symptoms. Importantly, PrP^{Sc} is only detectable in tonsil in vCJD, and not other forms of human

prion disease studied. The PrP^{Sc} type detected on Western blot in vCJD tonsil has a characteristic pattern designated type 4. A positive tonsil biopsy obviates the need for brain biopsy which may otherwise be considered in such a clinical context to exclude alternative, potentially treatable diagnoses. To date, tonsil biopsy has proved 100 % specific and sensitive for vCJD diagnosis and is well tolerated.

12.7   Iatrogenic CJD (iCJD)

CJD can be transmitted within a species and across species by experimental techniques such as intracerebral administration of infected brain and other tissues. There is often considerable resistance to transmission between species. However, as discussed above, there have been examples of accidental transmission between humans and even between another species and man (e.g. vCJD). We will now discuss intraspecific transmission in man in more detail.

While there have been a handful of intraspecific transmissions in man from neurosurgery (5 cases), cortical electroencephalography (2 cases), and corneal transplants (2 cases) two major causes of iatrogenic CJD have been identified viz: dural grafts and administration of contaminated human growth hormone to children. In addition, recently, transmission of vCJD by blood transfusion has been reported. Of particular interest is the fact that those few cases who developed CJD from intracerebral invasive procedures, develop a clinical picture similar to sCJD with predominantly cortical features while those receiving growth hormone systemically or dural grafts, with no intracerebral surgery, develop an initial ataxic illness with cerebellar features.

12.7.1   Dural Graft Associated CJD

There have been approximately 200 cases of CJD following dural grafting mostly from Japan. The majority of these cases received grafts produced from a single company before 1987. The first case was recorded in 1978 in the USA although the epidemic started later (1985). There is good evidence that the incidence is falling from a peak of about 20 cases in 1997 to 3 cases in 2005. The mean incubation period is 11 years (range 1.4–23 years). The initial symptoms are most frequently a cerebellar syndrome, especially ataxia of gait, rather than cerebral cortical symptoms although these features ultimately occur in most cases. There is no correlation between the site of the graft and the clinical picture. There are no good data on duration of disease but in general it is measured in months. As with most other types of CJD there is an excess of patients with homozygosity at codon 129, methionine being disproportionately represented. In a recent paper from Japan, where MM homozygosity at codon 129 is almost universal, there is evidence of at least two different pathologies occurring with equal frequency, one with and one without plaques. The first has a slower clinical evolution than the latter.

12.7.2 Growth Hormone Associated CJD

Growth hormone administration to children has resulted in a number of cases of CJD. All the cases have received hormones from pooled cadaver pituitary glands, a manufacturing process that ceased in 1985, when recombinant material became available. In the manufacturing process many hundreds or thousands of pituitaries were pooled thereby greatly increasing the chance of contamination from an infected cadaver.

The total number of cases recorded by 2006 was 194 with the majority occurring in France (107), UK (51) and USA (26). However in the UK cases are still occurring at a frequency of 0–6 per year and the total number of known cases is currently 77 (2014). The primary diagnosis requiring hormone replacement was idiopathic growth hormone deficiency or post surgery for hypothalamic or pituitary tumours in most cases. When the UK population was reviewed in 2003 the relative risk of getting iCJD from growth hormone injection was maximal at 9–10 years of

age and the lifetime risk at that time was about 3.5 %. In 2007 the mean incubation period worldwide, assuming a midpoint of administration as the time of infection, was 15 years (range 4–36 years). In the UK analysis of the products used suggests that one (Wilhelmi) was that most likely implicated although the data are not conclusive. The methods of preparation differed with different products worldwide but which of the various steps in these processes resulted in persistence of infective prions is not clear, a situation reminiscent of the situation in cattle supplementary feed manufacture and transmission of BSE.

As growth hormone was only administered in children the mean age of these patients is younger than for any other form of CJD except vCJD and rarely IPD. Patients typically present with an ataxia and subsequently develop some cortical features. The disease evolves over a period of months, death typically occurring within 12–18 months. Homozygosity at codon 129 is over represented in these cases but interestingly 129VV comprises the majority of the early UK cases whilst in the USA and France it is 129MM. The reason for this is unclear but a plausible explanation is that in the UK a 129VV infected donor contaminated the product whereas in the other countries it was 129MM, a more frequent phenotype in the general population. However, of great interest is the late appearance 129MM cases in the UK and the disappearance of 129VV cases (cf. kuru below).

12.7.3 Blood Transfusion Associated vCJD

There have been concerns that vCJD could be transmitted by blood transfusion. In sheep scrapie, which also has an extensive distribution of prions throughout the lymphoreticular system, transmission has been demonstrated. Surveillance of blood transfusion records linking these to the CJD registry revealed a case of vCJD in a patient who had received a transfusion just over 3 years before developing vCJD, the blood having come from an asymptomatic person who 4 months later developed. Two more cases have now been identified (one unpublished) in which a recipient of blood products from asymptomatic donors who later developed vCJD. One had received a large volume of red blood cells, platelets and FFP for a colectomy 6 years before becoming symptomatic and the donor had developed symptoms 20 months after donation. In these two cases the donor was the same.

Two additional cases of transmission of prions but who did not have symptoms of vCJD are known. One was an elderly patient who received blood from a donor who subsequently developed vCJD. She only had PrP^{Sc} detectable in the lymphoreticular system and died of an unrelated cause. The other was a patient with haemophilia who had received multiple transfusions of blood products, none of which was known to come from vCJD donor, who was shown to have PrP^{Sc} in the lymphoreticular tissue but not the CNS. Interestingly the three vCJD cases were all 129MM as were the donors but the cases of asymptomatic infection the patients were both 129MV. At present there are only a small number of persons thought to be at risk from transfusion sourced from patients who subsequently developed vCJD. However, as the true prevalence of prion infection in the community is unknown it is not possible to give an accurate assessment of the risk of a single or multiple transfusions of blood or blood products.

12.7.4 Secondary Prophylaxis After Accidental Exposure

Certain occupational groups are at risk of exposure to human prions, for instance neurosurgeons and other operating theatre staff, pathologists and morticians, histology technicians, as well as an increasing number of laboratory workers. Because of the prolonged incubation periods to prions following administration to sites other than the central nervous system (CNS), which is associated with clinically silent prion replication in the lymphoreticular tissue, treatments inhibiting prion replication in lymphoid organs may

represent a viable strategy for rational secondary prophylaxis after accidental exposure. There is hope that progress in the understanding of the peripheral pathogenesis will identify the precise cell types and molecules involved in colonization of the organism by prions. The ultimate goal will be to target the rate-limiting steps in prion spread with much more focused pharmacological approaches, which may eventually prove useful in preventing disease even after iatrogenic and alimentary exposure. A proof of principle of immunoprophylaxis by passive immunization using anti-PrP monoclonals has already been demonstrated in mouse models.

12.8   Kuru

Kuru is a fatal, predominantly ataxic disease confined to a remote region of Papua New Guinea. First recognised at the turn of the twentieth century it was clearly defined by Alpers in the 1950s and subsequently shown by Gajdusek to be transmissible to other primates by intracerebral inoculation and later to other animals.

Kuru predominantly affected women and children. The disease was transmitted at cannibalistic feasts where tissues with the greatest concentration of prions viz: brain, were preferentially eaten by the children and females, the males older than seven predominantly consuming muscle. The disease is a progressive ataxia and subsequent dementia developing over 1–2 years the patient ultimately becoming moribund but cognitive function is preserved. There is often a prodrome of headache.

Banning cannibalistic practices has resulted in a dramatic decline in the prevalence of kuru although a few cases may still occur. Interestingly, while the early cases were predominantly 129MM and 129VV, in the most recent examples heterozygotes are the majority some with extremely long incubation times (over 50 years). Some elderly women who atteneded cannibalistic feasts but did not get kuru possess a novel genetic resistance factor, G127V, unique to the Fore.

12.9 Investigations

12.9.1 Neuropsychology

Full cognitive assessment, which is a fundamental part of the neurological assessment, cannot be made by the clinician seeing the patient for the first time. It is important to obtain full assessment as soon as possible with a neuropsychologist to determine the nature of the cognitive defects. Repeated assessments to document change are important in trials of therapy bearing in mind that there can be a learning component if repeated too frequently. As was found in the PRION-1 trial, none of the instruments used in dementia trials are ideally suited for these cases as they often take too long to administer, omit certain cognitive assessments, give too much emphasis on others or are not sensitive to advanced stages of disease.

12.9.2 CT

CT scanning is an insensitive modality for diagnosis in CJD. Atrophy is apparent in some cases but this is usually a late feature. The greatest generalised atrophy is seen in CJD patients surviving several years. GSS patients (P102L mutation) have focal cerebellar atrophy in some cases. Enhancement does not occur.

12.9.3 Magnetic Resonance Imaging (MRI)

MRI is the most useful modality of imaging in CJD. High signal return from grey matter is characteristic of CJD except most inherited prion disease (IPD) and is usually most apparent on diffusion weighted images, less so on FLAIR and least on T2 weighted images but this is not an invariable rule. Diffusion weighted imaging (DWI) can be done at various b-values which conventionally is 1000 s/mm^2 but in some cases a 3000 s/mm^2 protocol is better. Apparent diffusion coefficient (ADC) maps should be calculated to confirm true restricted diffusion and remove T2-weighted 'shine through'. Enhancement with gadolinium does not occur in any type of CJD.

The distribution of the abnormal signal varies between different types of CJD. In sCJD there is usually high signal return from the basal ganglia, typically the caudate and anterior putamen. This may be asymmetrical. In addition thalamic signal is often abnormal and can be focal. In some patients the lateral complex returns high signal while in others the medial nuclei are more affected. The abnormality can include the posterior complex but invariably the thalamic signal is less intense than that from the caudate nuclei. Cortical 'ribboning' is found in many patients usually, but not invariably, in addition to the basal ganglia abnormality (Fig. 12.5). This is best seen on DWI and ADC maps. The distribution can be focal involving any part of the cortex; care must be taken in determining abnormality in areas of allocortex particularly the anterior cingulate and insula with 3 T scanning and with frontal cortex adjacent to the frontal sinuses. Nevertheless the cingulate abnormality often extends caudally and can be the sole abnormal cortical region. The cortical signal abnormality is usually asymmetrical. In a few patients cortical ribboning is the only abnormality. In many patients the body and tail of the hippocampus also returns high signal. Little is known about the progression of abnormal signal on serial MRI but it does become more extensive with time and the signal characteristics change.

In vCJD about 90 % of patients in a prospective series have high signal return from the pulvinar and medial areas of the thalamus particularly adjacent to the ventricle, the so called 'hockey stick' sign (Fig. 12.5). However, it is unclear when this sign develops and it is not infrequent that the initial scan is reported as normal but becomes clearly abnormal over a few months.

In growth hormone induced CJD the MRI typically shows diffuse thalamic signal change accompanied by increased signal from the tail of the hippocampus, superior cerebellar vermis and superior motor cortex, this latter region rarely being affected in other forms of CJD.

Fig. 12.5 (**a**) T2 weighted axial MRI in sCJD showing subtlety of increased cortical signal. (**b**) Diffusion Weighted Imaging (DWI) showing cortical ribbon in sCJD. (**c**) FLAIR images and (**d**) DWI showing high signal in the caudate, putamen, and less so from the thalamus in sCJD. (**e**) FLAIR images in iCJD showing cortical, caudate, putamen and thalamic high signal. (**f**) FLAIR images showing pulvinar sign in vCJD

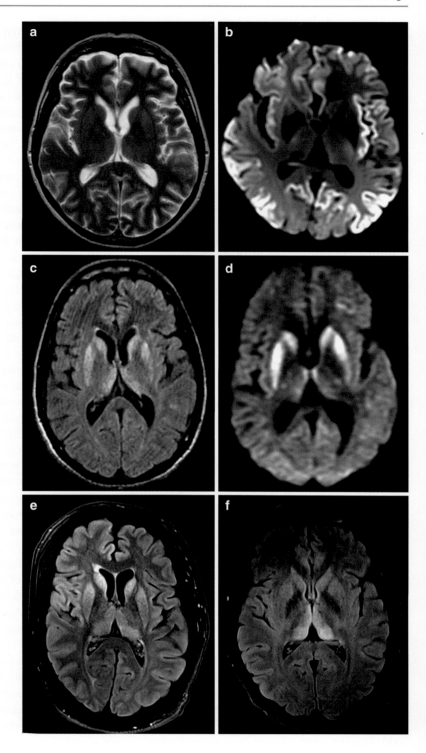

12.9.4 Electroencephalography

The EEG is abnormal in the majority of symptomatic patients with CJD. The most common abnormality is slowing of the background rhythm with predominant theta waves and loss of the normal alpha rhythm in many.

In sCJD a characteristic abnormality is repetitive (>5) bi- or triphasic periodic complexes occurring at 0.5–2 s intervals with <0.5 s variability between complexes and distributed widely over the cortex. They occur in up to 73 % of patients with the codon 129MM genotype at some time during the evolution of the disease. However the sensitivity declines if only a single EEG is obtained. The prevalence of periodic complexes increases with the age of the patient but decreases with disease duration. This abnormality occurs most frequently if myoclonus is present and there is phase locking between the complexes and the myoclonic jerks in many where the myoclonus is of cortical origin. This can be seen in the raw record if an electrode is placed over the affected part although back averaging may be required convincingly to demonstrate this phenomenon.

Periodic complexes are less frequent in sCJD patients with other polymorphisms at codon 129, especially valine homozygotes. The specificity of such complexes is fairly high but they do occur with a wide range of pathologies including those that mimic CJD such as metabolic disorders, especially hepatic coma, other neurodegenerative diseases and encephalitides, as well as stroke and tumours, conditions less likely to be confused clinically with CJD.

Epilepsy occurs in patients with sCJD and is said to be more common in some inherited types of CJD (E200K). It is uncommon in other forms of prion diseases. The majority of fits are major generalized convulsions. The EEG shows the typical changes associated with major convulsions if obtained during a fit and decreased activity post ictally. It may be difficult to separate periodic complexes from epileptic activity. Intravenous diazepines may help to distinguish the two with epileptic activity typically responding but this technique does not unequivocally distinguish between the two types of discharge.

12.9.5 Nerve Conduction Studies

Peripheral nervous system involvement is not common in prion diseases. However some of the inherited diseases do have abnormalities. The E200K mutation is also associated with a mixed axonal and demyelinating neuropathy in some cases. P102L patients also have clinical evidence of loss of thermal sensation on objective testing but this is probably centrally determined as peripheral nerve conduction and threshold tracking are normal.

Occasionally there is evidence of lower motor neurone destruction with fasciculation, fibrillation and small compound muscle action potentials. It is unclear how often this occurs, and in which patients, but it does appear to be rare.

12.9.6 Cerebrospinal Fluid Examination (CSF)

In all types of prion disease the CSF typically has a normal cell count of 0–2 cells/mm^3. A pleocytosis suggests an alternative diagnosis, particularly an inflammatory disorder. Total protein level is usually normal or only modestly elevated, and there is no evidence of intrathecal immunoglobulin synthesis.

The 14-3-3 proteins comprise a large family of intracellular proteins found in all eukaryotic cells, and constitute about 1 % of the total protein content of brain neurons. They are found in the CSF in a variety of conditions where there is rapid and extensive neuronal destruction. They are detected using a qualitative assay, giving a positive, negative or "weak positive" result. The 14-3-3 assay is included in the World Health Organization's diagnostic criteria for sporadic CJD (sCJD). The assay is typically positive in classical, rapidly progressive sCJD, with a sensitivity of 90–95 % for the MM1 subtype. However, it is less sensitive for longer duration cases, for younger patients, and for the acquired and the more slowly progressive inherited prion diseases. It is positive in only about 40 % of cases of variant CJD.

Interestingly, successive studies over the years have tended to show a reducing sensitivity of the 14-3-3 assay for CJD. This may well be related to the increasing recognition and inclusion of cases with atypical, more slowly progressive clinical features leading to more "false-negative" results in recent studies. There is some evidence that the 14-3-3 assay is more sensitive when performed at later stages of disease. It has therefore been suggested that in cases where there is continuing diagnostic uncertainty there may be a role for repeating the assay at a later stage if the first is negative. However, in practice this is often superseded by a decision either to obtain a definitive tissue diagnosis, or that further investigations are no longer appropriate.

The overall specificity of the 14-3-3 assay for prion disease is quite low, at around 70–80 %. In patients with clinically suspected CJD, false positive results occur most commonly when the final diagnosis is inflammatory or malignant (including CNS tumours and paraneoplastic syndromes). Other causes of a positive result include recent stroke, infective encephalitis and subacute sclerosing panencephalitis (SSPE), but these diagnoses can usually be ruled out clinically or on the basis of other tests. A raised CSF cell count has been shown to be highly significantly associated with an increased false positive rate, and should always prompt investigation for other causes. The specificity is not high enough for the test to have a role in screening unselected patients with dementia for prion disease.

S100b comprise a large family of calcium binding cytoplasmic proteins found in glia in the CNS, as well as widely outside the CNS. They are detected using a quantitative assay. Their levels are raised in the CSF in a large number of destructive diseases of the nervous system where there is extensive gliosis, including CJD. As with the 14-3-3 proteins, they are more likely to be raised in rapidly progressive disease, where sensitivity is around 90. However, the specificity is even lower than for 14-3-3, and in practice they rarely add any further useful diagnostic information.

Tau is a micro-tubule associated protein, which is found in increased levels in the CSF when there is destruction of neurons. In some disease states the Tau protein becomes hyperphosphorylated. The levels of total Tau and hyperphosphorylated Tau can be measured using quantitative assays. The total Tau (T-Tau) level in the CSF is elevated in a wide variety of degenerative CNS disorders, including Alzheimer's disease. It is increasingly used, in combination with CSF $A\beta_{42}$, as a diagnostic marker for Alzheimer's disease. In sCJD it can be elevated to a much higher level than in the more common slowly evolving degenerative disorders. If a high threshold is used, the sensitivity is again high for rapidly progressive CJD, and the specificity seems to be similar to that of the 14-3-3 assay. It has been suggested that CSF levels of hyperphosphorylated Tau (P-Tau) are particularly elevated in variant CJD (vCJD), such that the ratio of P-Tau to T-Tau is higher in vCJD than sCJD. This may have a role in helping to distinguish between these two conditions.

Various other proteins have been considered as CSF markers for CJD, including Neuron-Specific Enolase, prostaglandins and interleukins. However, these are less sensitive and specific than those above, and have little clinical utility. The limited data available on $A\beta_{42}$ in CJD suggest that it has little diagnostic significance.

Assays which rely on amplification of abnormal PrP are increasingly becoming available. The real-time Quaking Induced Conversion (RTQuIC) assay has proven to be the most specific and is abnormal in up to 90 % of sporadic CJD CSF samples. The assay relies of the conversion of recombinant PrP to abnormal forms by templating. The signal of conversion is measured by the binding of a fluorophore thioflavin T. These tests appear to have a high specificity and sensitivity but are still to be fully assessed.

12.9.7 Tissue Diagnosis

The only way to obtain a definite diagnosis of CJD, other than the inherited forms, is to obtain tissue. In sCJD brain biopsy or autopsy are required. In vCJD the lymphoreticular tissue is involved early in the evolution of the disorder. In the experience of the National Prion Clinic, tonsillar biopsy is diagnostic in all cases with symptomatic vCJD. It is not known when the tonsillar tissue first becomes involved but based on extrapolation from animal studies it is probably relatively early in the incubation period.

12.10 Therapy

There is no therapy that has been shown convincingly to alter the course of any form of prion disease. One trial of flupertine, in which a pacebo was also given, claimed a beneficial effect on certain clinical scores but not mortality; this trial was small and of borderline statistical significance. In PRION-1, a patient preference trial, quinacrine had no significant effect on survival or any clinical assessment variables. There have been a number of anecdotal reports concerning tetracycline derivatives claiming benefit but none is convincing, and a large randomised trial showed no benefit measure by survival. The glycosaminoglycan pentosan administered intraventricularly to animal models of prion disease has been shown to have a small beneficial effect. It has been given to a small number of patients with a variety of types of CJD and long survival has been described in some vCJD patients. However confounding factors such as parenteral feeding and aggressive management of coincident infection may partially or completely account for this increased survival.

There are no other properly conducted trials of putative therapeutic agents.

Administration of monoclonal antibodies or small molecules which interfere with conversion of PrP^c to PrP^{Sc} have been trialled in mouse models of CJD and show some benefit if given prophylactically during the incubation period after intraperitoneal injection of prions.

Some types of symptomatic therapy have been beneficial. This particularly applies to myoclonus (levetiracetam, valproate and clonazepam), aggression (risperidone), agiatation (diazepines) and hallucinations (centrally acting anticholinesterases). Other symptoms such as insomnia and rigidity are usually resistant to treatment with the standard agents. Supportive therapy, including various forms of parenteral nutrition and vigorous treatment of intercurrent infections may prolong survival but have little effect on quality of life measures.

Good nursing care in conjunction with symptomatic therapy and liaison with carers and relatives is mandatory in these diseases.

Further Reading

Collinge J. Prion diseases of humans and animals: their causes and molecular basis. Annu Rev Neurosci. 2001;24:519–50.

Collinge J. Molecular neurology of prion disease. J Neurol Neurosurg Psychiatry. 2005;76(7):906–19.

Mead S. Prion disease genetics. Eur J Hum Genet. 2006;14(3):273–81.

Zerr I, Kallenberg K, Summers DM, Romero C, Taratuto A, Heinemann U, et al. Updated clinical diagnostic criteria for sporadic Creutzfeldt-Jakob disease. Brain. 2009;132:2659–68.

Managing Neuropsychiatric Symptoms of Neurodegenerative Diseases

13

Joseph Trettel, Zeina Chemali, and Kirk R. Daffner

13.1 Introduction

A review of the worldwide incidence of dementia has estimated that a new case is diagnosed every 3 s. The World Alzheimer Report (2015) has estimated the prevalence of dementia to be over 46.5 million globally and projects that this will double every 20 years. Developing countries such as India, China and other south Asian and Pacific nations will see the greatest rise in incidence. It is estimated that in the United States alone approximately 470,000 individuals over the age of 65 will have newly diagnosed Alzheimer disease in 2014.

Dementia is a costly disease. According to Alzheimer's disease International, the estimated global annual cost of dementia was USD 604 billion in 2010. This number has increased to USD 818 billion in 2015. For perspective, this was equiv-

J. Trettel
Department of Neurobehavioral Medicine,
Gaylord Hospital,
Wallingford, CT, USA

Z. Chemali
Departments of Neurology and Psychiatry,
Massachusetts General Hospital, Massachusetts
Eye and Ear Infirmary, Harvard Medical School,
Boston, MA, USA

K.R. Daffner (✉)
Center for Brain/Mind Medicine, Department
of Neurology, Brigham and Women's
Hospital, Harvard Medical School,
Boston, MA, USA
e-mail: KDAFFNER@PARTNERS.ORG

alent to 1.1 % of the world's gross domestic product at that time. Although the direct costs of dementia care are often emphasized, one also needs to be concerned about the toll that caring takes on providers. Most people with dementia are still cared for at home by family members. The physical, psychosocial, and financial burdens of the caregiver need to be taken into consideration as well. The disease burden and cost of care are heightened even more when the patient suffers from neuropsychiatric symptoms associated with dementia. It is with these points in mind that this chapter was written. Our goal is to help the clinician and caregiver identify the neuropsychiatric symptoms associated with dementia and cognitive decline, offer treatment plans to address them, and if no cure is available, provide strategies for symptomatic relief with available drugs, highlighting the benefits and risks of use. Finally, we consider caregivers and caregiver burden and examine how dementia impacts the quality of life of all involved in the system of care.

13.2 Behavioral and Psychological Symptoms of Dementia

Behavioral and psychological symptoms of dementia (BPSD), also referred to as neuropsychiatric symptoms, represent a heterogeneous group of behaviors and psychiatric symptoms occurring in patients with different types of

© Springer International Publishing Switzerland 2016
O. Hardiman, C.P. Doherty (eds.), *Neurodegenerative Disorders: A Clinical Guide*,
DOI 10.1007/978-3-319-23309-3_13

dementia. More than 50 % of individuals with dementia suffer from BPSD, with 90 % of patients experiencing at least one symptom at some point in their disease course. BPSD increase the risk for injury to oneself and others, often necessitating acute interventions. Symptoms are distressing for patients and their caregivers, and are often the reason for placement into residential care. The development of BPSD is associated with a more rapid rate of cognitive decline, greater impairment in activities of daily living (ADLs), and a diminished quality of life (QOL).

The causes of BPSD are complex, often due to multiple etiologies, and appear to vary across cultures and countries. These include neuroanatomical (e.g., limbic or frontal network degenerations), neurochemical (e.g., deficiencies in various neurotransmitters), psychological (e.g., premorbid personality), social (e.g., caregiver factors and changes in the environment), and complications of other medical conditions (e.g., pain and delirium). Dysregulation of cholinergic function correlates with memory problems, while deficits in serotonin, noradrenalin, and GABA have been associated with depression, anxiety, and aggression. In addition, symptoms often co-occur and may share the same neuroanatomical correlates, although the underlying pathology may differ. For example, apathy and disinhibition in AD are both associated with frontal lobe dysfunction, while visual hallucinations and Capgras misidentification delusions observed in dementia with Lewy bodies (DLB) are associated with a reduction in function and metabolism of neurons in the posterior visual cortices.

During the last few years, the field has advanced to recognize the importance of BPSD, correctly diagnose them, and promptly treat them as part of the dementia syndrome. For example, there has been growing awareness of disinhibition as well as lack of personal concern and insight in frontotemporal dementia (FTD); visual hallucinations, mental status fluctuations, and sleep disturbances in DLB; apathy, anxiety, and depression in early-stage Alzheimer's disease (AD); and delusions, hallucinations, agitation, and aggression in the late stages of AD. In FTD and DLB, for instance, the behavioral problems may precede the cognitive ones by years.

Although specialists in the field are getting a better grasp of the neuropsychiatric problems associated with dementia, most patients are still managed within primary care systems that must deal with challenging medical and psychiatric issues. The behavioral and psychological presentations of dementia in patients increase utilization of medical services and cost of care; complicate clinical management of other comorbid diseases, especially involving cardiovascular or infectious processes, delirium, or falls; and cause family members to experience excessive anxiety, depression, sleep problems, and fatigue. Unfortunately, dementia-related symptoms often are under-recognized by primary care physicians. Patients may end up receiving medications with potential side-effects (e.g., anticholinergics). Co-morbid processes associated with alterations in mental status may not be identified and instead, patients are frequently treated with neuroleptics.

Improving the care for such vulnerable patients requires supporting the primary care system with resources. This includes dementia care managers, access to and coordination with interdisciplinary dementia specialists, a feasible dementia screening process, and a thorough diagnostic work-up that considers the etiology of the dementia, after the exclusion of other causes, such as drug-induced delirium, pain, or infection. At a systems level, physician education may have a significant impact on identifying and appropriately treating these conditions.

When facing BPSD, care planning should involve psychosocial treatments for both the patient and family. Although BPSD may respond to environmental and psychosocial interventions, pharmacotherapy is often required for more severe presentations. Below, we will review these issues in more detail.

13.3 Dementing Illnesses

BPSD are manifestations of dementing illnesses. Dementia affects multiple cognitive and functional, and impairs, if not debilitates, social functioning and quality of life. The list of dementing illnesses is extensive (Table 13.1). Since much of

Table 13.1 Causes of dementia

Neurodegenerative
Alzheimer disease
Frontotemporal dementia
Dementia with Lewy bodies
Huntington disease
Corticobasal degeneration
Progressive supranuclear palsy
Multisystem atrophy
Argyrophilic brain disease
Wilson disease
Hallevorden–Spatz disease
Mitochondial diseases
Kuf disease
Metachromatic leukodsytrophy
Adrenoleukodystrophy
Vascular
Vascular dementia
Hypoxic/ischemic injury
Post-CABG
CADASIL (cerebral autosomal dominant arteriopathy with subcortical infarcts and Leukoencephalopathy
Inflammatory/infectious
Multiple sclerosis
Syphilis
Lyme
HIV
Creutzfeldt–Jakob disease
Primary CNS vasculitis
Vasculitis secondary to other autoimmune disorders (i.e., lupus)
Sarcoid
Chronic meningitis (i.e., tuberculosis, cryptococcus, etc.)
Viral encephalitis (i.e., HSV)
Whipple disease
Systemic lupus erythematosus
Sjögren syndrome
Metabolic/toxins
Hypothyroid
Vitamin B_{12}
Thiamine deficiency (Wernicke–Korsakoff)
Niacin deficiency (pellagra)
Vitamin E deficiency
Uremia/dialysis dementia
Addison/cushing
Chronic hepatic encephalopathy
Heavy metals
Alcohol

Table 13.1 (continued)

Neoplastic
Tumor (depends on location)
Paraneoplastic limbic encephalitis (anti-Hu)
Acute and chronic sequelae of brain radiation (acute and subacute encephalopathy, radiation necrosis, diffuse late brain injury)
Chemotherapy
Lymphomatoid granulomatosis

Adapted from Daffner and Wolk (2010)

This list is not exhaustive, as any brain injury can result in dementia depending on location. Some diseases could be under multiple categories

CNS central nervous system, *HSV* herpes simplex virus, *CABG* coronary artery bypass graft, *HIV* human immunodeficiency virus

this book is devoted to elucidating the different dementing syndromes, only a few examples will be highlighted here. The main purpose of this section is to provide a broader context in which to consider BPSD.

Alzheimer's disease (AD) is the most common degenerative dementia and causes a progressive decline in cognitive and functional status. Episodic memory deficits are the predominant initial complaints in most cases. However, deficits in attention, visuospatial processing, naming/language, and executive functions may be present. Over the course of the illness, non-memory cognitive domains become progressively more involved and patients often deteriorate to the point at which they can no longer perform their activities of daily living, recognize family members, and maintain continence. The main pathologic findings of AD are amyloid plaques (an extracellular accumulation of Aβ[beta]), neurofibrillary tangles (intracellular, paired helical structures composed of hyperphosphorylated tau), synaptic loss, and eventually neuronal death. There is a reduction in the availability of acetylcholine (ACh) from loss of cholinergic neurons, which is associated with memory and other cognitive deficits. Other neurotransmitter systems also are disrupted.

Mild cognitive impairment (MCI) is believed to reflect the transition between normal aging and dementia, often due to AD pathology. Originally, MCI was defined in terms of relatively isolated memory deficits in the setting of preserved general cognitive and functional abilities. More recent formulations have categorized the syndrome into amnestic and non-amnestic subtypes, and specified the number of domains involved (single and multiple-domain). The neuropsychiatric aspects of MCI have only recently begun to receive attention. In studies involving specialty memory clinics, patients have tended to convert from MCI to AD at a rate of 10–15 % per year compared to the 1–2 % conversion of age-matched controls. However, in epidemiological studies, the rates of conversion are lower, and 20–40 % of patients may eventually "revert to normal" on subsequent evaluations. At autopsy, many patients who were diagnosed with amnestic-MCI have had neurofibrillary tangles in the hippocampus and entorhinal cortex, with variable findings of amyloid plaques in the neocortex. These findings are felt to be consistent with the idea that MCI often represents a transitional period to AD.

Behavioral variant frontotemporal dementia (bvFTD) is the most frequent form of the set of syndromes under the general rubric of frontotemporal lobar degeneration. Behavioral variant FTD is the second most common cause of neurodegenerative dementia in the presenile years. Patients with bv-FTD exhibit salient changes in personality and behavior that can range from apathy to disinhibition. Patients are frequently inappropriate and lack both insight and empathy. Tests of frontal executive function often are impaired (with relative sparing of memory storage and visuospatial function), but may not be abnormal when the disease is primarily limited to the medial aspects of frontal lobes, sparing the dorsolateral cortices.

Pathologically, tauopathies and TDP-43 proteinopathies make up approximately 90 % of cases of FTD. Taupathies include Pick's disease, corticobasal syndrome, and progressive supranuclear palsy. In bvFTD, pathology has an early anatomical predilection for medial frontal regions of the brain, including the frontoinsular and orbitofrontal cortices, which likely accounts for the prominent changes in personality and behavior that can occur early in the disease course. Neurochemically, deficiencies have been found

in the serotonin and dopamine systems, with relative sparing of the cholinergic and noradrenergic (NA) systems. It remains unclear if these changes reflect the loss of modulatory projection neurons, or a local reduction in synapses that secrete these transmitters. In situ animal models suggest that it is likely a combination of both mechanisms.

DLB appears to be the second most common form of neurodegenerative dementia in older patients, with Lewy body pathology found in up to 35 % of dementia cases. DLB often presents with fluctuations in cognition, visual hallucinations, and mild extrapyramidal features. The hallucinations tend to be well formed (e.g., animals or people). Cognitive impairments most often involve the realms of executive function, attention, speed of processing, and visuospatial abilities. Memory is disrupted at the level of encoding and retrieval, and tends to be less severe than clinical AD. REM sleep behavior disorder and depression are relatively common. The clinical overlap with Parkinson's disease associated dementia (PDD) is considerable and differentiating one from the other often is arbitrary. Pathologically, cortical Lewy bodies (spherical, intracytoplasmic, eosinophilic, neuronal inclusions containing α[alpha]-synuclein and ubiquitin proteins) are found in these patients. The temporal cortex and limbic structures are prominently involved. In addition, plaque and tangle pathology often is observed in these patients, with roughly half reaching pathologic criteria for AD. Neurochemically, cholinergic deficits are more pronounced in DLB than AD, which may explain why cholinesterase inhibitors tend to have a greater therapeutic benefit in DLB.

Huntington's disease (HD) is a fatal neurodegenerative disorder associated with severe BPSD. HD is rare with an estimated prevalence of 4–10/100,000 in Western countries. Symptom onset is early (i.e., 35–45 years) and follows an autosomal dominant pattern of inheritance. Pathologically HD is characterized by an abnormal expansion of CAG repeats in the Huntington's gene on chromosome four producing a neurotoxic protein. The initial and rapid loss of striatal neurons leads to choreiform movements and severe psychiatric disturbances. As the disease evolves to include the cerebral cortex and other subcortical structures, cognitive impairment may be subtle, typically presenting as a dysexecutive syndrome. Ultimately, multiple cognitive domains are impacted and most patients develop the 'HD Triad' of abnormal movements, psychiatric disturbances, and dementia (Walker 2007). Death occurs 15–20 years after symptom onset.

Vascular dementia (VaD) is often cited as the second most common form of dementia, with estimates ranging from 10 % to more than 33 % of all dementia cases. Vascular dementia represents the clinical end-product of vascular injury to the brain from a range of etiologies, including leukoariosis, small-vessel infarcts, multiple cortical strokes, or a single, strategically placed stroke. Multiple lacunar infarcts or significant white matter disease (Binswanger disease) can lead to apathy, frontal network impairment, and corticospinal and bulbar signs. Large-vessel strokes result in syndromes specific to the site of the lesion, such as amnesia, aphasia, agnosia, etc. The coexistence of vascular injury and AD pathology is extremely common (with some reports suggesting occurrence in more than 50 % of cases diagnosed with vascular dementia). Often, such cases are labeled as a "mixed dementia". Particularly pertinent is the observation that vascular events seem to hasten the onset and increase the severity of clinical AD, which makes it very difficult to accurately estimate the actual prevalence of vascular dementia. Not surprisingly, the risk factors for vascular dementia are believed to be the same as those for stroke, including hypertension, diabetes, high cholesterol, and atherosclerosis.

13.4 Spectrum of Neuropsychiatric Symptoms in Neurodegenerative Diseases

Recently (2012), the International Psychogeriatric Association (IPA) published the 'The IPA Complete Guide to Behavioral and Psychological Symptoms of Dementia' for academic and clinical specialists who manage and study BPSD. Aside from defining roles that clinicians play in the management of BPSD, these guidelines highlight the diversity of BPSD and review currently accepted, evidenced-based approaches to treatment. Notwithstanding, there remain several challenges and disagreements currently encountered in the literature regarding the neuropsychiatric and behavioral symptoms seen in dementia. For example, can BPSD be divided into syndromes that cluster as psychosis, agitation, and mood disorders? Should clinicians group together disparate symptoms if patients present with many different ones that have various underlying etiologies? An important issue is that clinicians and nursing home providers often lack formal screening batteries to appropriately identify the symptoms. Regardless of where one stands on these debates, there is clear evidence that BPSD increase the rate of institutionalization, caregiver distress, and the cost of care.

The study of BPSD has been challenging, as researchers have had difficulty accurately quantifying symptoms in trials. Dividing by subtypes of dementia has had limited benefit. For example, research comparing AD and VaD has found that behavioral dysregulation did not differ by subtype of dementia but rather by severity of the disease process. The majority of well-controlled studies on pharmacologic management of BPSD have been conducted on cohorts of AD patients. In some cases (e.g., PDD and DLB) the underlying neurobiology of BPSD is likely quite different from that of AD. Nevertheless, at this point it is most useful to extrapolate from the available data to make evidence-based treatment decisions, regardless of the underlying neurodegenerative process. There are exceptions to this approach, which will be discussed below.

There is frequently dissociation between the quasilinear decline in cognitive function and the expression of BPSD suggesting possible independent pathophysiological mechanisms. Neuropathologic and neuroimaging data suggests that BPSD reflect regional involvement verses diffuse brain pathology. In AD, for example, increased plaque and tangle burden in frontal and limbic areas correlates with psychotic and affective symptoms, while involvement of the anterior cingulate is associated with apathy and depression. As pointed out by Cassanova et al. (Cassanova et al. 2011), the complex interplay of neuropathology with neurochemical, premorbid psychiatric history, environmental, social, and genetic factors will influence the expression of BPSD. Few studies have demonstrated a consistent relationship between the emergence of specific BPSD and the natural course of the disease. However, some trends have been noted. For example, in comparing the onset of BSPD before and after the diagnosis of AD was made, Jost and colleagues (1995) found a progression of symptoms, in which depression, social isolation, anxiety, and suicidal ideation were among the first to arise. Later in the disease, irritability, agitation and aggression, loss of social comportment (e.g., inappropriate sexual behavior), and psychotic phenomena, including hallucinations and delusions, were commonly observed. This trend is evident when comparing BPSD in patients who are treated in outpatient settings with those in patients requiring inpatient hospitalization for behavioral reasons.

Currently, there are no medications approved by the US Food and Drug Administration (FDA) for the treatment of BPSD. The judicious use of high-dose, high-potency neuroleptics and anticonvulsants remains popular among inpatient providers despite these risks, while outpatient providers are more likely to utilize SSRIs, cholinesterase inhibitors, and low-dose, low potency neuroleptics to manage symptoms. Further complicating BPSD management, few accepted standards for non-pharmacological treatments exist. Many practitioners consider the guidelines established by the 'Expert Consensus Panel for Using Antipsychotic Drugs in Older Patients' (Alexopoulos et al. 2004), the 'American Geriatrics Society Guide to Management of Psychotic Disorders and Neuropsychiatric Symptoms of Dementia in Older Adults' (2011), and the 'IPA guidelines to BPSD' (Draper et al. 2012) to be good starting points. Nevertheless, many treatments are initiated on an empirical basis; trial and error is often the rule rather than the exception.

Below, we outline the most common neuropsychiatric symptoms in neurodegenerative diseases

Table 13.2 Most common neuropsychiatric symptoms based on informant report using the NPI-Q

Delusions
Hallucinations
Agitation
Depression
Anxiety
Euphoria
Apathy
Disinhibition
Irritability
Aberrant motor behavior
Sleep disturbance
Appetite disturbance

Adapted from Cummings (1997) and Kaufer et al. (2000)

Table 13.3 Behaviors with poor response to drugs

1. Wandering
2. Pacing
3. Attempting to leave
4. Disruptive vocalizations
5. Incontinence
6. Failure to bathe

Adapted from Omelan C. Approach to managing behavioural disturbances in dementia. Can Fam Physician. 2006;52:191–9

that are captured by the *Neuropsychiatric Inventory* (NPI; (Cummings 1997); Table 13.2). Many symptoms are extremely difficult to target with the currently available psychotropic medications (Table 13.3). For simplicity, we divide the BPSD into symptom clusters that are widely recognized in general neuropsychiatry (e.g., affective, psychotic, vegetative, etc.). Particular emphasis is placed on the underlying neuroanatomy and neurochemistry that correlates with symptoms. More comprehensive reviews focusing on the neurobiology and functional anatomy of BPSD can be found elsewhere (e.g., (Geda et al. 2013)).

13.4.1 Affective Symptoms

Loss of neurons in the dorsal raphe nuclei has been implicated in the development of depression in normal aging and AD. These neurons synthesize and release serotonin. They are segregated into multiple paramedian nuclei that project to a myriad of brain regions implicated in mood disorders such as limbic, peri-limbic, and frontal areas of the cerebral cortex. Emerging evidence suggests that there is a 'normal' age-related loss of dorsal raphe neurons. This predisposes the elderly to depression. This effect appears more robust in AD patients. PET imaging used to examine metabolic activity of dorsal raphe neurons in AD patients has shown a reliable decrease in activity beyond age-matched controls. Alterations in serotinergic tone have been implicated in several other BPSD that include apathy, agitation and aggression, and sleep changes. Some studies have also reported a decrease in NA in the locus coerulus in depressed patients with AD. Others have found increased NA activity in target areas, e.g., frontal and limbic cortex, perhaps to compensate for dysfunction elsewhere in the nervous system.

Findings such as these are difficult to interpret for a number of reasons. Neuromodulatory projection neurons from the brainstem project diffusely throughout the brain. In *all* instances, noradrenergic and serotonergic projections ascending to limbic and cortical structures are regionally unique. They employ various postsynaptic mechanisms and target different types of neurons, as well as different 'compartments' of those target neurons. The result is a complex, region-specific-effect of serotonin and noradrenalin. For example, noradrenergic transmission in the prefrontal cortex stimulates the release of dopamine, but has no effect on dopamine release in parietal and occipital corticies. Similarly, the effect of serotonin on cortical activity is highly variable, owing to the tremendous diversity of pre- and post-synaptic serotonin receptors. Exactly how this contributes to the BPSD is not known, but certainly impacts the pharmacologic approach used to target specific symptoms.

The superior frontal regions have been anatomically implicated in depression in normal controls and patients with AD and VaD. Several other areas that include the anterior cingulate, parahippocampal gyrus, amygdala, hypothalamus and limbic striatum are likely to be involved as well. The role of interoceptive, humoral, and sensory inputs to limbic circuitry remains unexplored in neurodegenerative diseases.

Depressed mood of varying intensity occurs in 30–40 % of patients with dementia. It is one of the most common BPSD and may develop at any stage of the disease. Depression is co-morbid with AD, DLB, VaD, PDD, and corticobasal syndromes (CBS). Recently, these symptoms have become of greater interest to clinicians and researchers. Depression was found to alter function, often preceding mild cognitive impairment (MCI) and heralding the transition to dementia. Some studies have even supported the association of biomarkers, such as Troponin and S100β (beta), with depression, while others reported that up to 1/3 patients with dementia and BPSD had prominent depressive symptomatology. A high association has been found between depression in dementia and symptoms of irritability, disinhibition, agitation, and anxiety.

Euphoria is medically recognized as a state of exaggerated sense of elation and well-being, most frequently associated with bipolar-spectrum disorders as well as damage to the anterior portions of the right hemisphere. An overexcited and elated mood could be a marker of frontal dysfunction and is often a sign of FTD. The affective disorders of BPSD are generally non-specific and can mimic hypomanic and manic states. Euphoria often precedes memory deterioration in FTD, for example. Once dementia has progressed, the identification of a hypomanic component becomes more difficult, as mental deterioration predominates.

13.4.2 Apathy/Behavioral Inertia

Symptoms of apathy in AD correlate with higher neuronal loss and an increased density of tangles in frontal areas. Similar patterns are seen with the accumulation of Lewy bodies in the same cortical regions. Neurochemically, multiple transmitters have been implicated, including a reduction in cortical NA and decreased dopaminergic and cholinergic signaling. Neuroimaging studies of apathy in Alzheimer's disease have demonstrated atrophy and hypoperfusion of the anterior cingulate and orbitofrontal cortex.

Apathy is commonly seen in AD, VaD, progressive supranuclear palsy (PSP) and FTD. The term apathy is being used with increasing frequency in both neurology and psychiatry. However, its definition varies. Some consider it a symptom of other major psychiatric disorders, whereas others view it as a syndrome of its own. Apathy is a disorder involving motivation rather than mood, and exists on a continuum between abulia and akinetic mutism. Apathy has been characterized by reduced goal-directed behavior (in domains of cognition, emotional expression, and self-generated, voluntary purposeful behavior). Behaviorally, apathy can be seen as an increase in behavioral inertia. In other words, the neural resources required to engage in a given act are greater than what the individual is volitionally willing to expend.

There is strong evidence that apathy is a common finding in AD. The MMSE and other brief cognitive screens do not measure apathy. Clinically, there can be a co-occurrence of apathy and agitation, or apathy and depression. Several apathy scales (see below) can be administered to either patients or caregivers to ascertain a quantitative measure of apathy. In some studies, apathy is cited as the most common BPSD in AD. For example, a study by Craig and colleagues (2005) enrolled 435 patients with AD and concluded that apathy and indifference were the most frequent symptoms at 76 %, followed by aberrant motor behavior (65 %), appetite changes (64 %), irritability (63 %), and agitation/aggression (58 %). Apathy has been shown to be associated with a decline in ADLs and a predictor of conversion to dementia in MCI patients. Although the current data were obtained from randomized controlled trials (RCTs) that did not investigate apathy, per se, it has been readily noted that apathy/indifference are moderately distressing to caregivers. Treatment with cholinesterase inhibitors and/or psychosocial interventions are the only available modalities for treating apathy in AD that have been shown to have some efficacy. The use of stimulants or 'stimulating' SSRIs (e.g., fluoxetine) has become a common practice, but supporting data are limited. Medications will be discussed in more detail in subsequent sections.

13.4.3 Anxiety

The pathophysiologic origins of anxiety are unclear. The disorder frequently co-occurs with depression. In individuals without dementia, a distributed network including the amygdala, medial prefrontal cortex, bed nucleus of the stria terminalis, and more ventral regions of the hippocampus have been implicated in the induction and maintenance of anxious states. There is evidence that modulating serotonergic transmission can affect anxiety. In addition, agents that increase GABAergic tone (e.g., benzodiazepines) can shift the delicate balance of cerebral excitation and inhibition towards the latter, leading to less anxious states. More studies are needed to pinpoint the neurobiology of this common symptom in BPSD and to determine if the underlying neurobiology differs significantly from what is observed in cognitively intact individuals.

Anxiety often occurs in AD, PD, and VaD. However, anxiety is rarely studied alone in medication trials for neurodegenerative diseases. It is usually coupled with depression and together form the 'affective dyad' in BPSD. Anxiety is often associated with irritability, aggression, agitation, and pathological crying. Some experts conceptualize anxiety as being on one end of a behavioral spectrum, with aggression at the other, while agitation lies in between the two, representing a transitional state between internal tension and outwardly-directed action. It has been challenging to quantify anxiety as a single variable. Refusal to bathe and attend to self-care have been attributed to anxiety. Repetitive sentences with senseless content also may be a sign of anxiety. However, these symptoms may result from any number of BPSD.

13.4.4 Agitation and Aggressive Behavior

As suggested above, agitation and aggression represent a continuum of behaviors that, in

Table 13.4 Behavior as a form of communication about underlying processes: BPSD and common mimickers

1. Review possible physical contributions (i.e., pain and infections)

2. Rule out delirium

3. Check for dehydration

4. Look at the patient's medication list (for drug-drug interactions and anticholinergic side effects)

5. Look for contributing environmental factors (noise, change of caregivers etc.)

6. Consider psychiatric diseases such as depression and anxiety

7. Sleep difficulties

8. Consider unwitnessed falls and resulting fracture or hematoma

general, are out of proportion to the inciting stimulus (internal or external). Greater agitation in AD correlates with more neurofibrillary tangles in the bilateral orbitofrontal and left anterior cingulate cortices. Chemically, the disruption of serotonin systems appears to be relevant, as symptoms partially respond to SSRIs that are used as a first-line treatment to target aggression, followed by neuroleptics to counter disruption in the dopaminergic system. In studies of non-demented psychiatric patients, lower levels of the serotonin metabolite 5-HIAA in the CSF are the most strongly correlated neurochemical changes seen in aggressive patients.

Agitation is commonly observed in AD and bvFTD. In these diseases, it manifests as restlessness, pacing, fidgeting, increases in directed and non-purposeful motor activities, and abnormal vocalizations such as verbigeration or yelling. It is the most common symptom in AD accompanied by aggression. Aggression is expressed as verbal insults, shouting, hitting, and throwing things. Needless to say, both agitation and aggression necessitate an increase in personal care assistance, and at least at their onset, should prompt a complete metabolic and structural work-up to rule out any acute reversible causes (Table 13.4).

Aggression/rage reactions and irritability are complex behaviors that frequently lead to assessment by physicians. Aggressive symptoms can be divided into physically aggressive symptoms, such as hitting, biting, punching, grabbing, and

kicking; and verbally aggressive symptoms, such as yelling, cursing, and anger outbursts. Aggression is associated with FTD and the later stages of AD, VaD, and DLB. It can be influenced by environmental and physical factors, such as pain or changes in the environment, to name a few. It was recently demonstrated by a research team in England that systematically treating pain significantly reduced the frequency and intensity of aggressive acts in nursing home patients with moderate to severe dementia. Interestingly, empirical prescribing of analgesics reduced the overall severity of BPSD, suggesting that carefully screening for pain in patients with impaired communication can lead to an improvement in overall behavioral symptomatology.

Aggression is associated with increased use of psychotropics, augmented caregiver burden, and greater likelihood of transfer to nursing homes or other long-term care facilities. A large epidemiological study of community dwelling and nursing home residents reported by Lyketsos and colleagues (2002) found that 30 % of dementia patients are considered agitated or aggressive. 'Rage reaction' can also occur in patients with dementia. It manifests as a sudden emotional/physical response disproportionate to the stimulus. This behavior can be explosive, unpredictable, and very difficult for caregivers to manage safely.

13.4.5 Psychotic Symptoms

In AD patients there is an association between psychosis and the density of neurofibrillary tangles in the middle frontal, superior temporal, and inferior parietal areas, even after accounting for Lewy body pathology. Neurochemically, a significant decrease in hippocampal serotonergic activity, hyperactivity of dopamine, and intact noradrenaline in the substantia nigra were implicated. Involvement of these regions and modulatory systems (i.e., serotonin, dopamine, and acetylcholine) have been implicated in psychotic symptoms in non-degenerative neurologic disease as well, including delirium and formal thought disorders on the schizophreniform spectrum.

In general, psychotic phenomena become more common in the late stages of dementia. Ascertaining the underlying etiology can be difficult; symptoms such as delusions frequently co-occur with changes in affective state and cognition. La Salvia and Chemali (2011) have argued that deficits in social cognition may be a unifying principle that can explain the emergence of psychotic symptoms late in life. Delusions are extremely common in patients with AD and create significant caregiver distress. In the natural course of the disease, up to 73 % of AD patients will develop at least one non-systematized delusion. They also occur in patients with DLB, VaD, and PDD. Incidence rates in VaD are similar to that in AD; data on incidence in DLB and PPD are lacking. The most common delusion patients have is that other people are stealing from them; themes of abandonment and sexual infidelity are also common. Physical aggression can often be an indication that paranoid delusions are present.

Hallucinations occur commonly in dementia. Similar to primary psychotic disorders, alterations of dopamine transmission have been implicated in the etiology of hallucinations in neurodegenerative disorders. This is consistent with the higher incidence of hallucinations seen in DLB and PDD, compared to late-stage AD. In dementia patients, hallucinations in all sensory modalities appear to be less responsive to traditional D2-receptor antagonism. This finding may reflect an as-of-yet unidentified difference in the underlying neurobiological basis of hallucinosis in dementia compared to cognitively intact patients. Hallucinations in DLB and PDD are particularly difficult to treat and the D2 blockade typically exacerbates the motor manifestations of the disease and worsens cognitive function. Hallucinations frequently predict a rapid rate of decline and have been correlated with severity of dementia and aggression.

Misidentification syndromes as seen in Capgras (i.e., a familiar person becomes an imposture) and Fregoli (i.e., people dressed up as others) are often seen in DLB and FTD. The response patients have to the delusions may lead to aggressive behavior. Moreover, these delusions are often very distressing for caregivers when they are the 'object' of the delusion.

13.4.5.1 Neurovegatative Symptoms

Sleep disturbances are often found in early stages of DLB, with REM disorders and disrupted sleep-wake cycles, although these may occur in other dementias, especially with increasing severity of the disease. Abnormal REM sleep behavior can predate the onset of cognitive symptoms in DLB by several decades. Appetite and eating disturbances are often seen in FTD. Hyper-orality and carbohydrate craving may herald this disease. Patients may choke on what they are eating as they cannot gauge the quantity of food they put in their mouth. Sense of satiety appears to be lost, as is the capacity for the appropriate experience of disgust. Disturbance of satiety and disgust have been linked to dysfunction of the frontoinsular cortex.

13.4.5.2 Other Symptoms

Behaviors such as chanting, pacing, and repetitive tapping may be symptoms of underlying anxiety or may occur alone. Wandering is one of the most common and troublesome symptoms of BPSD, with a prevalence rate of up to 53 %. Wandering can be seen as aimless walking, trying to leave the house, leaving the premises to go to unfamiliar, and sometimes dangerous areas, and shadowing the caregiver. Delirium in patients with BPSD can exacerbate symptoms. Delirium itself can lead to BPSD and needs to be ruled out as a cause of alterations in behavior. Often this behavioral change comes on abruptly. Of note, risk factors for the development of delirium include advancing age, cognitive impairment, and dementia.

13.5 Neuropsychiatric Symptoms in MCI

Data from the Alzheimer's disease Neuroimaging Initiative (ADNI) suggests that many of the symptoms endorsed by patients with dementia on the NPI-Q are observed in MCI patients at rates that are higher than in the general population of cognitively intact controls, but at lower rates than in AD patients. Some behaviors characteristic of moderate and severe AD, such as wandering, pacing, abnormal vocalizations, and pseudobulbar affect were not observed in MCI. In addition, disruptions in appetite seem to occur at similar rates in both MCI and AD. However, the nature of these changes is likely quite different between the two groups. Neuropsychiatric symptoms in cognitively normal older adults, including depression, apathy, irritability, anxiety, and agitation have been associated with increased risk of progression to MCI (Geda et al. 2014).

13.6 Assessment and Testing of Presence/Absence of Neuropsychiatric Symptoms

Although neuroimaging, functional imaging, and CSF biomarkers are readily available and are used to help diagnose different types of neurodegenerative disorders, clinicians continue to rely heavily on quantifying deficits using neuropsychological testing and standardized behavioral scales. More than 30 scales are available for use to measure BPSD. Some of the most commonly used include:

- Cohen-Mansfield Agitation Inventory (CMAI): Examines 29 types of agitated behaviors.
- Neuropsychiatric Inventory (NPI) and its version for Nursing Homes (NPI-NH): Assess 12 behavioral issues.
- Behavioral Pathology in AD (BEHAVE-AD) scale: Structured around the clinical psychiatric interview. Assesses 25 abnormal behaviors in seven different domains of psychosis, affective disorders, aggressiveness and diurnal rhythm changes.
- Cornell Scale for Depression in Dementia (CSDD): Developed to assess signs and symptoms of major depression in patients with dementia during the week preceding the interview. Because some of these patients may give unreliable reports, the CSDD requires an interview with an informant. Each item is rated for severity on a scale of 0–2 (0 = absent, 1 = mild or intermittent, 2 = severe). Scores >10 suggest probable major depression; scores >18, definite major depression; and scores <6 indicate absent depression.

- Apathy Evaluation Scale (AES): Includes 14 items on initiation, motivation, and goal-directed behaviors that are rated by the patient's relative or care provider. Scores on each item vary from 0 to 3, with higher scores indicating more severe apathy. An alternative is the Starkstein Apathy scale; both measures capture similar behavioral phenomena.

13.7 Treatment

Management of dementia should focus on the maintenance of function and independence for the person with the disease. Current symptomatic treatments for dementia have only modest efficacy. An international group of caregivers, organizations, and professionals with expertise in dementia developed a consensus statement that recommended that medication trials should state clear, pre-defined diagnostic and severity criteria as well as outcome measures (i.e., functional and executive capacity). It was suggested that to be complete, health economic measures should be incorporated as secondary outcomes in all future Phase III trials, with analysis of cost-effectiveness and clinical outcome. Although current drugs for AD may reduce the amount of family caregiver time required, the treatment may have a negative impact on the time spent with patients, and reduce their opportunity for connectedness, crucial for wellbeing. As the population of older adults grows across the world, their empowerment may impact the political establishment and lead to a change in the economics of treatment in dementia. One example is increased caution about the use of neuroleptics, and more stringent regulations with black box warnings as well as documentation of side-effects and duration of treatment. There are several factors that should be considered before starting any psychotropic medication (Table 13.5).

13.7.1 Neuroleptics

Several neuroleptics have been investigated in older adults with psychosis, and studies have shown some benefit in select groups of patients,

Table 13.5 Questions to ask before starting a medication

1. What is the targeted behavior to be treated?
2. Is a drug really necessary?
3. Have alternative non-pharmacological methods been tried?
4. Was informed consent sought? (If patient is not capable of providing consent, was caregiver asked?)
5. Which drug to use?
6. What is its lowest therapeutic dose?
7. When will the treatment plan be reassessed?
8. Are side effects checked for and treatment plan adjusted accordingly?
9. Is this the most cost-effective choice?

Modified from Avorn and Gurwitz (1995)

but with various side effects and risks, including increased mortality and cardiovascular and cerebrovascular events. Neuroleptic use is common in both community-dwelling older adults and nursing home residents to address symptoms of psychosis and/or BPSD. In community dwelling adults aged 40–64 living in the United States, an average of 620,000 individuals, annually, were found to be prescribed neuroleptics during an 8-year study period (51.9 % typical neuroleptics and 50.4 % atypical neuroleptics). That number increases in the 65 and older population, where approximately 1 million individuals per year are prescribed atypical antipsychotics. In the United Kingdom, almost 18 % of older adults in contact with a mental health provider are prescribed neuroleptics, mostly second-generation (atypical neuroleptics). In many cases these medications are used for their sedating properties, not for antipsychotic treatment, per se. Of note, there is an ongoing movement in many nursing homes around the United States to reduce, and even eliminate, the use of neuroleptics for dementia patients, and progress is being made in reaching goals set forth by national agencies.

Neuroleptics that have been examined in randomized clinical trials (RCTs) for the treatment of BPSD include haloperidol, risperidone, quietapine, olanzapine, and aripiprazole. To our knowledge, there have been no RCTs of clozapine for treatment of BPSD, though data on its use in older adults with schizophrenia are available.

All antipsychotics carry a black box warning of higher risk of all-cause mortality and cerebrovascular events in elderly patients with dementia. In a systematic review of 17 RCTs, including 5377 patients with BPSD who had been on aripiprazole, olanzapine, risperidone, quetiapine, ziprasidone, and haloperidol, it was found that the risk of death in drug treated patients was 4.5 % vs. 2.6 % in placebo treated patients who also had BPSD. It was later found that haloperidol had the greatest mortality rates. Subsequently, this warning has been expanded to cover all first- and second-generation neuroleptics.

In addition, data suggest that neuroleptics further impair cognition and can lead to a more rapid course of clinical deterioration, with falls and recurrent respiratory and urinary tract infections cited often. When considering their use, the risks and benefits of treatment should be carefully considered and discussed with both caregivers and involved family. Finally, the provider might bear in mind that antipsychotics are *not indicated* for wandering, restlessness, uncooperativeness, vocalizations, insomnia, or other behaviors that do not represent a risk of harm to self or others. While these behaviors can certainly be problematic, the authors do not feel that they warrant the added dangers of neuroleptic treatment unless a clear risk of harm is documented.

Risperidone appears to have the most support for the treatment of agitation and aggression in dementia. In five RTCs involving predominantly AD patients, including the BEHAVE-AD study of over 600 nursing home patients, risperidone has been shown to have modest but significant efficacy. The incidence of EPS in dementia patients treated with risperidone is dose dependent and most estimates range from 10 to 30 % (multiple studies). In the Clinical Antipsychotic Trials of Intervention Effectiveness-Alzheimer's Disease (CATIE-AD) trial, a 12-week multicenter randomized placebo-controlled trial investigating the efficacy of olanzapine, quetiapine, and risperdone in AD patients with BPSD, there was no significant difference between patients treated with an atypical neuroleptic and a placebo in terms of clinical response. Additional analyses in the CATIE-AD trial revealed modest efficacy of risperidone for treating psychosis, total NPI score, and hostility. In contrast, olanzapine was efficacious only for treating hostility, most likely due to its sedating effects, whereas quitiapine was not found to be effective on any measure. Interestingly, citalopram appears to be at least as effective as risperidone for treating agitation and psychosis in AD, VaD, mixed dementia, DLB, and Dementia NOS.

The AGIT and DART-AD (Ballard et al. 2008, 2009a, b, c, d) trails did not find a benefit of neuroleptic use verses placebo over a 6-month treatment period. However, a randomized double blind trial of continued treatment of 112 AD patients in long-term care facilities with risperidone vs. placebo beyond 6 months found a greater relapse rate (agitation and psychosis) for placebo (48 %) vs. risperidone (15 %). Subanalyses in the DART study also reveled some benefit of risperidone for patients with a total NPI score >15, suggesting that patients with a high symptom burden may benefit from long-term treatment. Aripiprazole has been shown to have modest efficacy in treating AD-related psychosis and agitation in several RCTs (Reviewed by De Deyn et al. 2013), and in general is well tolerated. The efficacy of aripiprazole in treating psychosis and abnormal movements in HD has been well established.

Quetiapine is widely used in both in- and out-patient settings for its mild sedating effects at hypnotic doses (i.e., < 100 mg) as well as an augmentation strategy for mood disorders at higher doses. The latter is a result of its actions on numerous serotonin receptors throughout the brain. In many US hospitals, quetiapine is unfortunately considered a first line agent for insomnia in the elderly even though it has a myriad of receptor affinities and potential side-effects. Despite its common use for BPSD, quetiapine has been associated with greater global deterioration and its efficacy in treating agitation appears no better than placebo or the cholinesterase inhibitor, rivastigmine. One exception is in the treatment of psychotic symptomatology in PDD and LBD. Lower D2 receptor affinity is essential to avoid exacerbation of parkinsonism; quitiapine

and clozapine are generally considered the safest of the neuroleptics, although their potent anticholinergic properties may limit their use by worsening cognition and gait stability.

The first generation neuroleptics enjoy frequent use in the inpatient setting due to routes of administration and rapid onset of action. However, in treating BPSD, haloperidol was found to increase overall morbidity and mortality in four RCTs. A report from the US Medicare and Medicaid database of over 75,000 patients demonstrated greater morbidity and mortality risk associated with haloperidol use compared to risperidone. Based on current evidence, the authors do not encourage the use of first generation antipsychotics. There are, however, some situations when their use may be the best treatment option. This often occurs on inpatient psychiatric units where late-stage dementia patients can become very aggressive and pose a considerable risk of harm to self or others. Intramuscular administration of low-potency, highly sedating agents, such as chlorpromazine, may be temporarily effective and avoid patient and/or caregiver harm. Appropriate fall precautions and routine monitoring of cardiac conduction intervals (i.e., QTc) must be clearly in place in such circumstances.

Lastly, a common issue that arises in dementia care involves the impact of discontinuing neuroleptic treatment, often because of possible adverse effects. Studies of neuroleptic discontinuation first appear in the early 1990s (e.g., (Fitz and Mallya 1992)). Many early studies found that the discontinuation of neuroleptics did not have a significant impact on behavioral outcomes such as agitation and psychosis. However, many of these studies were plagued by inconsistencies in symptom assessment, duration of treatment (i.e., some patients were on neuroleptics for >3 years), and the discontinuation of multiple psychotropics simultaneously. More recently, a well designed study by Devanand and colleagues (2012) demonstrated that discontinuation of risperidone was associated with an increased risk of relapse in patients with Alzheimer's disease who had psychosis or agitation and who responded to risperidone therapy over 4–8 months.

13.7.2 Cholinesterase Inhibitors

Acetylcholinesterase inhibitors (AChE-I) are alternative treatments to neuroleptics. Cholinergic neurons projecting to cortical and limbic structures are predominantly found in the nucleus basalis (of Meynart). Acetylcholine appears to generally facilitate cognitive function, especially episodic memory. Disruption of cholinergic systems contribute to different behaviors, such as psychosis, depression, agitation, and personality changes.

AChE-I have been shown to produce secondary benefits in BPSD. More than 30 RCTs have been published regarding the use of ACH-I in the treatment of BPSD, with treatment periods ranging from 6–12 months. The medications are generally well tolerated. Gastrointestinal symptoms were the most common including nausea, vomiting, and diarrhea. Bradycardia and syncope need to be closely monitored. The pooled evidence suggests sustained benefits for anxiety, depression and apathy, but no benefit for agitation and aggression over 24 weeks of study. Efficacy may vary among agents and differ across individual patients. There has been scant investigation employing head-to-head trials. The majority of studies have used donepezil. Drug benefits were easier to demonstrate for moderate-to-severe BPSD compared with mild-to-moderate symptoms. A large meta-analysis found that AChE-I offer a small but significant improvement in multiple BPSD compared to placebo. Also of note, the withdrawal of donepezil at 6 weeks has been associated with increased overall NPI scores.

Galantamine is a specific reversible AChE-I. It also works on nicotinic receptors to potentiate cholinergic neurotransmission. There is some evidence demonstrating that galantamine has positive effects on ADLs and behavior. A 2001 Cochrane data analysis noted seven RCTs for galantamine addressing these issues.

Many reports examining the impact of rivastigmine on behavior (as a secondary endpoint) have been open label studies. They have shown some efficacy in treating behavioral disturbances in patients with a wide range of dementias, including AD, VaD, FTD, mixed dementia, DLB, PDD, and schizophrenia with dementia. A number of case reports have suggested that rivastigmine is particularly beneficial for behavioral disturbances in DLB and FTD, but this has not been confirmed in controlled studies. An additional benefit of rivistigmine is the option of transdermal administration that seems to reduce GI side effects. In summary, additional research is needed to more clearly establish the efficacy of AChE-I on the BPSD. They appear to be beneficial for anxiety, depression, and apathy, but not for *acute* agitation and aggression.

13.7.3 Memantine

Memantine is complex drug with several actions in the brain that deserve mention. At NMDA receptors, it acts as a low-affinity, non-competitive antagonist that shows voltage-dependent binding. Physiologic release of glutamate in the presence of substhreshold depolarization will displace memantine, suggesting that its effects on the glutamate system are probably related to limiting excitotoxicity rather than modulating synaptic glutamate signaling, per se. In addition, memantine is a weak D2 agonist, $5-HT_3$ antagonist, and a weak antagonist at several nicotinic Ach receptors. In animal models, memantine-induced NMDA antagonism has been shown to enhance activity of histamine neurons and increase levels of brain-derived neurotrophic factor (BDNF) in the hippocampus and parahippocampal areas. This further implicates NMDA antagonism with improved cognition often observed in AD patients treated with memantine.

Individual studies, meta-analysis, and pooled analysis showed benefit from the use of memantine to target mild to moderate irritability, lability, agitation, aggression, and psychosis over 3–6 months. There is very little evidence that it is useful for acute agitation. Results from the Memantine for Agitation in Dementia (MAGD) were recently presented at the International Conference on Alzheimer's disease. This large placebo-controlled RCT did not show a reliable benefit. Memantine was well tolerated, but studies are still needed in patients with moderate-to-severe agitation to determine its efficacy in treating BPSD. A Cochrane review indicated little effect of memantine for symptoms in VaD and failed to show any benefit in PDD and DLB.

13.7.4 Antiepileptic Drugs

Anticonvulsants and 'mood stabilizers' (carbamazepine, valproic acid, gabapentin, lamotrigine, topiramate, oxcarbazepine) have been studied in the treatment of BPSD and "non-cognitive" symptoms of dementia. Among these medications, only carbamazepine has demonstrated efficacy in the treatment of the BPSD in controlled studies. Two small RCTs of 6 weeks or less suggested a potential benefit for treating agitation. *Post hoc* meta-analysis did show improvement in scores on the Clinical Global Improvement and Brief Psychiatric Rating Scales. Significant adverse events of carabamazepine have been reported in the elderly, including sedation, hyponatremia, and cardiac toxicity. In addition, carbamazepine is a strong hepatic CYP450 inducer; elderly patients on multiple medications may be at higher risk of drug-drug interactions.

A number of open label studies and case reports yielded promising results with valproic acid for the treatment of BPSD. However, five published controlled studies have failed to demonstrate that it was a useful treatment modality for BPSD. The continued use of valproic acid likely reflects its accepted utility as a mood-stabilizing agent in general neuropsychiatric populations. However, more studies need to be conducted on the role of valproic acid in preventing or treating BPSD.

Evidence that gabapentin treats BPSD is still very preliminary. The drug is well tolerated when used for this purpose, but no controlled study has been conducted to provide evidence of its efficacy, despite case reports and open label studies showing encouraging results. There are two case reports in which gabapentin was used in the context of agitation in DLB. It has not been shown to have any efficacy in other types of dementia. Two recent case reports seem to indicate some effi-

cacy of lamotrigine in BPSD. This drug may have neuroprotective effects by reducing the hyperactivity of neurons in the hippocampus and parahippocampal gyrus. The concurrent use of lamotrigine and valproic acid should be avoided due to hepatic interactions and an increased risk of adverse side effects, including Stevens-Johnson syndrome. Topiramate has shown promising results in one open study in BPSD. However, given its potential negative side effects on cognition, it cannot be recommended for routine use. No clinical study has been published studying oxcarbazepine in the treatment of BPSD. In general, this drug is better tolerated than carbamazepine, but can induce severe and more frequent hyponatremia. Moreover, it has considerably less mood stabilizing properties than carbamazepine. In summary, with the exception of carbamazepine, the off label use of antiepileptic agents cannot be recommended for the treatment of BPSD.

13.7.5 Antidepressants

Depression, anxiety, apathy, and agitation may have an underlying neurobiological profile that would make the use of serotinergic antidepressants in BPSD a reasonable choice. These symptoms respond to modulation of serotonin transmission in general psychiatric patients, and several structures with high densities of serotonin receptors including the medial and dorsolateral prefrontal and anterior cingulate cortices have been implicated in the pathophysiology, among a myriad of others.

The evidence for selective serotonin reuptake inhibitors (SSRIs) is encouraging but still at an early stage. Citalopram (Celexa) has been the most frequently studied SSRI, in part because of its selective binding profile for the serotonin transporter and partly because of its low cost compared to the more potent, purified enantiomer, escitalopram (Lexapro). The Citalopram for Agitation in Alzheimer Disease study (CitAD) remains one of the most influential investigations to date. In AD patients treated with both nonpharmacological psychological treatments and citalopram, significant improvement was found on the

Neurobehavioral Rating Scale agitation subscale (NBRS-A) and the modified Alzheimer Disease Cooperative Study – Clinical Global Impression of Change (mADCS-CGIC) after 9 weeks of treatment. There were improvements in multiple secondary measures as well, including a decrease in caregiver distress. However, prolongation of the QT interval (doses ≥30 mg) and mild worsening of overall cognitive function was observed. Sertraline has shown to be beneficial for agitation and is often used to treat the behavioral dyscontrol related to bvFTD. This SSRI has mild dopaminergic activity at doses over 75 mg and this may partly explain its efficacy in FTD. A meta-analysis on trazodone failed to show sufficient efficacy. However, in bvFTD, one small RCT by Liebert and colleagues in 2004, indicated that trazodone improved neuropsychiatric symptoms. Side-effects, especially sedation, were frequent.

Antidepressants that augment NA (i.e., TCAs) have been used to target apathy, depression, and anxiety. However, anticholinergic side-effect profiles can render these impractical for use in treating the BPSD. No RCT trials have been carried out on the combined serotonin/noradrenaline reuptake inhibitors such as duloxetine, venlafaxine and milnacipram. To date, the likelihood that the noradrenergic system has a role to play in BPSD has led to the use of lipophilic beta-blockers to address aggression and agitation in patients with dementia. These agents have demonstrated effectiveness in brain-injured patients, some of whom also show cognitive benefit from AChE-I. Nevertheless, their efficacy remains to be determined.

Mirtazapine has been used successfully in one case report by Raji and Brady, and its antecdodal use to treat BPSD is growing. Like atypical neuroleptics and trazadone, the sedating properties of mirtazapine in low doses (e.g., ≤7.5 mg) seem to be the psychopharmacologic property being utilized. One SSRI that should generally be avoided is paroxetine because of its strong anti-cholinergic and anti-histiminergic profile. If a patient does show a good response to an agent with anti-cholinergic effects, co-treatment with an AChE-I may offset some of these effects. In summary, citalopram has the best evidence to date for treating a broad range of BPSD beyond anxiety and depression.

13.7.6 Benzodiazepines

Benzodiazepines are to be used only on an as needed basis and for severe agitation over short periods of time. As previously discussed, patients can develop paradoxical reactions, become more agitated, and have worsening of cognitive symptoms. As benzodiazepines are being titrated, there is often a period of worsening agitation. This may represent a paradoxical reaction or the effects of cumulative cognitive compromise and resultant behavioral dysregulation. There may be other detrimental effects of using benzodiazepines. In a recent case control study, a correlation between the use of benzodiazepines and the development of AD was suggested (Billioti-de-Gage et al., 2014). Although these results are intriguing and potentially worrisome, this study does not establish a causal link between benzodiazepines and dementia. Replication in other cohorts will be needed to define the relationship between benzodiazepine use and the progression from MCI to AD.

In summary, pharmacotherapy for the treatment of BPSD has substantial limitations as well as potential benefit. However, several factors should be taken into account. First, whenever feasible, a non-pharmacological approach is always considered the first line treatment (see below). These are more labor intensive, but lack side effects, *per se*, and may actually be more efficacious for targeting the problem behavior/symptom. Second, to date, most studies in the literature are the ones that show positive effects. Negative trials may be less likely to be published. This may bias our choices of treatment for BPSD. Third, given the inclusion/exclusion criteria of clinical trials, most tend to enroll "better behaved" patients, making it difficult to evaluate the treatment effect in the most difficult patients with BPSD. Fourth, agitation and aggression often co-exist with depression and psychosis. Segregating the various BPSD into logical 'symptom clusters' will require more knowledge about the neurobiological basis of these

Table 13.6 Drugs to avoid

1. Those causing orthostatic hypotension and anticholinergic effects:
(a) Typical low-potency antipsychotics: chlorpromazine
(b) TCA: amitryptiline
(c) Anticholinergic drugs: benztropine
(d) SSRI: paroxetine
2. Those causing EPS:
(a) High-potency antipsychotics
3. Those causing paradoxical agitation:
(a) Benzodiazepine

Table 13.7 Charting behaviors before starting a drug

Use of **A**ntecedents-**B**ehavior-**C**onsequences (A-B-C) method may help identify temporary patterns of behavioral decompensation. Although this method may be helpful early in the disease process, it may lose its efficacy as the disease progresses in severity. Nonetheless, it is easy to implement and may curtail the use of powerful medications for a some time. The ABC paradigm is often conceptualized and documented as follows:
1. Date and time behavior occurred
2. Antecedents (What was the trigger?)
3. Behavior (What happened?)
4. Consequence (What was the response?)

Adapted from Omelan (2006)

symptoms. Fifth, biomarkers are needed, especially concerning pathologies in which our knowledge is limited and where response to treatment has been variable. A significant advancement in this area has been the establishment of normative values for CSF amyloid and tau proteins, as well as specific findings on FDG-PET studies (e.g., posterior cingulate hypometabolism). The authors concur with the adage 'start low, go slow', but would add that when a medication trial is initiated it should proceed unless significant side effects emerge. In other words, "start low and go slow, but go". Moreover, it is wise to assess treatment frequently over time with validated psychometrics that can be administered by other providers and caregivers. Vigilant monitoring of side effects is crucial in this population as they are often unable to articulate unpleasant sensations or experiences. Lastly, avoid drugs that are known to cause side effects (Table 13.6), and engage family members and caregivers in the treatment of the patient whenever possible.

13.8 Non-pharmacologic Management of BPSD

In addition to medications, there are numerous other evidence-based treatments for the management of BPSD. Some of these include aerobic exercise, personalized music, reminiscence, 'pleasant activities' with and without social engagement, and alterations in the structure of the patient's support/caregiver network, among others. Some of these will be highlighted below.

Livingston and colleagues (2005) reviewed more than 160 studies examining the impact of psychotherapy, including the brief psychosocial therapy (later investigated in the CALM-AD trial), music therapy, aromatherapy use, light therapy, and education of nurses and family members. Some psychosocial interventions appear to have specific therapeutic properties over and above those due to the benefits of participating in a clinical trial. The effect sizes were small-to-moderate, with a short duration of action. They work when implemented systematically by a seasoned staff. For example, learning the ABC Model (Antecedents, Behaviors, Consequences) was useful to reduce unwanted behaviors (Table 13.7). Also, when the "unmet needs" paradigm is addressed, some negative behaviors were ameliorated. The unmet needs point to the fact that people have inappropriate behavior when their emotional and physical needs are not met. The "stress threshold model" views dementia as a reduced capacity to cope with stress, leading to more behavioral outbursts.

Project ACT is an RCT designed to test the effectiveness of a non-pharmacological home-based intervention to reduce BPSD and caregiver distress. It targeted 272 diverse family caregivers who provided in-home care to persons with moderate-stage dementia with one or more behavioral disturbances. Services involved nurses and occupational therapists going to see families over 13 visits and working with family members to identify and resolve triggers to behaviors (miscommunication, complex commands, high and unrealistic expectations). The study found that teaching caregivers coping strategies, either individually or in a group, improved caregiver level of stress and psychological wellbeing. Selwood and colleagues (2007) found excellent evidence for the efficacy of therapy centered on the patient's behavior to lessen caregiver burden and help with BPSD in patients both immediately, and for up to 32 months.

Similarly, Mittelman and colleagues (2007) conducted a RCT of usual care vs. an enhanced social work counseling and support intervention (six sessions of individual and family counseling, support group participation, and continuous availability of telephone counseling, as needed). They found that over the 9.5-year study period, the intervention for spouse-caregivers was associated with a 28.3 % reduction in the rate of nursing home placement of the patients with dementia (median difference between groups in time to nursing home placement was 557 days). Improvements in caregivers' satisfaction with social support, symptoms of depression, and response to patient behavior problems accounted for 61.2 % of the beneficial impact of the intervention.

More recently, Gitlin and colleagues (2012) employed a case-based assessment of symptoms to propose an algorithm for implementing the best non-pharmacologic approaches. These can be either behavior-targeted or more generalized. They identified five general 'domains' where modification can lead to improvement of BPSD: (1) activities, (2) caregiver education and support, (3) communication, (4) simplified environment, and (5) simplify tasks. The authors would direct the reader to their manuscript (Gitlin et al. 2012) for numerous examples of behavioral modifications in each domain.

Early-onset alzheimer dementia (EOAD) presents a unique constellation of challenges for families, patients, and providers. Approximately 5 % of Americans diagnosed with AD had symptoms prior to age 65. Previously the dominant form of AD, opposed to its 'senile' counterpart, EOAD has reemerged as an important area of investigation. Between 25 and 65 % of EOAD patients have a non-amnestic syndrome. Deficits with spatial cognition, executive control, attention, praxis and focal parietal signs can predominate the clinical presentation. EOAD patients frequently develop a neuropsychiatric prodrome (e.g., depression, apathy, irritability, etc) prior to quantifiable disturbances in cognition, leading to misdiagnoses and inappropriate treatment. Children of patients suffer emotionally and physically when parents become incapacitated or unable to care for them. Family members grow fearful of developing the illness and need considerable guidance in exploring the ramifications of genetic testing. Employers are put in a difficult situation when the patient can no longer carry out his or her job. Early onset dementia causes substantial economic burdens and has a profound impact on family systems. Treatment of early onset dementia, like any other dementia, should revolve around quality of life (QOL). Addressing early psychiatric symptoms and frequent assessment of cognitive function essential.

13.9 Multidimensional Treatment of Patients with BPSD: A Better Quality of Life

The best way to address disorders as complex as BPSD is to take the problem as a whole and understand the burden it creates for the patients, their caregivers, and their treatment team. Biomedical, psychological, and social aspects of BPSD should be considered in the context of maintaining the highest QOL possible that emphasizes respect and dignity to the elders. It should aim to make patients comfortable, sparing the patient and his/her system of care as much as possible from disease burden, ageism, and pain. There are high levels of stress, distress, and psychological illness in family caregivers of individuals with dementia. Practitioners are well advised to identify these signals and work hard to alleviate them. Discussion about end-of-life care should be addressed early in the process and the wishes of the patient made clear, when possible, before cognitive decline precludes meaningful and thoughtful decision-making.

Conclusion

In summary, neuropsychiatric and behavioral symptoms are extremely common in dementia. They cause considerable suffering and distress to patients and their caregivers. Quality of life is undermined and there is a greater probability of nursing home placement. There has been increased investigation and understanding of some of the neurobiological mechanisms underlying these disorders, augmenting the likelihood of developing more effective treatment interventions. Awareness of the nature of BPSD has grown, which can facilitate a more systematic approach to the identification, evaluation, and treatment of neuropsychiatric impairments. Social and behavioral interventions can be effective tools and are associated with fewer "side-effects" than medication. Practitioners and families alike should be vigilant in detecting early signs and symptoms that may represent initial stages of early onset dementia.

Pharmacologic treatment of depression, anxiety, and cognitive impairments with pharmacotherapy has been shown to have a modest beneficial impact on the lives of patients. In general, neuroleptic medications should only be used to manage severe behavioral disorders or psychosis in patients for whom less risky interventions have failed. In many cases, the authors would support limiting the use of antipsychotics to treat psychosis, unless there are no alternatives for maintaining patient and caregiver safety. Under such circumstances, patients need to be closely monitored to determine if treatment is yielding benefits and to assess ongoing risks. Cardiovascular function should be routinely monitored. For most BPSD, including agitation, aggression, and mood disturbance, citalopram currently has the strongest evidence base. That said, the armamentarium of available medications to selectively target specific BPSD needs to expand. Investment in ongoing research is necessary to discover more effective interventions for these devastating symptoms.

Acknowledgements The authors would like to acknowledge the generous support from the Wimberly family, the Muss family, and the Mortimer/Grubman family. We would also like to thank Nancy Donovan, M.D. and Sarah Fackler, M.A. for their helpful suggestions.

Suggested Reading

Alexopoulos GS, Streim J, Carpenter D, Docherty JP, Expert Consensus Panel for Using Antipsychotic Drugs in Older Patients. Using antipsychotic agents in older patients. J Clin Psychiatry. 2004;65 Suppl 2:5–99.

Ballard C, Brown R, Fossey J, Douglas S, Bradley P, Hancock J, James IA, Juszczak E, Bentham P, Burns A, Lindesay J, Jacoby R, O'Brien J, Bullock R, Johnson T, Holmes C, Howard R. Brief psychosocial therapy for the treatment of agitation in Alzheimer disease (the CALM-AD trial). Am J Geriatr Psychiatry. 2009a;17:726–33.

Ballard C, Hanney ML, Theodoulou M, Douglas S, McShane R, Kossakowski K, Gill R, Juszczak E, Yu LM, Jacoby R. The dementia antipsychotic withdrawal trial (DART-AD): long-term follow-up of a randomised placebo-controlled trial. Lancet Neurol. 2009b;8:151–7.

Ballard C, Margallo-Lana M, O'Brien JT, James I, Howard R, Fossey J. Quality of life for people with dementia living in residential and nursing home care: the impact of performance on activities of daily living, behavioral and psychological symptoms, language skills, and psychotropic drugs. Int Psychogeriatr. 2009c;21:1026–30.

Ballard CG, Gauthier S, Cummings JL, Brodaty H, Grossberg GT, Robert P, Lyketsos CG. Management of agitation and aggression associated with Alzheimer disease. Nat Rev Neurol. 2009d;5:245–55.

Ballard C, Lana MM, Theodoulou M, Douglas S, McShane R, Jacoby R, Kossakowski K, Yu LM, Juszczak E, Investigators DART AD. A randomised, blinded, placebo-controlled trial in dementia patients continuing or stopping neuroleptics (the DART-AD trial). PLoS Med. 2008;5(4):e76.

Billioti de Gage S, Moride Y, Ducruet T, Kurth T, Verdoux H, Tournier M, Pariente A, Bégaud B. Benzodiazepine use and risk of Alzheimer's disease: case-control study. BMJ. 2014;349:g5205.

Campbell N, Ayub A, Boustani MA, Fox C, Farlow M, Maidment I, Howards R. Impact of cholinesterase inhibitors on behavioral and psychological symptoms of Alzheimer's disease: a meta-analysis. Clin Interv Aging. 2008;3:719–28.

Cassanova M, Starkstein S, Jellinger K. Clinicopathological correlates of behavioral and psychological symptoms of dementia. Acta Neuropathol. 2011;122(2):117–35.

Chahine LM, Acar D, Chemali Z. The elderly safety imperative and antipsychotic usage. Harv Rev Psychiatry. 2010;18(3):158–72.

Craig D, Mirakhur A, Hart DJ, McIlroy SP, Passmore AP. A cross-sectional study of neuropsychiatric symptoms in 435 patients with Alzheimer's disease. Am J Geriatr Psychiatry. 2005;13:460–8.

Cummings J. The neuropsychiatric inventory: assessing psychopathology in dementia patients. Neurology. 1997;48(Suppl):10–6.

Cummings JL, Mega M, Gray K, Rosenberg-Thompson S, Carusi DA, Gornbein J. The neuropsychiatric inventory: comprehensive assessment of psychopathology in dementia. Neurology. 1994;44:2308–14.

Daffner K, Wolk D. Behavioral neurology and dementia. In: Samuels MA, editor. The manual of neurologic therapeutics. Philadelphia: Lippincott, Williams, and Wilkins; 2010.

Devanand DP, Mintzer J, Schultz SK, Andrews HF, Sultzer DL, de la Pena D, Gupta S, Colon S, Schimming C, Pelton GH, Levin B. Relapse risk after discontinuation of risperidone in Alzheimer's disease. N Engl J Med. 2012;367(16):1497–507.

De Deyn P, Drenth AF, Kremer BP, Oude Voshaar RC, Van Dam D. Aripiprazole in the treatment of Alzheimer's disease. Expert Opin Pharmacother. 2013;14(4):459–74.

Draper B, Brodaty H, Finkle S. The IPA Complete Guides to BPSD: Specialists Guide. International Psychogeriatric Association (IPA). 2012.

Finger E, Daffner K. Behavioral and cognitive neurology. In: Burneo J, Demaerschalk B, Jenkins M, editors. Neurology – an evidence based approach. New York: Springer Science; 2012.

Fitz D, Mallya A. Discontinuation of a psychogeriatric program for nursing home residents: psychotropic medication changes and behavioral reactions. J Appl Gerontol. 1992;11:50–63.

Forstl H, Burns A, Levy R, Cairns N, Luthert P, Lantos P. Neuropathological correlates of behavioural disturbance in confirmed Alzheimer's disease. Br J Psychiatry. 1993;163:364–8.

Gauthier S, Cummings J, Ballard C, Brodaty H, Grossberg G, Robert P, Lyketsos C. Management of behavioral problems in Alzheimer's disease. Int Psychogeriatr. 2010;22(3):346–72.

Geda Y, Schneider LS, Gitlin LN, Miller DS, Smith GS, Bell J, Evans J, Lee M, Porsteinsson A, Lanctôt KL, Rosenberg PB, Sultzer DL, Francis PT, Brodaty H, Padala PP, Onyike CU, Ortiz LA, Ancoli-Israel S, Bliwise DL, Martin JL, Vitiello MV, Yaffe K, Zee PC, Herrmann N, Sweet RA, Ballard C, Khin NA, Alfaro C, Murray PS, Schultz S, Lyketsos CG, Neuropsychiatric Syndromes Professional Interest Area of ISTAART. Neuropsychiatric symptoms in Alzheimer's disease: past progress and anticipation of the future. Alzheimers Dement. 2013;9(5): 602–8.

Geda YE, Roberts RO, Mielke MM, Knopman DS, Christianson TJ, Pankratz VS, Boeve BF, Sochor O, Tangalos EG, Petersen RC, Rocca WA. Baseline neuropsychiatric symptoms and the risk of incident mild cognitive impairment: a population-based study. Am J Psychiatry. 2014;171(5):572–81.

Gitlin LN, Kales HC, Lyketsos CG. Non-pharmacologic management of behavioral symptoms in dementia. JAMA. 2012;308(19):2020–9.

Gitlin LN, Winter L, Dennis MP, Hauck WW. A non-pharmacological intervention to manage behavioral and psychological symptoms of dementia and reduce caregiver distress: design and methods of project ACT3. Clin Interv Aging. 2007;2:695–703.

Jost B, Grossberg G. The natural history of Alzheimer's disease: a brain bank study. J Am Geriatr Soc. 1995;43(11):1248–55.

Kaufer D, Cummings JL, Ketchel P, Smith V, MacMillan A, Shelley T, Lopez OL, DeKosky ST. Validation of the NPI-Q, a brief clinical form of the neuropsychiatric Inventory. J Neuropsychiatry Clin Neurosci. 2000;12(2):233–9.

La Salvia E, Chemali Z. A perspective on psychosis in late life and deficits in cognition. Harv Rev Psychiatry. 2011;19(4):190–7.

Livingston G, Johnston K, Katona C, Paton J, Lyketsos C, The Old Age Task Force of the World Federation of Biological Psychiatry. Systematic review of psychological approaches to the management of neuropsychiatric symptoms of dementia. Am J Psychiatry. 2005;162(11):1996–2021.

Lyketsos CG, Lopez O, Jones B, Fitzpatrick AL, Breitner J, DeKosky S. Prevalence of neuropsychiatric symptoms in dementia and mild cognitive impairment: results from the cardiovascular health study. JAMA. 2002;288(12):1475–83.

Mittelman M, Roth D, Clay O, Haley W. Preserving health of Alzheimer caregivers: impact of a spouse caregiver intervention. Am J Geriatr Psychiatry. 2007;15(9):780–9.

O'Connor DW, Ames D, Gardner B, King M. Psychosocial treatments of behavior symptoms in dementia: a systematic review of reports meeting quality standards. Int Psychogeriatr. 2009;21:225–40.

Porsteinsson AP, Drye LT, Pollock BG, Devanand D, Frangakis C, Ismail Z, Marano C, Meinert CL, Mintzer JE, Munro C, Pelton G, Rabins PV, Rosenberg PB, Schneider LS, Shade DM, Weintraub D, Yesavage J, Lyketsos CG, CitAD Research Group. Effect of citalopram on agitation in Alzheimer disease: the CitAD randomized clinical trial. JAMA. 2014;311(7):682–91.

Rodda J, Morgan S, Walker Z. Are cholinesterase inhibitors effective in the management of the behavioral and psychological symptoms of dementia in Alzheimer's disease? A systematic review of randomized, placebo-controlled trials of donepezil, rivastigmine and galantamine. Int Psychogeriatr. 2009;21:813–24.

Salzman C, Jeste DV, Meyer RE, Cohen-Mansfield J, Cummings J, Grossberg GT, Jarvik L, Kraemer HC, Lebowitz BD, Maslow K, Pollock BG, Raskind M, Schultz SK, Wang P, Zito JM, Zubenko GS. Elderly patients with dementia-related symptoms of severe agitation and aggression: consensus statement on treatment options, clinical trials methodology, and policy. J Clin Psychiatry. 2008;69:889–98.

Selwood A, Johnston K, Katona C, Lyketsos C, Livingston G. Systematic review of the effect of psychological interventions on family caregivers of people with dementia. J Affect Disord. 2007;101:75–89.

The IPA complete guide to the biological and psychological symptoms of dementia: specialists guide. Northfield: International Psychogeriatric Association; 2012.

Wadsworth L, Donovan N, Lorius N, Locascio J, Rentz D, Johnson K, Sperling R, Marshall G. Neuropsychiatric symptoms and global functional impairment along the Alzheimer's continuum. Dement Geriatr Cogn Disord. 2012;34:96–111.

Walker FO. Huntington's disease. Lancet. 2007; 369(9557):218–28.

World Alzheimer Report 2015: The Global Impact of Dementia. An analysis of prevalence, incidence, cost and trends. http://www.alz.co.uk/research/world-report-2015.

HIV and Other Infectious Causes of Dementia

14

Patricia McNamara, Lilia Zaporojan,
Colin P. Doherty, Robert F. Coen, and Colm Bergin

14.1 Human Immunodeficiency Virus

In 2013 an estimated 35 million people worldwide were living with HIV. HIV is a blood borne virus. It can be transmitted sexually, through the use of contaminated needles in the intravenous drug using (IVDU) population, from mother to child and via infected blood products. HIV is a lentivirus which is a member of the retroviridae family. It is a single-stranded, positive-sense, enveloped RNA virus. Its hallmark is the reverse transcription of viral RNA to DNA. The DNA is then integrated into the host's genome as a provirus. The genetic diversity of HIV is due to its high viral replication rate along with its ability to recombine. This genetic diversity has been classified into subtypes called clades. In Europe and North America the most common clade is subtype B while subtype C is the dominant form in Africa and Asia. Viral tropism refers to the cell types that a virus can infect. When the HIV protein, gp120, binds to CD4 cells or macrophages it opens up a binding site allowing for attachment via two chemokines. Viruses which attach via the chemokine receptor CCR5 are called R5-tropic viruses and they primarily infect macrophages. X4-tropic viruses attach via the chemokine receptor CXCR4 and primarily infect primary CD4 T-cells. Viruses which can use

P. McNamara
Academic Unit of Neurology,
Trinity Biomedical Sciences Institute,
Dublin, Ireland

L. Zaporojan
Academic Unit of Neurology,
Trinity College, Dublin, Dublin, Ireland

C.P. Doherty (✉)
Department of Neurology, St. James's Hospital,
Dublin, Ireland

Academic Unit of Neurology,
Trinity College Dublin, Dublin, Ireland
e-mail: colinpdoherty@gmail.com

R.F. Coen
Memory Clinic, Mercer's Institute
For Research on Aging, St James's Hospital,
Dublin, Ireland

Department of Gerontology, Trinity College Dublin,
Dublin, Ireland

C. Bergin
Department of Infectious Diseases,
St. James's Hospital, Dublin, Ireland

Department of Clinical Medicine,
Trinity College, Dublin,
Dublin, Ireland

© Springer International Publishing Switzerland 2016
O. Hardiman, C.P. Doherty (eds.), *Neurodegenerative Disorders: A Clinical Guide*,
DOI 10.1007/978-3-319-23309-3_14

both chemokines are called dual or mixed tropic viruses. After binding, gp41 then facilitates fusion of the host cell membrane and the viral membrane thus releasing the virus into the host cell cytoplasm and allowing the infective cycle to begin. HIV primarily infects CD4 positive T cells, macrophages and dendritic cells thereby suppressing the infected individual's immune system and predisposing them to opportunistic infections and some malignancies. It is recommended to commence highly active anti-retroviral therapy (HAART) in patients with cognitive impairment in the setting of HIV irrespective of CD4+ count.

14.2 HIV and Cognitive Impairment

Many terms have been used to describe cognitive impairment or dementia secondary to HIV over the years, including sub-acute encephalitis, AIDS dementia complex, HIV encephalopathy and HIV-1 associated cognitive/motor complex. The most recent term, HIV Associated Neurocognitive Disorders (HAND), was introduced by the American Academy of Neurology (AAN) in 2007 (Table 14.1; Fig. 14.1).

14.3 Prevalence of Cognitive Impairment in HIV

Prior to the introduction of HAART up to 20 % of patients with AIDS developed HIV dementia and it was associated with a high mortality rate with a mean survival of 6 months to 1 year after the development of dementia. Prior to HAART mild neurocognitive impairment was described in 30 % of patients with asymptomatic HIV disease and in up to 50 % of patients with AIDS defining illnesses. The incidence of HIV associated dementia has declined in the post-HAART era to approximately 2 %, however cognitive impairment continues to be an ongoing clinical issue despite good virological control of HIV. Prevalence rates of 20–50 % of HAND have been demonstrated in large prospective studies.

Table 14.1 AAN diagnostic criteria for HAND

HIV associated asymptomatic neurocognitive impairment (ANI)

1. Acquired impairment in cognitive functioning, involving at least two ability domains, documented by performance of at least 1 standard deviation below the mean for age-education-appropriate norms on standardised neuropsychological tests. The neuropsychological tests must survey at least the following abilities: verbal/language, attention/working memory, abstraction/executive, memory (learning, recall), speed of information processing, sensory-perceptual, motor skills

2. The cognitive impairment does not interfere with everyday functioning

3. The cognitive impairment does not meet criteria for delirium or dementia

4. There is no evidence of another pre-existing cause for the ANI

HIV associated mild neurocognitive disorder (MND)

1. Acquired impairment in cognitive functioning, involving at least two ability domains, documented by performance of at least 1.0 standard deviation below the mean for age-education-appropriate norms on standardised neuropsychological tests. The neuropsychological tests must survey at least the following abilities: verbal/language, attention/working memory, abstraction/executive, memory (learning, recall), speed of information processing, sensory-perceptual, motor skills

2. The cognitive impairment produces at least mild interference in daily functioning (at least one of the following):

   (a) Self-report of reduced mental acuity, inefficiency in work, homemaking or social functioning

   (b) Observation by knowledgeable others that the individual has undergone at least mild decline in mental acuity with resultant inefficiency in work, homemaking or social functioning

3. The cognitive impairment does not meet criteria for delirium or dementia

4. There is no evidence of another pre-existing cause for the MND

HIV associated dementia (HAD) (Fig. 14.1)

1. Marked acquired impairment in cognitive functioning, involving at least two ability domains, typically the impairment is in multiple domains, especially in learning of new information, slowed information processing, and defective attention/concentration. The cognitive impairment must be ascertained by neuropsychological testing with at least two domains 2 standard deviations or greater than demographically corrected means

(continued)

Table 14.1 (continued)

2. The cognitive impairment produces marked interference with day-to-day functioning (work, home life, social activities)
3. The pattern of cognitive impairment does not meet criteria for delirium
4. There is no existing evidence of another, pre-existing cause for the dementia

14.4 Neuropathology of HIV

HIV is neuroinvasive, neurotropic and neurovirulent. HIV enters the brain through infected monocytes and lymphocytes. They are used as a "Trojan horse" mechanism to cross the blood brain barrier. HIV has been found in the cerebrospinal fluid (CSF) of patients during seroconversion, suggesting that HIV enters the CNS early in the course of infection. Neurons are not infected directly by HIV. Microglial cells and macrophages are the primary targets for productive HIV infection within the CNS as they both possess receptors for CD4 and CCR5. Microglia cells act as the brain's native immune response cells. Astrocytes are also infected by HIV despite their lack of receptors for viral attachment but in a more restricted fashion.

HIV can cause an inflammatory reaction upon entry to the CNS which may be manifested

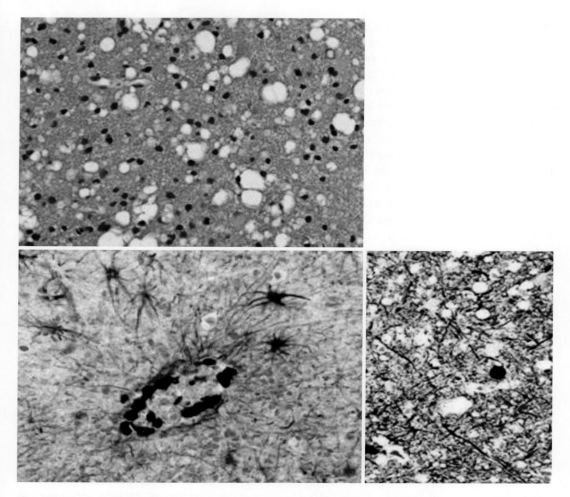

Fig. 14.1 *Top*: vacuolar leukoencephalopathy; *bottom right*: shows perivascular CD8 T lymphocytes, *Bottom left*: shows axonal injury; Histology slides courtesy of Prof Michael Farrell (Department of Neuropathology, Beaumont Hospital, Dublin, Ireland)

by a T cell reaction with vasculitis and lepto-meningitis. There is upregulation of MHC class II antigens, increased number of microglial cells found and increased production of cytokines. Perivascular microglia are likely involved early in infection and the parenchymal microglia become involved in the later stages of infection. The chemokine receptor CCR5 is the dominant receptor used within the brain. There is proliferation of astrocytes and intense perivascular lymphocytic and macrophagic infiltration has been seen at autopsy which has been postulated to be related to immune reconstitution inflammatory syndrome (IRIS).

The pathognomonic feature of HIV encephalitis (HIVE) on histological examination is the presence of multinucleated giant cells. These cells are the fusion of infected and uninfected microglia and macrophages and they stain positively for HIV antigens. Together they provide evidence of productive infection by HIV within the CNS. This pathological feature was present in 20–50 % of patients who had autopsies performed in the first 15 years of the HIV epidemic. HIVE has a predilection for the basal ganglia and white matter and affects the neocortical grey matter, cerebellum and brainstem to a lesser extent. Other pathological features of HIV include myelin pallor, axonal loss, microglial nodules and gliosis. There is also disruption of the blood brain barrier and apoptosis of astrocytes. This leads to dendritic and neuronal loss (Fig. 14.2; Table 14.2).

14.5   Risk Factors for HAND

Risk factors include a low nadir $CD4^+$ T-cell count, older age, substance abuse, lower educational level, co-infection with hepatitis C, CCR2 polymorphisms, the 2578G variant of CCL2 (MCP-1), TNF-α 308A allele and systemic features such as low haemoglobin, constitutional symptoms and a low body mass index. Apolipoprotein E status, particularly in older patients, has been associated with HAND in some studies.

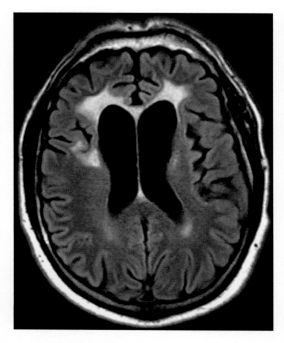

Fig. 14.2 Bifrontal white matter hyperintensities (seen on FLAIR) in a patient with HIV dementia and vacuolar leukoencephalopathy on the same patient's brain biopsy. MRI courtesy of Dr Niall Sheehy (Department of Radiology, St James's Hospital, Dublin, Ireland)

14.6   Functional Consequences of HAND

HIV-associated dementia remains an independent predictor of time to death. Functional impairment in the areas of work assessment, finances, medication management, cooking and shopping has been demonstrated. Unemployment is higher.

14.7   Clinical Features in the 1980s of HAND

Patients exhibited disturbance in cognitive, behavioural and motor function. Patients complained of forgetfulness, loss of concentration, difficulty recalling recent events and losing their train of thought. Motor symptoms included lower limb weakness, loss of balance and abnormal co-ordination. Apathy and social withdrawal were the most common behavioural symptoms. It

Table 14.2 Summary of neuropathogenesis

Neuropathology	
Pathological findings	Lymphocytic meningitis
	Multinucleated giant cells with encephalitis
	Perivascular lymphocytic and macrophagic infiltration
	Myelin pallor
	Axonal loss
	Microglial nodules
	Gliosis
Inflammatory and immune activation	**Effects and roles**
Activated macrophages and monocytes	Release viral gene products and proinflammatory cytokines
	CD163 is a marker of activated macrophages
	Expansion of CD14$^+$/CD16$^+$ monocytes
	Migration of CD16$^+$ cells across BBB increased by fractalkine
	TNF + VCAM-1 increase membrane bound fractalkine
	IFN-γ and ICAM-1 decrease membrane bound fractalkine
CD8$^+$ T Cells	CD8 encephalitis
	Loss of specific cytotoxic CD8 immune response in aging
Microbial translocation	Increased LPS induces monocyte activation and trafficking into CNS
	LPS induces expression of E-selectin and VCAM-1 on macrophages
Neurotoxic and neurodegenerative mechanisms	**Effects and roles**
Viral proteins	
Gp120	Toxicity of blood brain barrier
	Activates protein kinase C
	Cytotoxicity requires presence of IFN-γ and p38 MAPK
	Degradation of ZO-1 and ZO-2
	Dysfunction of nigrostriatal dopaminergic system
	Alters glutamate signalling + Ca^{++} homeostasis
Tat	Affect tight junction proteins
	Decreases expression of occludin, ZO-1, ZO-2
	Increases trafficking of monocytes into CNS
	Neuronal cell death and excitotoxicity – partially dependent on NMDA receptors
	Neuronal apoptosis increased by *tat* and TNF-α
	Mitochondrial dysfunction
Vpr	Disrupts Ca^{++} homeostasis
	Impairs glutamate signalling
Nef	Apoptosis of brain microvascular endothelial cells
	Causes neuronal damage mediated by MCP-1
Platelet activating factor	Increases glutamate release
	Increases vulnerability of neurons to dendritic alterations
Neopterin	Elevated in CSF and remains mildly elevated even with viral suppression
	Induces release of QUIN
	Correlates with release of reactive oxygen species by macrophages
QUIN	Excitotoxic agonist at NMDA receptors
	Forms free radicals
	Correlates with cerebral atrophy

(continued)

Table 14.2 (continued)

Monocyte chemoattractant protein 1 (MCP-1)	Upregulated in HIVE
	Associated with poorer outcomes
	Mediates neuronal death caused by *nef*
Astrocytes	Astrocytosis – feature of HIVE
	Astrocyte apoptosis propagates macrophage activation and causes loss of neurotrophic support for neurons
Synaptodendritic injury	Retraction of dendritic spines, dendritic beading and aberrant sprouting
	Disrupts normal communication and impairs axonal transport
	NFL is a marker of axonal injury
HAART	Mitochondrial dysfunction
	Beading and pruning of dendrites
	Destabilisation of neuronal Ca^{++} homeostasis and a reduced response to glutamate
	Increase NO production
Aging	Decreased levels of amyloid-beta
	Normal or low levels of tau
	Neuritic α-synuclein expression in substantia nigra

was consistent with a subcortical dementia given the prominent psychomotor slowing and the absence of cortical signs such as aphasia and apraxia. The neuropathological findings supported this hypothesis given the predominance of white matter and subcortical nuclei pathology. One study demonstrated increased rates of neuropsychological impairment at each successive stage of HIV infection. The domains most often affected were attention, speed of information processing and learning efficiency and they suggested that this pattern was consistent with earliest involvement of subcortical or fronto-striatal brain systems.

14.8 Changes in HAND Pre and Post HAART

In the post-HAART era more cortical findings have been demonstrated. Impairment in learning and memory and executive function are more predominant than the subcortical impairments in motor skills, cognitive speed and verbal fluency that were common in the pre-HAART era. Some studies have shown that recall, working memory and attention have been stable across the two time periods whilst others have demonstrated an improvement in

attention, verbal fluency and visuospatial skills, but there was a deterioration in learning efficiency and complex attention.

14.9 Neuropsychological Findings in HAND

Impairment in motor skills and information processing has been evident in HAND since the early 1980s. Bradykinesia and bradyphrenia were prominent features. Older HIV positive adults were more impaired on the motor scale of the Unified Parkinson's Disease Rating Scale compared to HIV negative age, gender and ethnicity matched controls, especially on measures of bradykinesia, hypomimia, action/postural tremor and hand agility. Motor slowing in HIV infection has also been assessed using timed gait test, finger tapping and manual dexterity. Impaired performance on tests of information processing speed could arise from a variety of deficits including attention, visuoperception, working memory, praxis and motor skills.

Episodic memory impairment is a sensitive indicator of HAND. Deficits are most consistent with a mixed encoding and retrieval profile however there is considerable heterogeneity in the memory profile of HIV infection but most support a frontal-striatal conceptualization of verbal memory performance in the setting of HIV infection. This pattern of mixed encoding and retrieval issues is characterised by impaired immediate and delayed free recall but relatively better performance on tasks of recognition. Impairment of the hippocampal system as well as the prefrontal system during episodic encoding in HIV positive patients has been demonstrated during a functional MRI study. This suggests that there is hippocampal involvement in addition to the role of the fronto-striatal circuits in the memory profile of HIV.

Attentional deficits have been shown in the areas of response inhibition, divided attention and visual attention. HIV positive patients usually score lower on executive tasks such as the Stroop Colour Word Test, Trail Making Test Part B and the Wisconsin Card Sorting Test.

Visuospatial deficits were not seen prominently in early studies of HAND however deficits were noted in spatial abilities that relied on the integrity of the fronto-striato-parietal networks such as egocentric spatial tasks. Abnormalities were noted in spatial attentional tasks. A recent study demonstrated deficits on tasks of mental rotation and hierarchical pattern perception in HIV and these are tasks which depend highly on parietal function. Mental rotation was explored further in a subsequent study and HIV positive patients made more errors on the task than did HIV negative controls. The errors were associated with poorer performance on tasks of executive function and working memory suggesting that the fronto-striatal-parietal networks were disrupted. Impairment of numerical and spatial cognition has been demonstrated in HIV infection through tasks of mental number line bisection, physical line bisection and physical number line orientation. This again provided evidence for disruption of fronto-striato-parietal networks in HAND.

Verbal fluency is impaired in patients with HIV associated dementia (HAD) with significantly more impairment on letter fluency and relatively intact category fluency. In a meta-analysis of verbal fluency in HIV mild word generation deficits were evident with similar impairments in both letter and category fluency.

Effect size increased with advancing HIV disease severity.

14.10   MRI Features of HAND

Early volumetric studies in the 1980s and early 1990s demonstrated global cerebral atrophy with ventricular enlargement and prominent involvement of basal ganglia and white matter. The particular predilection for basal ganglia was in keeping with the subcortical nature of HIV dementia. In the post HAART era and with the evolution of imaging techniques more extensive atrophy has been demonstrated affecting both nigro-striatal and fronto-striatal circuits and frontal, parietal, temporal and occipital cortices. Hippocampal atrophy has also been demonstrated. Nadir CD4 count and duration of infection have been shown to correlate with atrophy of the parietal, temporal and frontal lobes and the hippocampus whilst plasma HIV RNA levels correlated with atrophy of basal ganglia. The pattern of HIV-associated brain loss may be changing from a predominantly subcortical disease to a more cortical disease in the post-HAART era.

14.11   DTI Findings in HAND

DTI has been shown to be a very sensitive method for the detection of white matter abnormalities. Overall the studies in HIV have shown increases in mean diffusivity (MD) and decreases in fractional anisotropy (FA). Abnormalities in FA and MD are not related to specific white matter pathology but are sensitive markers of white matter integrity. Patients on HAART have been shown to have higher FA values suggesting better white matter integrity compared to HIV positive patients naïve to therapy. Another study demonstrated that HIV positive patients naïve to HAART had higher radial diffusivity (RD) measures in inferior cingulate, occipital forceps and superior longitudinal fasciculus indicative of myelin disruption while HIV positive patients with AIDS had higher axonal diffusivity (AD) measures, indicative of axonal compromise, in posterior callosal regions, fornix and superior cingulate bundle.

14.12 Role of Amyloid and Tau in HAND

HIV disrupts the clearance of beta-amyloid. Gp120 induces release of TNF-α and IL-1β from microglia and these cytokines stimulate increased cleavage of amyloid precursor protein (APP) by β and γ secretases. The HIV protein *tat* inhibits neprilysin and increases the aggregation of beta-amyloid$_{(1-42)}$ into neuronal endolysosomes through endocytosis. The results of analysis of tau and beta-amyloid$_{(1-42)}$ levels in CSF in HAND have been conflicting. Most studies have shown decreased beta-amyloid with normal phosphorylated tau.

14.13 Syphilis

Neurosyphilis was a common cause of dementia until the discovery of penicillin at the turn of the twentieth century. The causative organism is the spirochaete *treponema pallidum*. Usually dementia is a manifestation of the late stages of the disease although neurosyphilis can occur at any stage. Dementia may occur in meningovascular syphilis, general paresis, tabes dorsalis or due to a focal gumma.

General paresis develops 10–25 years after initial infection but can occur as early as years in 5–10 % of those untreated for early syphilis. It has a poor prognosis without treatment and in the pre-penicillin era resulted in death within an average of 2.5 years. General paresis manifests initially as depression, mania, psychosis, personality changes, memory deficits and impaired judgment with insidious progression to frank dementia. The characteristic Argyll-Robertson pupil (small, asymmetric, irregular pupils that respond to accommodation and convergence but do not react to direct light) may be present. Other common neurological findings are facial and limb hypotonia, reflex abnormalities, dysarthria, tongue and hand intention tremor, and rarely other movement disorders.

CSF abnormalities are characterised by elevated protein levels, a lymphocytic pleocytosis and a positive VDRL (Venereal Diseases Research Laboratory) test. Neuroimaging may show atrophy, most commonly of the frontal and temporal lobes with dilatation of the lateral ventricles. Pathologically, there is atrophy of the frontal and temporal lobes with sparing of the motor, sensory, and occipital cortices, and dilatation of lateral ventricles. The cerebellum and basal ganglia can also be affected in rare cases. There is evidence of chronic meningitis, most intense over the atrophic areas. Spirochetes have been found in the grey matter, microglial cells and endothelial cells, but not in the white matter.

Diagnosis involves screening for serum non-treponemal tests: VDRL and RPR (Rapid Plasma Reagin) and serum treponemal tests: Fluorescent Treponemal Antibody Absorption (FTA-ABS); Treponema Pallidum Particle Agglutination Assay (TPPA); Syphilis Enzyme Immunoassay (EIA) should be performed. The nontreponemal tests may be non-reactive in late neurosyphilis, but the treponemal tests remain reactive for life regardless of treatment. CSF analysis should be performed in patients with a known history of syphilis displaying neurologic or ophthalmic signs, evidence of tertiary syphilis affecting other parts of the body, treatment failure at any stage of disease, HIV infection with late latent syphilis or syphilis of unknown duration to evaluate the possibility of neurosyphilis. Serum rapid plasma reagin (RPR) titre has been shown to be useful as a surrogate marker of neurosyphilis.

All patients with confirmed neurosyphillis should be treated. The goal of treatment is to prevent further progression and to reverse the symptoms. The latter may not be achieved in parenchymal neurosyphilis. Treatment is with penicillin or ceftriaxone or doxycycline in those who are allergic to penicillin but all attempts should be made to treat patients with penicillin including desensitisation as doxycycline is a static antibiotic. Follow up lumbar puncture is recommended every six months thereafter until CSF abnormalities have resolved although following RPR titres has also been recommended as some groups have shown a relationship between normalisation of RPR and resolution of CSF abnormalities. Retreatment is recommended if CSF remains abnormal by 2 years after treatment.

Although, the tertiary form of syphilis became very rare in the antibiotic era, its rates remain to be observed after the re-emergence of syphilis with the start of the HIV epidemic in the 1980s. Since 2000 rates of syphilis have been increasing in the US, Europe and Australia. The rates of primary and secondary syphilis increased annually from 2001 reaching a peak of 5.3 cases per 100,000 population in the United States in 2013. The rates of late and late latent syphilis remained unchanged through the end of 2012 in the US, but could potentially increase worldwide in the future due to the re-emergence of syphilis since 2000 and the potential for late presenters or patients who failed to comply with full treatment protocols or who were re-infected and did not represent for treatment. It is extremely important to bear in mind that while dementia due to syphilis usually occurs in the later stages, neurosyphilis can occur at any stage of syphilis and all patients presenting with cognitive impairment or dementia should be investigated for syphilis.

14.14 Toxoplasmosis

Toxoplasmosis is caused by an obligate intracellular protozoon Toxoplasma gondii. It is one of the most common parasite zoonoses that infects up to a third of the world's population. Toxoplasmosis is acquired by ingestion of contaminated food or water or by eating undercooked meat. It can also be transmitted vertically. Primary infection is asymptomatic in most immunocompetent individuals or may cause mild symptoms however, in immunocompromised individuals, it can have severe manifestations including encephalitis, hepatitis and myocarditis. Toxoplasmosis remains the most common opportunistic CNS infection in patients with AIDS although rates have declined with the advent of HAART but many patients still present late with

low CD4 counts or live in resource poor countries with limited access to testing and HAART. Primary prophylaxis is recommended in HIV positive patients with CD4 counts less than 100/μl.

Toxoplasmic encephalitis in HIV appears to be almost exclusively caused by reactivation of latent infection. Clinical presentation can vary from acute onset of a confusional state to a sub-acute insidious process that evolves over days or weeks. Patients may present with focal motor deficits, cranial nerve disturbances, speech impairment, movement disorders, cerebellar signs, seizures, neuropsychiatric symptoms, lethargy, apathy, memory impairment or frank dementia. Sometimes focal neurological findings are associated with constitutional signs such as fever and general malaise. If left untreated, it will progress to seizures, stupor and coma. Encephalitis can be the sole presentation of toxoplasma infection in immunocompromised individuals or may be associated with toxoplasma chorioretinitis, pneumonitis or multi-organ involvement.

CT or MR brain imaging will typically show multiple ring enhancing lesions with a predilection for cortical grey matter and basal ganglia with perifocal oedema. Sometimes TE can manifest as diffuse encephalitis or a single focal contrast-enhancing lesion (Fig. 14.3a, b). Detection of the parasite on a biopsy sample is required for a definitive histological diagnosis but diagnosis is usually made on clinical and radiological features. If there is no improvement of clinical and/or radiological features after 2 weeks of empiric treatment then biopsy is recommended. Treatment is usually with pyrimethamine and sulfadiazine co-administered with folinic acid to prevent the haematologic complications of pyrimethamine therapy. Clindamycin, atovaquone and trimethoprim/sulfamethoxazole may also be used.

14.15 Cryptococcosis

Cryptococcosis is caused by one of two fungus species, *Cryptococcus Neoformans* and *Cryptococcus Gattii*. Cryptococcus is a worldwide fungus and is spread by bird droppings. It is not

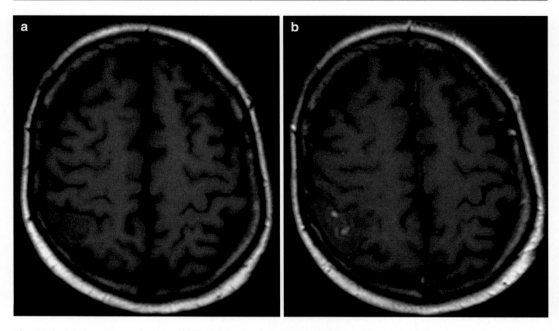

Fig. 14.3 (**a**) Hypointense lesions on T1-weighted axial MRI in CNS Toxoplasmosis demonstrating enhancement on post-contrast imaging (**b**)

transmissible from person to person. In immuno-competent hosts cryptococcus may colonise the airways and have an asymptomatic course or may cause cough, pleuritic pain, low grade fever, malaise, and weight loss. In immunocompromised individuals, especially those with a defective cell response (AIDS, Hodgkin's lymphoma, sarcoidosis, those receiving chronic steroid treatment or immunosuppressive therapy after solid organ transplant) it can spread from the lungs to the CNS and cause potentially fatal cryptococcal meningitis or meningoencephalitis. Cryptococcal meningitis due to *C. neoformans* usually occurs in immunocompromised hosts although there are rare case reports of infection amongst immuncompetent hosts. It causes approximately one million infections per year. *Cryptococcus gattii* is more associated with infections in immunocompetent hosts. In the past it was associated with Eucalyptus trees in tropical and subtropical climates and causing low incidences of disease in immunocompetent hosts, but since 1999 infections are increasing in Pacific Northwestern America also.

Cryptococcus meningitis has an insidious onset and may go on for weeks to years. The most common symptoms are headache and altered mental status, including personality changes, disorientation, lethargy, obtundation and coma. It can cause hydrocephalus, dementia, seizures and focal neurological deficits. Dementia caused by cryptococcal meningitis or meningo-encephalitis can clinically mimic Alzheimer's type dementia (with insidious onset and progressive cognitive impairment over a few years) or vascular type dementia (progressive memory impairment which begins within weeks after a stroke like episode).

In the CNS, cryptococcus has a predilection for the subarachnoid space and perivascular spaces. Here it grows extensively causing cystic distension of perivascular spaces. Post = mortem brain sections have a "Swiss cheese" appearance. On MR brain imaging these cystic lesions can be mistaken for subcortical lacunar infarcts or enlarged Virchow-Robin spaces. MRI can also reveal meningeal enhancement, communicating hydrocephalus, leptomeningeal nodules or may show no pathology (Fig. 14.4). CSF shows a lymphocytic pleocytosis, elevated protein and low glucose. CSF opening pressure is often

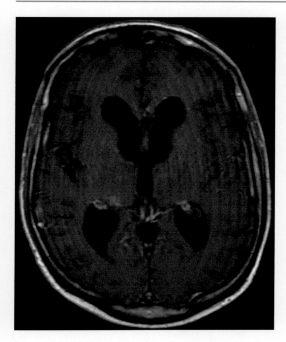

Fig. 14.4 Criptococcal ventriculitis in an immune-compromised patient. Post-contrast T1-WI reveals dilated ventricles and enhancement of choroid plexuses in keeping with ventriculitis and choroid plexitis

elevated. India ink test is used to detect cryptococci but is only positive in 25–50 % of patients. Detection of cryptoccocal antigens in the CSF by latex agglutination tests is the most sensitive diagnostic test for cryptococcal meningitis or meningoencephalitis. Intravenous Amphotericin B combined with oral formulations of flucytosine is recommended for treatment of cryptococcal CNS disease.

14.16 Whipple's Disease

Whipple's disease is a very rare condition caused by *Tropheryma Whippelii*. The annual incidence of the disease since 1980 has been approximately 30 cases per year. It usually presents with gastrointestinal and systemic symptoms including diarrhoea, malabsorption with steatorrhea, weight loss, fever, lymphadenopathy and arthritis. CNS involvement occurs in 5–40 % and presents with psychosis, insidious memory loss leading to dementia, seizures and sudden onset of focal

motor deficits. The classic triad of CNS Whipple's disease is cognitive impairment, ophthalmoplegia and myoclonus. The myoclonus type that is considered most specific for Whipple's disease is oculo-masticatory myorhythmia (continuous rhythmic convergence movements of eye with concurrent masticatory muscle contractions) but a series from the Mayo Clinic in 2005 of 11 patients with CNS Whipple's disease found only one patient had that. That series demonstrated a wide variety of symptoms and signs including memory loss, ataxia, corticospinal tract signs, visual disturbance, dysarthria, supranuclear gaze palsy, hallucinations, parkinsonism, insomnia, hypersomnia, myoclonus, dystonia, postural tremor and myopathy.

In the CNS, Tropheryma whippelii has a predilection for limbic structures. MR brain imaging can show mesial temporal lesions with peripheral contrast enhancement and oedema, with or without mass effect. Diagnosis is confirmed by finding diagnostic periodic acid-Schiff (PAS) positive macrophages in intestinal or brain biopsy samples. Tropheryma Whippelii can be seen within these macrophages on electron microscopy. Whipple's disease requires long term antibiotic therapy which should include an antibiotic that crosses the blood-brain barrier. Treatment may be with IV ceftriaxone initially and subsequently long term oral antibiotics such as co-trimoxozole.

14.17 Hepatitis C

Viral hepatitis C constitutes a major public health concern affecting approximately 200 million people worldwide. Hepatitis C Virus (HCV) is a single stranded RNA virus of the Flaviviridae family, genus Hepacivirus. It is transmitted sexually, vertically, through infected blood products and by sharing needles in intravenous drug abusers. About 15–45 % of HCV infected individuals spontaneously clear the virus. The remaining 55–85 % will go on to develop chronic hepatitis C infection. Prevalence of chronic HCV in most European and North American countries is reported to be between 0.5 and 2 %. The main sequelae of chronic HCV infection are primarily hepatic: chronic hepatitis, cirrhosis and hepatocellular carcinoma. Neurological complications have been described in a large number of patients and range from peripheral neuropathy to cognitive impairment. Cognitive dysfunction, characterized by forgetfulness, attention and concentration difficulties, poor word recall, and impaired psychomotor speed, has been documented in 13–50 % of HCV infected individuals.

Cognitive dysfunction in HCV infection has long been attributed to liver disease, specifically cirrhosis and hepatic encephalopathy. However, recent studies indicate that approximately one-third of patients experience cognitive impairment in the absence of cirrhosis and its occurrence is unrelated to viral load, genotype or history of substance misuse. HCV RNA has been isolated in post-mortem brain tissue and in the CSF of HCV infected individuals. Brain cells harbouring HCV have been identified as CD68-positive microglial macrophages. HCV can replicate in peripheral blood mononuclear cells, therefore, it is possible that the virus is introduced to CNS via a "trojan horse" mechanism where it induces an inflammatory cascade.

Neuroimaging studies in patients with chronic hepatitis C and cognitive dysfunction show altered structure and function of several neuronal systems, including the frontal neocortex, basal ganglia, and connecting white matter tracts. Diagnosis of HCV infection is made by finding a positive serum HCV antibody and then HCV RNA viral load and genotype. Antiviral HCV treatment is available and the decision to treat is based on assessment of viral and host factors, including staging of liver disease. Vibration-controlled transient elastography (VCTE) with FibroScan® is comparable to liver biopsy and thus obviates the need for liver biopsy in most cases.

The prevalence of HCV among HIV positive patients is around 35 % in the United States and Europe and can be as high as 80–90 % in the intravenous drug using population. Studies have confirmed that HIV co-infection accelerates the natural course of chronic hepatitis C and progression to liver cirrhosis and therefore increases the risk of hepatocellular carcinoma. There is no clear evidence yet that HCV co-infection in HIV-positive patients increases the risk of developing cognitive impairment.

Conclusion

HIV has evolved into a chronic disease with the advent of HAART. Although the incidence rates of HIV associated dementia have decreased significantly in the post HAART era, it is evident that a milder spectrum of neurocognitive disorders is still quite prevalent. The exact aetiology of HAND remains to be fully elucidated despite many advances in our understanding of this disorder. The role of on-going inflammation and immune activation in the aetiology of HIV related cognitive impairment is intriguing and may exist despite viral suppression in the primary blood compartment. Whether the on-going inflammation and immune activation are as a direct result of primary HIV infection in the CNS, a consequence of the CNS being a reservoir for on-going HIV replication despite adequate viral suppression in the primary blood compartment or as a consequence of HAART remains a subject of great interest and debate. Whatever the mechanism of the initial inflammatory insult, there is evidence that low level inflammation continues even in those who are virally suppressed and does not require a continuous viral presence. It is most likely that the initial upregulation of inflammation and immune activation stems from a number of sources and pathways. This inflammatory cascade may then induce excitotoxicity resulting in neurotoxicity. This may be contributed to by HAART and also directly by HIV and its viral proteins. The neuropathogenesis of HIV is multifactorial and is probably the result of the interaction of all these factors that contributes to the development of HAND.

Normal function of the brain requires a delicate balance between neuroprotective and neurodegenerative processes. These are tightly regulated to maintain normal neuronal function and it is likely that HIV disrupts this balance through many potential mechanisms as evidenced above. This has implications for therapeutic interventions as it will be necessary for any successful intervention to be able to block or reverse the damaging effects of HIV, its resultant inflammatory cascade and neurodegenerative mechanisms without causing further disruption to this fine balance. This challenge is not unique to HAND but is also faced by researchers in the wider neurodegenerative field. Future challenges include establishing the exact aetiology of HAND, discovery of reliable biomarkers for its diagnosis and establishing therapies, both for those with HAND and for those HIV positive patients at risk of developing HAND.

Other issues contributing to HIV and cognitive impairment include an ageing population, late presenters and increasing survival. An ageing population, both in terms of older patients presenting with new HIV infections and those living and ageing with HIV infection, present unique challenges in terms of their risk of cognitive impairment. They will also be at risk of developing cognitive impairment due to other causes including Alzheimer's disease and vascular dementia therefore the importance of understanding the neuropsychological profile of HAND and developing reliable biomarkers for the diagnosis of HAND will be critical in distinguishing it at an early stage from other causes in order to ensure the correct diagnosis is established and management can therefore be tailored accordingly. Cardiovascular disease and stroke are increased in HIV infection and these factors will also contribute to the increasing risk of cognitive impairment in an ageing HIV positive population. With increased survival people will live with the effects of HIV on their cardiovascular and central nervous systems for longer with the resultant ongoing inflammatory response that will increase their risk of cognitive impairment. They will also be exposed to considerably longer durations of HAART. Patients presenting late with low CD4 counts will be at increased risk of opportunistic infections and HAND.

Screening for cognitive impairment in all HIV positive patients is of utmost importance with longitudinal follow up of all patients clinically although this can be difficult in clinical settings without adequate resources but it must be developed as part of any HIV service and there are multiple short screening tools available which are easy to use. Referral to a specialist neurology service should be sought for those who are found to have a positive screen for cognitive impairment. Given that over 30 million people worldwide are living with HIV and up to half of them may experience cognitive impairment it necessitates resource planning to ensure that these patients are identified, treated and monitored from a cognitive perspective as well as an infectious standpoint and emphasises the importance of ongoing research to establish therapeutic interventions and guidelines.

In general one must be increasingly aware of infectious causes of cognitive impairment with changing demographics worldwide: an ageing population with resultant immune paresis, increased travel, unusual hobbies which expose people to potential pathogens, increasing number of sexual partners, changing structure and dynamic of sexual relationships whereby many people no longer conform to one monogamous relationship lifelong and increasing worldwide use of biologic agents and monoclonal antibodies for the treatment of many systemic diseases which increase the risk of opportunistic infections. It will be imperative to consider infectious causes of cognitive impairment and rapidly progressive dementias in order to establish a diagnosis and initiate treatment as early as possible to ensure the best outcome.

Further Reading

Anthony IC, Bell JE. The neuropathology of HIV/AIDS. Int Rev Psychiatry. 2008;20(1):15–24.

Antinori A, Arendt G, Becker JT, Brew BJ, Byrd DA, Cherner M, et al. Updated research nosology for HIV-associated neurocognitive disorders. Neurology. 2007;69(18): 1789–99.

Byrnes III EJ, Li W, Lewit Y, Ma H, Voelz K, Ren P, et al. Emergence and pathogenicity of highly virulent Cryptococcus gattii genotypes in the northwest United States. PLoS Pathog. 2010;6(4):e1000850.

Ghanem KG. Neurosyphilis: a historical perspective and review. CNS Neurosci Ther. 2010;16:157–68.

Ibanez-Valdes L, Foyaca-Sibat H, Mfenyana K, Chandia J, Gonzalez-Aguilera H. Neuropsychiatry manifestations in patients presenting cryptococcal meningitis. Internet J Neurol. 2004; 5(1).

Lescure FX, Moulignier A, Savatovsky J, Amiel C, Carcelain G, Molina JM, et al. CD8 encephalitis in HIV-infected patients receiving cART: a treatable entity. Clin Infect Dis. 2013;57(1):101–8.

Masters MC, Ances BM. Role of neuroimaging in HIV-associated neurocognitive disorders. Semin Neurol. 2014;34(1):89–102.

Matthews BR, Jones LK, Saad DA, Aksamit AJ, Josephs KA. Cerebellar ataxia and central nervous system whipple disease. Arch Neurol. 2005;62(4):618–20.

Monaco S, Ferrari S, Gajofatto A, Zanusso G, Mariotto S. Review article HCV-related nervous system disorders. Clin Dev Immunol. 2012: Article ID 236148, 9 pages. doi: 10.1155/2012/236148.

Montoya JG, Liesenfeld O. Seminar. Toxoplasmosis. Lancet. 2004;363:1965–76.

Morris KA, Davies NW, Brew BJ. A guide to interpretation of neuroimmunological biomarkers in the combined antiretroviral therapy-era of HIV central nervous system disease. Neurobehav HIV Med. 2010;2:59–72.

Navia BA, Jordan BD, Price RW. The AIDS dementia complex: I. Clinical features. Ann Neurol. 1986a;19(6):517–24.

Navia BA, Cho ES, Petito CK, Price RW. The AIDS dementia complex: II. Neuropathology. Ann Neurol. 1986b;19(6):525–35.

Rahejaa AA, Luia YW, Pinzon-Ardilab A, Limc RP, Sparrb SA. Use of diffusion-weighted imaging in recurrent central nervous system Whipple's disease: a case report and review of the literature. Clin Imaging. 2010;34:143–7.

Woods SP, Moore DJ, Weber E, Grant I. Cognitive neuropsychology of HIV-associated neurocognitive disorders. Neuropsychol Rev. 2009;19(2):152–68.

Neuroinflammatory Disorders

15

Lisa Costelloe, Jean Fletcher,
and Denise Fitzgerald

15.1 Epidemiology, Demographics, and Clinical Features

15.1.1 Demographics and Epidemiology of Multiple Sclerosis

Multiple Sclerosis (MS) is a chronic autoimmune demyelinating disease that is the commonest cause of non-traumatic neurological disability in young adults affecting more than 2.3 million individuals worldwide. Disease onset is usually in the third or fourth decade, but 2 % of patients with multiple sclerosis present before age 10 years, and 5 % before age 16 years.

Though its exact aetiology remains unknown it is likely due to a combination of environmental triggers in genetically susceptible individuals. Early seminal studies of MS established that the incidence of the disease increased with distance from the equator (Fig. 15.1). Kurtzke classified

L. Costelloe (✉)
Department of Neurology, Beaumont Hospital,
Dublin, Ireland
e-mail: lisacostelloe@beaumont.ie

J. Fletcher
Schools of Medicine and Biochemistry
and Immunology, Trinity College, Dublin,
Dublin, Ireland

D. Fitzgerald
Queens University, Belfast, Ireland

different parts of the world according to their prevalence of MS. High prevalence regions had more than 30 cases per 100,000 population, intermediate prevalence had 5–30 cases, and low prevalence areas had less than 5 cases. This may be explained by the genetic composition of the population but environmental factors such as sunlight exposure and Vitamin D as well as infections are also potential explanatory factors. Early migration studies also suggest an environmental influence when it was established that immigration before the age of 15 lead to a reduced risk for the development of MS in immigrants from Northern Europe settling in South Africa.

However, recent evidence suggests that this latitude gradient in MS incidence may be decreasing. This may be partly due to lifestyle changes leading to decreased sunlight exposure and Vitamin D deficiency. Another possible explanation is the so-called hygiene hypothesis. It is thought that exposure to infections in early childhood has a protective effect against the later development of autoimmune diseases. As socioeconomic factors lead to decreased childhood infections, thus autoimmunity in adulthood may be increasing over time. It has long been known that MS is about twice as common in women compared to men. Similarly however, it has recently been reported that the female- to-male ratio of MS is increasing over time. One study reported the female-to-male ratio increased from approximately 2 for patients diagnosed in

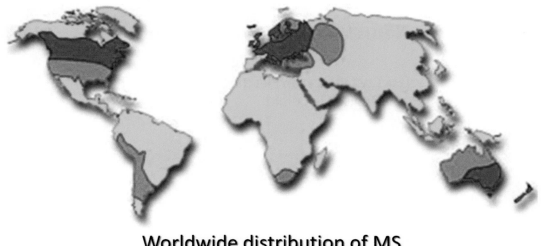

Worldwide distribution of MS

■ Higher than 30/100,000

■ Between 5/100,000 and 30/100,000

□ Below 5/100,000

Fig. 15.1 Global prevalence of multiple sclerosis- people per 100,000 with MS

1940 to 4 for those diagnosed in 2000. The cause of the observed rise in this ratio remains unclear though increased smoking in women during the twentieth century is one putative contributing factor. Though MS is thought to affect Caucasians more than other racial groups, a recent US study found that the risk of developing MS was higher in black women when compared to white women though the risk did not differ between men of various ethnicities.

15.1.2 Clinical Course and Subtypes of Disease

Multiple Sclerosis can develop in many forms, the most common of which is relapsing remitting MS (RRMS), characterised by discrete attacks or relapses followed by remissions. A relapse represents the development of a new neurological symptom or worsening of a pre-existing symptom that persists for greater than 24 h and is not associated with infection. Relapses are usually followed by a period of complete or incomplete remission of variable duration. MS is characterised by this relapsing-remitting onset in about 85 % of cases. When a patient initially presents with a first relapse and does not yet meet criteria for MS, this is said to be a clinically isolated syndrome (CIS).

Eventually, remissions are of shorter duration, relapse associated disability accumulates, and the patient enters a progressive disabling phase. About 80 % of relapsing remitting cases will progress to secondary progressive MS (SPMS) within two decades. The secondary progressive stage is characterised by a slow disease progression as irreversible disability is gradually accrued. Its onset is usually determined retrospectively. The mean time interval for conversion from RRMS to SPMS is 10.4 years. Relapses persist in around 40 % of cases during the progressive phase. The primary progressive MS subtype (PPMS) is present in 15–20 % of MS cases and is characterised by at least 1 year of relapse free progression at onset. There are no remissions as the patient suffers a progressive decline in function. A slowly developing motor onset is more typical of PPMS however it can also be characterised by progressive ataxia. Between 15 and 20 % of MS patients will prove to have a benign form of multiple sclerosis, remaining fully functional in all neurological systems more than 10 years after disease onset. Acute MS, or Marburg's disease, is thankfully very rare. It is characterised by rapid disease progression and an exceptionally severe course usually leading to death within a few years of onset.

15.1.3 Clinical Features

MS is a clinically heterogenous disease and almost any neurological symptom can occur during the course of the illness. The symptoms and signs of multiple sclerosis merely reflect the functional anatomy of impaired conduction due to demyelination in the optic nerves, brain, and spinal cord. A number of clinical presentations are very typical of MS. A specific and characteristic sensory symptom seen in MS is the "useless hand syndrome" where one hand is functionally impaired due to proprioceptive loss. Acute bilateral internuclear opthalmoplegia (INO), Lhermitte's symptom, Uthoff's phenomenon, unilateral facial myokimia, bilateral trigeminal neuralgia, and unilateral remitting optic neuritis, are all also suggestive of MS when occurring in young adults. Among the commonest chronic symptoms of the disease are fatigue and depression, bladder irritative problems and urinary retention, limb weakness and spasticity, sensory symptoms, neuropathic pain, and cognitive impairment. Paroxysmal symptoms such as trigeminal neuralgia and tonic spasms can also frequently occur.

15.2 Pathology and Aetiology of MS

15.2.1 Pathology

The pathological hallmark of MS is demyelination. It is caused by inflammation targeting the myelin sheath and is associated with the formation of focal lesions within the CNS known as *plaques*. The classic acute MS plaque is characterised by perivascular infiltration of activated macrophages and T lymphocytes. The pathology of the acute plaque is heterogenous and four different patterns have been described based on myelin protein loss, the location and extension of the plaque, the pattern of oligodendrocyte destruction, and the involvement of complement components. The pattern may not be static within a given individual, and more than one pattern can be observed in the same patient. Partial remyelination of plaques occurs to a variable extent. Severe demyelination results in axonal loss and damage to surrounding oligodendrocytes.

The classical view of MS as a disease that exclusively affects the white matter has more recently been refuted. Pathological studies and modern MRI modalities have convincingly demonstrated diffuse pathology in both the normal appearing white matter (NAWM) of the brain and spinal cord, as well as cortical demyelination affecting the grey matter in MS patients. This diffuse pathology is seen even at very early stages of disease.

MS is believed to start with activation and proliferation of autoreactive CD4+ T helper lymphocytes in the periphery. These cells then migrate across the blood brain barrier (BBB), recognise auto-antigens, and initiate inflammation via the production of pro-inflammatory cytokines. This inflammatory cascade cumulates in damage to the myelin sheath, oligodendrocytes, and axons. It is an extremely complex process involving multiple cell types, cytokines, and co-stimulatory molecules. In the progressive stage of the disease less active inflammation is observed and disability is thought to occur due to degenerative changes. Nonetheless, oligodendrocyte progenitor cells (OPCs) capable of remyelination have been observed in the white matter plaques of chronic MS patients suggesting that remyelination may be possible even in the late stages of disease. This represents an encouraging therapeutic target for treatment of progressive MS.

15.2.2 Genetics of MS

MS is not inherited in a Mendelian fashion and is likely to be polygenic. There is however a familial recurrence rate of about 15 %. The age-adjusted risk is higher for siblings (3 %), parents (2 %), and children (2 %) than for second degree and third-degree relatives. Recurrence in monozygotic twins is around 35 %. Linkage studies in multiplex families have confirmed that variation within the major histocompatibility complex (MHC) has the greatest individual effect on risk. A large genome wide association study (GWAS) has recently replicated this finding and has identified at least another 29 susceptibility loci. Immunologically relevant genes are significantly overrepresented among those mapping close to these loci confirming that MS is primarily an immune mediated disease.

15.2.3 Environmental Factors and MS

Migration studies, geographical variation in disease rates, and high rates of discordancy in identical twins suggest that environmental agents must play a role in the pathogenesis of MS. The role of Vitamin D status in MS has gained importance in recent years as both epidemiological and experimental data increasingly suggest that Vitamin D deficiency plays an importance role in both MS pathogenesis and disease activity. A case control study involving seven million US military personnel with stored serum found that lower risk of MS was associated with higher levels of 25-hydroxyvitamin D. This effect was interestingly seen in white people but not in black or Hispanic people. A study that included 42,0000 people found that significantly fewer people with MS are born in November and significantly more are born in May, a fact that is putatively linked to the Vitamin D status of the mother during gestation. It has been shown that Vitamin D levels are significantly lower in relapsing remitting MS patients compared to controls and are also lower in patients experiencing disease activity compared to those in remission. A recent study demonstrated that a 50-nmol/L (20-ng/mL) increment in average serum 25-hydroxyvitamin D levels within the first 12 months of disease predicted a lower relapse rate,

a lower rate of T2 lesion accumulation on MRI, and a lower rate of yearly brain atrophy from months 12–60. This suggests that vitamin D deficiency is a strong predictor of future relapse activity and disease progression.

With respect to lifestyle factors only smoking has emerged as a moderate risk factor for MS. More recently childhood obesity has been highlighted as a possible risk factor for later development of MS. Over the years several transmissible agents have been implicated as possible causes of MS though to date no infectious trigger has been definitively identified. In recent times the leading candidates include Epstein-Barr virus (EBV) and Human Immunodeficiency Virus (HIV). The epidemiological data associated EBV infection with MS remains strong. We know that almost all patients with MS (>99 %) have evidence of prior EBV infection when compared to only about 90 % of controls. People who have had symptomatic EBV infection (infectious mononucleosis) are at increased risk of developing MS for up to 30 years after the original infection. In this large Danish cohort the ratio of observed: expected MS cases was 2.27. High titres of EBV antibodies predict a higher risk of MS than low titres and Hodgkin's lymphoma, another EBV associated condition, occurs more frequently in MS patients when compared to controls. None of these facts provide proof of causation but they do suggest a role for EBV in the pathogenesis of MS.

Though both MS and HIV are widely documented in the medical literature, only one case of co-existent MS and HIV infection has been documented. The individual in question was commenced on combination anti-retroviral therapy (cART) following which their MS remained quiescent for up to 12 years of follow up. It was postulated that the anti retroviral therapy may be coincidentally treating or preventing MS or that perhaps the HIV infection itself exerted some form of biological protection. This case report prompted further enquiry into this phenomenon. A large UK linkage study investigating the possible association between MS and HIV was recently reported. The relative risk of MS in people with HIV, relative to those without HIV, was

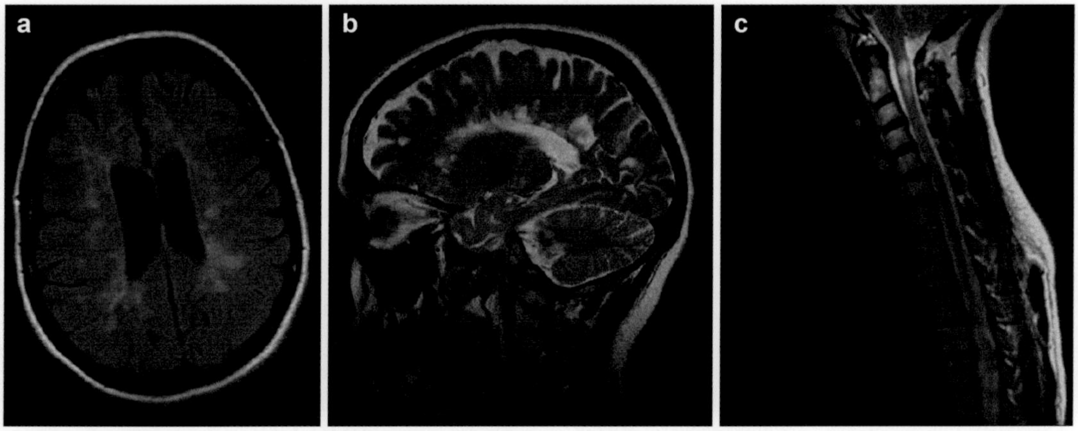

Fig. 15.2 MRI images typical of MS reproduced with patient permission. (**a**) Axial FLAIR image showing ovoid periventricular and juxta-cortical white matter hyper intensities, (**b**) sagittal T2 image showing "Dawson's fingers" perpendicular to the corpus callosum, and (**c**) a sagittal T2 spinal image demonstrating an MS plaque in the cervical cord

0.38. The magnitude of this effect (>60 %) is at the highest level of any prognostic risk factor reported to date. This finding may prompt future trials of anti-retroviral therapies in MS patients.

15.3 Current Diagnostic Criteria

The diagnosis of MS relies on providing evidence for dissemination of CNS lesions in both time and space, as well as excluding alternative diagnoses. MS is primarily a clinical diagnosis and there is no one test that is pathognomonic of the disease. However, the widespread availability of magnetic resonance imaging (MRI) has revolutionized the diagnostic workup and has led to earlier diagnosis of disease than ever before. Typical MRI findings in MS patients include ovoid lesions located perpendicularly to the corpus callosum (Dawson's fingers), in the juxtacortical white matter, in the cerebellum, brainstem, and cervico-thoracic spinal cord (see Fig. 15.2). Fluid attenuated inversion recovery (FLAIR) is the most sensitive imaging sequence for these white matter abnormalities. Active plaques that are associated with disruption of the blood brain barrier enhance with administration of paramagnetic contrast agents such as gadolinium.

The McDonald criteria are a set of diagnostic criteria for MS that incorporate the clinical characteristics of the disease alone or in combination with MRI features. These criteria were first introduced in 2001 by an international panel and were revised in 2005 and most recently in 2010 (see Table 15.1). To demonstrate dissemination of lesions in space (DIS) using MRI, one or more T2 lesions must be seen in areas typical of MS; namely the periventricular, juxtacortical or infratentorial white matter or within the spinal cord. Dissemination of lesions in time (DIT) can be demonstrated using MRI when a new T2 and/or gadolinium enhancing lesion develops relative to a baseline MRI scan. Alternatively, the simultaneous presence of asymptomatic gadolinium enhancing and non-enhancing lesions at any time is sufficient to demonstrate DIT.

Examination of the cerebrospinal fluid (CSF) is also a useful ancillary investigation in suspected multiple sclerosis cases. In MS intrathecal synthesis of oligoclonal immunoglobulin G (IgG) bands are found in approximately 90 % of patients. A simultaneous blood sample is required to demonstrate the intra-thecal origin of the bands as the passive transfer of bands from the systemic circulation is of no diagnostic value. Isoelectric focusing and immunodetection of oligoclonal bands (OCBs) is the gold standard technique used to identify intrathecal antibody synthesis. A raised IgG index is also suggestive of MS but is not as sensitive or specific as the presence of OCBs.

Table 15.1 2010 revised McDonald criteria for the diagnosis of multiple sclerosis

Clinical presentation	Additional information needed to make MS diagnosis
2 or more relapses Objective clinical evidence of 2 or more lesions with history of prior relapse	None, clinical evidence will suffice. MRI brain is still desirable
2 or more relapses Objective clinical evidence of 1 lesion	Dissemination in space demonstrated by MRI or await further relapse implicating a different CNS site
1 relapse Objective clinical evidence of 1 lesion	Dissemination in space demonstrated by MRI or await 2nd relapse implicating a different CNS site And Dissemination in time demonstrated by MRI or a 2nd clinical relapse
Insidious neurological progression suggestive of primary progressive MS	One year of disease progression and dissemination in space demonstrated by 2 of the following: 1 or more T2 brain lesions typical of MS 2 or more T2 lesions in the spinal cord Positive CSF- OCBs and /or raised IgG index
Relapse- a new neurological symptom lasting at least 24 h in the absence of infection. There must be at least 30 days between onset of one relapse and onset of another	CSF- cerebrospinal fluid OCB- oligoclonal band

Reproduced and modified with permission of John Wiley and Sons from Polman et al. Diagnostic criteria for multiple sclerosis: 2010 Revisions to the McDonald criteria. *Annals of Neurology*. 2011;69:292–302

15.4 Differential Diagnosis and Syndromes That Overlap with MS

15.4.1 Neuromyelitis Optica (NMO)

NMO (Devic's disease) is an inflammatory demyelinating disease of the CNS that for many years was thought to be a variant of MS but is now known to be immunologically and pathologically distinct. Clinically it presents with optic neuritis and myelitis, often with a poor recovery and a relapsing course. MR imaging typically shows longitudinally extensive cord lesions, extending over three or more vertebral segments. Brain lesions can be clinically silent and are seen in about 60 % of patients often in the diencephalon and hypothalamus. Pathologically NMO is characterised by demyelination, neuronal loss, and often pronounced necrosis. The discovery of aquaporin-4 autoantibodies in 2004 (AQP4-Ab, also known as NMO-IgG) in the serum of patients with NMO represented a considerable advance in both the diagnosis and treatment of the disease and distinguished NMO from MS as an independent disease entity. The specificity of these antibodies is between 90 and 100 % in the correct clinical context. More recently, antibodies to myelin oligodendrocyte glycoprotein (MOG) have been reported in AQP4-Ab negative cases with a typical NMO phenotype. However, the exact diagnostic implications of this finding are still under investigation.

More women than men have NMO (ratio 9:1) and the median age of onset is more than 10 years older than in MS. Moderate pleocytosis in the CSF of NMO patients is seen more commonly than in MS and OCBs are only seen in about 30 % of cases. In NMO the CSF OCB status can change over time, which is uncommon in MS. More recently high concentrations of IL-6 have been found in the CSF of NMO patients which may help in differentiating it from other demyelinating diseases. Therapy should be initiated early in NMO and the therapeutic pathway is different from that of MS. Azathioprine and Rituximab are recommended as first line agents. Other immunosuppressant agents such as methotrexate, mycophenylate mofetil, and mitoxantrone are recommended as second line agents. Promising new therapies such as anti- AQP4-Ab and anti-IL-6 receptor biologicals are emerging.

AQP4-Ab have also been demonstrated in patients with clinical syndromes atypical of NMO such as brainstem syndromes including intractable vomiting, narcolepsy, neuroendo-crine disturbances, and olfactory dysfunction. The term "NMO spectrum disorders" is often used as an umbrella term for these varied presentations.

15.4.2 Acute Disseminated Encephalomyeltis (ADEM)

ADEM is an inflammatory demyelinating disorder that can often be considered in the differential diagnosis of an initial demyelinating event or clinically isolated syndrome (CIS). It can present with a number of clinical symptoms but usually includes encephalopathy as well as multifocal symptoms suggestive of an inflammatory disorder. ADEM differs from MS and NMO in that it is a monophasic illness that does not relapse and therefore does not require disease modifying therapy (DMT). A recent review has proposed a number of clinical, imaging, and laboratory features that are helpful in distinguishing ADEM from a first presentation of other inflammatory disorders. ADEM is seen much more commonly in the paediatric population but can also occur in adults. Unlike MS, it is often preceded by an infection or vaccination. It should be considered when there is a multifocal polysymptomatic presentation, encephalopathy, seizures, fever, headache, and bilateral optic neuritis. On CSF examination a lymphocytic pleocytosis is more commonly seen in ADEM than in MS and CSF OCBs are seen less frequently than in MS and often resolve when present in ADEM. MRI will often demonstrate large (1–2 cm) multifocal areas of T2 abnormality in the CNS white matter often with diffuse enhancement and grey matter involvement in addition. Periventricular involvement is less prominent than in MS. A brain biopsy is sometimes warranted when the diagnosis remains uncertain and the pathological hallmark of ADEM is perivenular inflammation with "sleeves of demyelination". Intravenous methylprednisolone is the most common treatment used in practice when an infectious aetiology has been excluded, IVIG may be an effective alternative.

Table 15.2 Differential diagnoses of progressive and relapsing forms of multiple sclerosis

Differential diagnosis of a progressive cord syndrome	Differential diagnosis of a relapsing CNS disorder
Tumour	**Vascular disease**
Intramedullary- glioma, ependymoma	CADASIL
Extramedullary- meningioma, neurofibroma	Cerebral amyloid angiopathy
Extradural- metastasis	Antiphospholipid antibody syndrome
Vascular- Dural arteriovenous malformation	Fabry's disease
Metabolic	**Vasculitis**
B12 deficiency	Behcet's disease
Copper deficiency	Neurosarcoidosis
Vitamin E deficiency	Sjogren's syndrome
Phenyketonuria	Susac's syndrome
Degenerative-	Sysyemic lupus erythematosus
Amyotrophic lateral sclerosis	Primary angiitis of the CNS
Infectious	**Mitochondrial disease**
HIV	MELAS
HTLV-1	**Chronic infection**
Syphilis	Lyme disease
Tuberculosis	Neurosyphilis
Schistosomiasis	HTLV-1
Inflammatory	HIV encephalitis
Neurosarcoidosis	Fungal/parasitic infections
Systemic lupus erythematosus	Whipple's disease
Paraneoplastic	CADASIL- Cerebral Autosomal Dominant
Genetic	Arteriopathy with
Hereditary spastic paraparesis	subcortical infarcts and leucoencephalopathy
Freidreich's ataxia	MELAS- Mitochondrial
Adrenomyeloneuropathy	Encephalopathy with Lactic Acidosis and
Toxic- Nitrous oxide	Stroke-like episodes

15.4.3 Differential Diagnosis of MS

Diagnostic criteria for MS emphasize that that an alternative explanation for the presentation must be considered and excluded before a diagnosis of MS can be made. International consensus based guidelines have been published to guide the clinical, laboratory, and imaging assessments of patients with possible MS in order to best exclude alternative diagnoses. The differential diagnosis of MS is wide and includes diseases that can mimic both relapsing and progressive neurological disturbances. These are outlined in Table 15.2 although such lists are always selective and incomplete.

Table 15.3 First- generation self-injectable disease modifying therapies for relapsing remitting MS

Drug	Interferon-beta 1b	Interferon-beta 1b	Interferon-beta 1a	Interferon-beta 1a	PegInterferon-beta 1a	Glatiramer acetate
Brand name	Betaferon	Extavia	Avonex	Rebif	Plegridy	Copaxone
Year approved	1993	2009	1996	2002	2015	1997
Dose	250 µg	250 µg	30 µg	22 or 44 µg	125 µg	20 mg or 40 mg
Route	SC	SC	IM	SC	SC	SC
Frequency	Every other day	Every other day	Once/week	3 times/week	once every 2 weeks	Daily or All days (40 mg) (20 mg)

SC subcutaneous, *IM* intramuscular

15.4.4 Disease Modifying Therapies (DMTs)

In the long-term management of MS, a number of disease modifying therapies (DMTs) are used to reduce the relapse rate and therefore reduce the amount of relapse- associated disability accumulated during the relapsing remitting phase of the illness. Several new DMTs have been developed in recent years many of which are more targeted and efficacious than their predecessors. Each of these agents have undesirable side effects and the risk benefit ratio of each therapy has to be considered for each individual patient. There is currently no DMT licensed for use in progressive MS and this remains a critical area of unmet need in MS therapeutics. In RRMS it is now recognised that there is a therapeutic "window of opportunity" during the first 5 years of the disease during which aggressive control of the inflammatory phase of the illness is of most benefit in the long term. It remains unclear to date whether early suppression of relapses and neuro-inflammation with any drug will ultimately prevent the onset of progressive disease.

15.4.5 "First- Generation" Self Injectable Therapies

The first DMTs to be licensed for use in RRMS were self administered injections given either subcutaneously or intramuscularly at a variable frequency depending on the specific agent used. The type 1 beta-interferons were the first immunomodulatory agents to be licensed for use in MS in 1993, and while they are used routinely in RRMS patients,

their precise mechanism of action remains to be elucidated. There are currently five commercially available beta-interferon preparations in clinical use (see Table 15.3). Glatiramer acetate (GA, Copaxone) is a synthetic peptide composed of four amino acids designed specifically to mimic the structure of myelin basic protein (MBP). MBP is the principle component of CNS myelin and is therefore a putative autoantigen in MS. Glatiramer acetate received US Food and Drug Administration (FDA) approval for use in MS patents in 1987. All these drugs have comparable efficacy, reducing the relapse rate by about a third, reducing the number of new brain lesions in RRMS patients, and slowing but not preventing the onset of disease progression. They have all established long-term safety but are limited by injection-related skin reactions, and flu-like side effects seen with the interferon-beta preparations. A PEGylated form of interferon-beta 1a plegridy with a longer half-life and a reduced dosing frequency (once every 2 weeks) has recently received a license in RRMS.

15.4.6 Oral DMTS

Three oral agents have been approved for use in relapsing MS: fingolimod, teriflunomide and dimethyl-fumarate (BG-12). Efficacy data from pivotal randomised controlled trials of these agents are summarized in Table 15.4

15.4.7 Fingolimod (Gilenya)

Fingolimod is a sphingosine- 1-phosphate (S1P) receptor agonist which binds to 4 of the 5

Table 15.4 Summary of efficacy data from pivotal controlled trials for recently developed disease modifying therapies for relapsing MS

Drug	Fingolimod	Dimethyl fumarate (BG-12)	Teriflunomide	Natalizumab	Alemtuzumab
Brand Name	Gilenya	Tecfidera	Aubagio	Tysabri	Lemtrada
Year approved	2010	2013	2012	2004, 2006	2014
Dose	0.5 mg	240 mg	7 mg or 14 mg	300 mg	12 mg
Route	PO	PO	PO	IV	IV
Frequency	Daily	Twice daily	Daily	Once every 4 weeks	Annually 5 doses year 1 3 doses year 2 and thereafter as required
Clinical relapse Relative RR	54 %	51 %	31 %	68 %	55 % (vs rebif 44)[a] 49 % (vs rebif 44)[b]
Disability progression Relative RR	30 %	38 %	26 % (14 mg dose only)	42 %	NS[a] 42 % (vs rebif 44)[b]

[a]CARE MS 1
[b]CARE MS 2

sphingosine receptors and acts as a functional antagonist. As such it prevents the egress of lymphocytes from lymph nodes and causes a relative lymphopenia. It also enters the CNS where it affects neurons and supporting glia that express S1P receptors. There is much recent interest in the possible neuroprotective role of fingolimod in addition to its anti-inflammatory effects. Adverse effects of the drug reflect the effects of lymphopenia as well as the fact that S1P receptors are expressed in other tissues including the heart and the retina. The risk of opportunistic viral infections, in particular varicella zoster infection is well described and it is recommended that immunity to VZV is documented prior to initiation of therapy. Due to its effects on cardiac smooth muscle, fingolimod is contraindicated in those with a history of cardiac problems. Bradycardia is nearly always observed but is rarely symptomatic. Cardiac monitoring is required for 6 h after the administration of the first dose. There is a 0.5 % risk of macular edema and opthalmological assessment is required 3 months after initiation of therapy. The risk is higher tin those with a history of diabetes mellitus or prior uveitis and such patients require annual ophthalmology review while on therapy.

15.4.8 Dimethyl-Fumarate (BG-12)

The mechanism of action of BG-12 remains to be fully elucidated but it is known to activate the nuclear-related factor 2 transcriptional pathway which reduces oxidative cell stress, as well as modulating nuclear factor κB which may have an anti-inflammatory effect. More than 30 % of patients will experience flushing (which may be mitigated by aspirin pre-medication or ingestion with food), as well as gastrointestinal side effects including abdominal pain and bloating, nausea and diarrhoea. These side effects tend to improve after the first month of therapy in the majority of patients. The risk of opportunistic infection with this agent was thought to be low however, a recent case of progressive multifocal leucoencephalopathy (PML) has been described in a patient on BG-12 for 4 years with chronic lymphopenia. PML is an untreatable brain infection which occurs due to re-activation of the John Cunningham (JC) virus in the context of profound immunosuppression. It remains to be seen whether or not PML will emerge as a long term side effect of BG-12 in a proportion of treated MS patients.

15.4.9 Teriflunomide

Teriflunomide is a derivative of leflunomide, a drug used in rheumatoid arthritis. It exerts its immunological effect by inhibiting dihydroorotate dehydrogenase, an enzyme required for pyrimidine synthesis in proliferating cells. It can cause potentially serious hepatotoxicity and as such requires fortnightly liver function testing after its initiation. A particular concern is that of teratogenicity. It is contraindicated in pregnancy and it is excreted in both breast milk and semen. Because of enterohepatic recirculation, it has an extended half-life and if pregnancy or serious side effects occur while on therapy it must be eliminated from the body using cholestyramine or activated charcoal over a period of several days.

15.4.10 Humanised Monoclonal Antibodies

The efficacy data from the pivitol randomised controlled trials for both natalizumab and alemtuzumab are summarized in Table 15.4

15.4.11 Natalizumab

Natalizumab is a humanised monoclonal antibody that selectively targets the α4- subunit of "very late antigen 4" or VLA4 which is expressed on the surface of lymphocytes and monocytes. In order for these cells to cross the blood brain barrier (BBB), VLA-4 must bind to its ligand on the surface of vascular endothelium. When natalizumab prevents this interaction, systemic lymphocytes cannot enter the CNS. The drug is generally well tolerated though infusion related hypersensitivity reactions can occur which should prompt testing for anti-natalizumab antibodies which if present necessitate treatment discontinuation.

When two natalizumab- treated patients developed PML in 2004, the drug was temporarily withdrawn from the market. It was re-introduced in 2006 and continues to be used with risk management guidelines for the development of PML. It is now known that PML is more likely to occur in patients who have positive anti-JC antibodies in the serum, in those who have had prior exposure to immunosuppressing drugs such as mitoxantrone or azathioprine (but not immunomodulators such as beta-interferons or GA), and after a duration of two years on therapy. More recently anti-JC antibody titres have been used to develop an "antibody index" which can also help to predict risk of PML. In JC negative patients, serology should be re-checked every 6 months and the patient re-counselled about increased PML risk if sero-conversion has occurred. Because of the risk of PML, natalizumab has been reserved for patients with highly active MS; namely those with very aggressive disease from the outset or those who have failed more benign therapies such as beta-interferons or GA. Disease activity is known to rebound within 3 months of natalizumab discontinuation and transition to another DMT should be considered early to try and negate this.

15.4.12 Alemtuzumab

Alemtuzumab is a humanised monoclonal antibody directed against the cell surface marker CD52 which is present on the surface of lymphocytes and monocytes. It causes a profound lymphopenia with B lymphocytes recovering to the lower limit of normal (LLN) within 6 months but T lymphocytes recovery to the LLN can be up to 1 year after a single dose. Alemtuzumab was the first MS DMT to be trialled compared to an active comparator (Rebif 44) rather than a placebo.

Somewhat surprisingly, serious infections are uncommon and PML has not been described to date. Mild viral infections including herpes virus infections are relatively common and antivirals such as acyclovir are recommended for 1 month after therapy. Secondary autoimmune conditions commonly occur, often several years after the standard dose of the drug has been administered. The process by which this secondary autoimmunity occurs is not completely understood, but circulating levels of IL-21 may play a role in its development. The commonest of these is autoimmune thyroid disease which occurs in about one third of treated patients, necessitating 3 monthly thyroid function testing for up to 4 years after the treatment. Idiopathic thrombocytopenic purpura (ITP) occurs in about 1 % and monthly platelet counts need to be checked on an ongoing basis as well as cautioning patients about bleeding complications. Goodpasteur's (anti-GBM) disease rarely occurs but is potentially life threatening and urine samples need to be followed for haematuria and proteinuria. Autoimmune cytopenias have also been rarely described.

Infusion reactions are common due to a cytokine release syndrome and pre-medication with intravenous steroids and anti-histamines is required. Neutralizing antibodies to alemtuzumab have not been clinically significant to date. Alemtuzumab has received a European Medicines Evaluation Agency (EMEA) license for active disease in RRMS patients and is generally reserved for the same type of patients with aggressive MS in whom natalizumab would be used. It has to date been rejected by the US Food and Drug Administration (FDA) based on its side effect profile.

15.5 Symptomatic Therapies

Disease modifying therapies have no effect on current neurological symptoms therefore symptomatic management and multidisciplinary neuro-rehabilitation are critical elements of MS management. People with MS usually have multiple symptoms, not all of which can be symptomatically managed. Common symptoms that are readily treatable include fatigue, depression, neuropathic pain, muscle spasms and spasticity, bladder irritative symptoms and urinary retention and some forms of sexual dysfunction. Recently a new drug called fampridine (Fampyra) has been licensed to improve walking speed in patients with all forms of MS. This is a sustained release formulation of 4-Aminopyridine that improves walking speed in about 25–30 % of patients who try it. The therapies commonly used to treat the commonest symptoms of MS are summarised in Table 15.5.

Symptoms that are less amenable to treatment include weakness, ataxia, cognitive impairment and visual loss. Input from physiotherapy and occupational therapy is invaluable particularly in dealing with various mobility problems either in

Table 15.5 Summary of pharmacological and non-pharmacological therapies for the common treatable symptoms of MS

Symptom	Drugs	Non-pharmacological therapies
Fatigue	Modafinil Amantadine	Graded aerobic exercise program
Spasticity and painful spasms	Baclofen Tizanidine Benzodiazepines	Physiotherapy IM Botulinum toxin (Botox) Intrathecal baclofen pump
Bladder Dysfunction	Overactivity: Anti-cholinergics- oxybutynin, solifenacin, tolterodine Intranasal desmopressin	Overactivity: Detrusor muscle Botox Retention: Intermittent self -catheterization (SIC) Suprapubic catheter
Erectile dysfunction	Phosphodiesterase inhibitors- sildenafil	Intracorporeal prostaglandin E1 injection Counselling
Neuropathic pain and paroxysmal symptoms	Amitryptiline Gabapentin Pregabalin Carbamazepine	
Depression	SSRI- citalopram SNRI- venlafaxine	Cognitive behavioural therapy (CBT)
Impaired walking speed	Fampridine	Physiotherapy occupational therapy

SSRI selective serotonin reuptake inhibitor, *SNRI* selective serotonin and noradrenaline reuptake inhibitor the context of a relapse or in patients with progressive disease. Vocational rehabilitation is particularly important in MS as it is a chronic disease of young people, many of whom are in the workforce. Other services such as speech and language therapy, psychology, psychiatry, pain medicine, urology, and palliative care may be involved in the care of an MS patient, depending on their individual needs.

15.5.1 Molecular Biomarkers

A biomarker is defined as "a characteristic that is objectively measured and evaluated as an indicator of normal biological processes, pathogenic processes, or pharmacologic responses to a therapeutic intervention". There have been a number of difficulties in identifying biomarkers for MS that are sufficiently sensitive and specific. The choice of the optimal biological fluid for use in screening potential biomarkers is a key issue. Given that MS pathology is localised to the CNS, CSF is the most appropriate biological fluid to sample for biomarker analysis. However CSF sampling is invasive and not always included in diagnostic procedures. On the other hand, while blood is much more accessible it is likely to be more difficult to detect CNS-specific biomarkers. CNS proteins can leak into the peripheral circulation when the blood brain barrier is permeable; for example during a relapse however this is not always the case and so the blood may not generally reflect the changes within the CNS. Furthermore, the high background levels of serum proteins can make it difficult to detect specific biomarkers at low concentrations. Additionally the heterogeneity between MS patients and also within the disease course of patients represents a significant hurdle to the search for reliable biomarkers for MS. Despite these drawbacks, a significant amount of research has been done in attempts to identify biomarkers that would undoubtedly be useful in diagnosing MS, identifying disease subtypes, monitoring disease progression and response to treatment. The progress made thus far in identifying different types of biomarkers for MS are discussed

below. In general the biomarkers that have been investigated for MS tend to be related to the two key processes that occur in MS; inflammation and neurodegeneration/axonal damage.

15.5.2 Biomarkers of Axonal Damage

Neurofilament (NF) has emerged as one of the most promising potential biomarkers for MS. NF is a protein that forms part of the axonal cytoskeleton, and therefore detection of neurofilament proteins or peptides within the CSF or blood is thought to be a reflection of axonal damage. NF occurs in two isoforms, NF light (NF-L) and NF heavy (NF-H). A number of studies have analysed NF proteins in CSF from RR and progressive MS patient cohorts and it has been suggested that NF-L may reflect axonal damage due to the acute inflammatory response during RRMS, while elevated NF-H may correlate with chronic irreversible damage during disease progression. A long term follow up study measured NF-L upon diagnosis and again on average 14 years later in 99 early MS patients. High CSF levels of NF-L were associated with conversion to SPMS, suggesting that NF-L could be used as a prognostic marker in early RRMS. NF-L levels in the CSF of 127 untreated MS patients were analysed and found to correlate with the lymphocytes and antibody in the CSF as well as with disease severity and lesions measured by MRI. NF-L levels in the CSF of 148 CIS and MS patients were significantly elevated compared with controls, and correlated with EDSS. A role for NF-L as a therapeutic biomarker was shown in a study where CSF levels of NF-L were measured prior to and after 1 year of natalizumab treatment. Both NF-L and NF-H levels were dramatically reduced after natalizumab treatment, whereas only NF-L was significantly lower for patients in remission.

Interestingly, NF-H levels increased with age in both healthy controls and CIS/RRMS patients. In addition NF-H levels were higher during relapse in CIS and RRMS patients and correlated with EDSS but not with any of the CSF inflammatory markers examined. NF-H has been shown to reflect axonal damage as early as the CIS stage, since CSF NFH levels in 67 CIS patients correlated with both physical disability and change in brain volume but not with change inT2 lesion load. These studies indicate that NF–L and NF-H are useful CSF biomarkers for MS that may be associated with inflammatory and neurodegenerative processes respectively.

15.5.3 Auto-Antibodies

Evidence of a role for B cells and antibodies in MS is accumulating, and auto-antibodies specific for a range of brain antigens have been identified in MS patients. These auto-antibodies have potential use as biomarkers. As mentioned above, the presence of antibody OCB in CSF has for many years been used in the diagnosis of MS. However more recent efforts have focused on identifying specific auto-antibodies. Initially myelin antigens were considered to be the most likely target of auto antibodies in MS and indeed myelin-reactive antibodies were detected in the CSF from CIS, RRMS and SPMS patients. Although the antibodies correlated with disease activity measured by MRI, they were not MS specific since they could also be detected in OND and healthy controls. A number of other studies have identified auto antibodies specific for myelin proteins MOG, MBP and PLP, however a lack of consensus has lead to the view that myelin antigens may not be the main auto antibody target in MS. It has now emerged that antibodies are targeted to a range of cells in the brain including neurons, oligodendrocytes, astrocytes and even infiltrating immune cells.

The pathogenic role of auto-antibodies targeting the Aquaporin-4 channel in astrocytes in NMO patients has already been discussed above. However auto antibodies against another channel, the potassium channel KIR 4.1, were detected in approximately half of MS patients tested and were absent in healthy controls , suggesting that auto antibodies to KIR 4.1 may be a useful biomarker in a subset of MS patients.

As discussed above, there has recently been much interest in the possible role of neurofilament as a biomarker, reflecting axonal damage. However auto antibodies against neurofilament may also be potential biomarkers. Auto antibodies to NFL have been associated with axonal loss and disease progression. In addition anti-NFL antibodies in CSF were associated with progression from CIS to MS. Studies using serum rather than CSF showed elevated auto antibodies for NFL in PPMS but not RRMS patients. Auto antibodies specific for other neuronal antigens including gangliosides and tubulin have also been detected in MS patients. However these auto antibody biomarkers specific for neuronal antigens do not seem to be specific for MS as they are also detected in a range of other neurological conditions. In summary, no single auto antibody can yet be used as a biomarker for MS, and it is likely that screening patient samples with panels of antigens may be required. A further hurdle to the use of auto antibodies as biomarkers is the fact that their specificity for MS has mostly been demonstrated in the CSF rather than serum.

15.5.4 microRNAs

In recent years there has been a significant interest in the use of microRNAs as biomarkers in a range of different diseases including MS. MicroRNAs are short non-coding RNA sequences that have the ability to regulate gene expression at the post transcriptional level, where their role is thought to be in the fine tuning of gene expression. The system is complex as over 2000 microRNAs have been identified to date and each of these can potentially regulate hundreds of genes involved in cellular processes. In addition, each mRNA sequence can be regulated by many different microRNAs. Thus analysis of microRNAs can yield important information on the mechanisms of disease as well as being potential biomarkers. MicroRNAs can be analysed in human bodily fluids including blood and CSF, however samples must be collected and stored under carefully controlled conditions as differences in sample processing has been shown to result in highly variable results. MicroRNAs can be analysed by a non-targeted approach using microarrays to analyse a large number of microR-NAs simultaneously, or by a more targeted approach using PCR to detect specific microR-NAs of interest. Overall, 33 different microRNAs have been reported to have altered expression in MS patients. However in many cases there has been a lack of consistency in the results between different studies, which may be accounted for by differences in sample processing or other technical factors. Thus only microRNAs which were shown to be altered in the same direction in more than one study are mentioned below.

Only one analysis of microRNAs expression in CSF from MS patients has been performed thus far. In this study, global microRNA profiling was performed on the CSF of 53 patients with MS and 39 patients with other neurologic diseases (OND), after which candidate microRNAs were validated by quantitative RT-PCR. MiR-922, miR-181c and miR-633 were found to be differentially regulated in patients with MS as compared with OND. Interestingly, miR-181c and miR-633 differentiated RRMS from SPMS disease courses with specificity up to of 82 % and a sensitivity of 69 %. However, while miR-181c was upregulated in CSF in the latter study, it was shown in a different study to be down-regulated in blood. The following microRNAs were found to be down regulated in at least 2 independent studies: MiR-16 was down regulated in B cells and whole blood from MS patients. MiR-20b was down regulated in MS whole blood MiR-140-5p was down regulated in B cells and whole blood from MS patients. Finally, miR-letg7 was down regulated in MS whole blood.

The following micro-RNAs were shown in more than one study to be upregulated in MS patients: MiR-19a was upregulated in Treg cells nd PBMC from MS patients. MiR-22 was upregulated in T cells and blood from MS patients. Interestingly the latter study also identified miR-145 as a biomarker strongly associated with MS in blood, serum and plasma which was consistent with an earlier study that found miR145 to the best single marker in distinguishing MS patients from controls. miR128 was upregulated in blood and naive T cells from MS

patients, with a suggested role in skewing the balance between Th1 and Th2 cells Mir-142-3p was upregulated in blood from MS patients and reduced in response to treatment with glatiramer acetate. MiR-146a was upregulated in blood and T cells from MS patients compared with controls. Mir-155 was upregulated in PBMC from MS patients compared with controls and SNPs in MiR155 were associated with MS. MiR-223 was upregulated in MS blood and Treg cells. MiR-326 has been shown to be upregulated in MS patients in 2 independent studies Interestingly miR-326 was also shown to regulate pathogenic Th17 cells in the EAE model since its knockdown inhibited Th17 cells and ameliorated disease.

Most of the studies above have used relatively small patient cohorts and will need to be independently validated in larger cohorts. In summary, microRNAs may have potential for use as biomarkers in MS but more research needs to be done particularly in terms of standardising assay protocols and validation of results in multiple MS cohorts before they can be used as biomarkers.

15.6 Important Recent Developments

15.6.1 B Cell Targeting

There have been many important clinical and research developments in what has been a fast-paced era of advances in understanding Multiple Sclerosis recently. One of the somewhat surprising outcomes was the clinically efficacy of targeting B cells in RR-MS, surprising in part because some of the common animal models of MS are centrally driven by T cells rather than B cells. This emphasises the need to use animal models appropriately and understand that models such as experimental autoimmune encephalomyelitis (EAE) are a collection of varied models and if a question of B cells is posed, an EAE model of B cell prominence should be utilised.

Clinical trial of Rituximab, a monoclonal antibody to CD20 expressed on B cells, demonstrated impressive reduction in relapse rates in RR-MS

Also encouraging was the fact that anti-CD20 depleted circulating B cells but left pre-B cells and follicle-resident plasmablasts relatively intact. This affords a degree of maintained humoral immunity for patients, thereby reducing the risk of serious adverse infectious events. This striking positive trial outcome prompted follow-on phase II trial with ocrelizumab, a humanised anti-CD20 antibody and Phase III trials for both RR-MS and PP-MS are ongoing. The fascinating aspect of the initial anti-CD20 trial outcome was the fact that the original rationale of targeting B cells in MS, to reduce pathogenic autoantibody production, is not the likely principal mechanism of efficacy. The rapid, almost immediate, reduction in gadolinium-enhancing lesions (indicative of active inflammation) observed is not in line with targeting production of long-lived plasmablasts and immunoglobulins. Much more likely is that effector functions of B cells in active immune responses such as antigen presentation, antigen transfer and co-stimulation of T cell responses are inhibited with depletion of CD20+ cells.

Another interesting aspect of the anti-CD20 targeting trial was the discovery of a small proportion of circulating mature T cells that express low levels of CD20 and would be targeted however it is not yet clear whether depletion of this subset contributes to the observed therapeutic effect in MS. It is important to note when discussing B cells in MS however that some B cell populations such as regulatory B cells (Bregs) exert protective effects by secreting anti-inflammatory cytokines such as IL-10 and promoting regulatory T cells As such targeting B cells in MS must be done selectively, as emphasised by the exacerbation of MS in a trial of atacicept which inhibits B cell growth factor binding.

15.6.2 Genome-Wide Association Studies (GWAS)

Originally, HLA alleles had been identified as possible genetic risk factors for susceptibility to MS in the 1970s. However a series of recent large-scale GWAS studies at multiple sites worldwide brought the number of susceptibility loci first to approximately 60 and most recently to 110. The vast majority of genes identified to date are associated with immune function which has strengthened the argument for a primary immune basis to MS pathogenesis. However, it is important to note that a gene regarded as an 'immune' gene may have a range of other, equally important biological roles in other systems. Over the past four decades the scope of genetic studies have developed to cohorts of tens of thousands of patients in largely unbiased screens.

Genome-wide association studies in MS have been heavily invested in since the development of this technology. Advances in molecular biology, automation, chemistry and affordability have facilitated this work which now occurs through large international collaboration and confirmation. The first GWAS study in MS was reported in 2007 with strong hits identified, and since validated, for genes encoding receptors for two key immune growth factors, IL-2 and IL-7 (IL-2R α and IL-7R α) amongst others. Despite the fact that this study was the first to study thousands of individuals, power was considered limited which informed the design of ensuing GWAS undertakings. The International MS Genetics Consortium (IMSGC) was established to overcome the feasibility and funding challenges of the larger cohorts required to progress GWAS research in MS. This brought together research centres worldwide that through 2 parallel studies collectively identified 56 candidate. In addition to validating previous loci such as HLA, IL-2R and IL-7R, this GWAS identified several candidates that conceptually match to other active research areas in MS. For example, CYP27B1 is a gene identified through this study which is involved in vitamin D metabolism and as discussed earlier, vitamin D deficiency is implicated in epidemiological studies in MS.

Most recently, studies from the IMSGC generated further candidate susceptibility loci bringing the total to 110, again, predominantly immune-associated genes based on an input of over 30,000 individuals. Interestingly, but perhaps not surprisingly, despite this deluge of new knowledge pertaining to genetic susceptibility loci, HLA retains the strongest relationship to disease susceptibility. GWAS research in MS which is not without detractors, has yielded an incredible wealth of data that must now be interrogated for context and relevance to exploit full value of these datasets to understand the genetic basis of MS.

15.6.3 Grey Matter Pathology

Another area that has revolutionised our thinking of MS is the growing field of research into grey matter pathology. Although MS was commonly referred to as a 'white matter disease', it is now widely accepted that lesions also frequently occur in grey matter and indeed, grey matter lesion perhaps make a greater contribution to disease burden and progression in patients.. These advances have arisen from careful neuropathological and imaging studies but it is noteworthy that early descriptions by Charcot in the nineteenth century included observation of grey matter pathology. The focus on white matter pathology was likely due to the technical difficulty in identifying demyelinated lesions in grey matter using classical histochemistry approaches.

Four main types of lesions in cortical grey matter have been classified by location and distribution based on whether lesions span to white matter and/or pial tissue. Grey matter lesions are more prominent in progressive MS than relapsing MS although it is possible that this may reflect enhanced resolution of lesions in grey matter in early disease phases. Grey matter lesions bear some similarity to white matter lesions characterised by myelin and oligodendrocyte loss however differences are clearly apparent also. In general, grey matter lesions tend to be less inflammatory with reduced immune cell infiltration, reduced expression of MHC II, reduced complement deposition and reduced blood-brain-barrier permeability. However, regional meningeal inflammation may be an underlying driver of cortical grey matter lesion development. Post-mortem analysis identified meningeal lymphoid follicles containing B cells associated with more extensive grey matter demyelination and atrophy. Such follicles were reported to occur in >40 % of SP-MS cases studied and associated with increased pace of permanent disability onset. It is likely that such follicles are a source of damaging cytokines, metabolites and pathogenic autoantibodies that act on underlying grey matter. Much remains to be understood about grey matter lesions and subpial lymphoid follicles however given such prominent in progressive MS, and the complete lack of disease-modifying therapies for progressive disease this will likely continue to be a topical area of active research.

15.7 Important Future Developments

The past 20 years has seen outstanding progress in the development of disease-modifying therapies for relapsing-remitting MS (discussed earlier), unprecedented in the field of neurology. Since the advent of the first interferon-beta modality clinicians now have up to ten approved DMTs for MS depending on the country with a choice of delivery routes as well as packed pipelines ready to deliver even safer and more effective treatments. By far, the most pressing therapeutic need in MS now is the development of disease modifying therapies for progressive MS and inhibiting the transition to progression. To date, all RR-MS DMTs have failed in trials of progressive disease, most likely due to the fact that each current agent is immunomodulatory, targeting the pathological activity of the immune system. Achieving disease modification in progressive disease, characterised by reduced or little inflammation, is a challenging goal given the pathological changes that occur with progressive MS but strides are being made toward achieving it.

Neuroprotection and neuroregeneration are two areas that hold great potentiation for inhibiting disease progression. Contrary to previous dogma, the CNS has profound regenerative capacity particularly in the case of regenerating myelin (remyelination). A pool of oligodendrocyte progenitor cells (OPC) persists in the CNS throughout life even into old age. Upon demyelination OPCs migrate to the site of damage, proliferate, differentiate into oligodendrocytes that engage exposed axons and regenerate myelin sheaths (Franklin and Ffrench-Constant 2008).

Regenerated myelin is thinner and has shorter internodes however, this is still sufficient to restore neurological function. Remyelination is extensive in early MS but declines with age and disease progression. Thus, a concerted effort has evolved to develop therapeutics that promote remyelination and clinical trials are underway. Up to 80 % of lesions that fail to remyelinate contain copious undifferentiated OPCs suggesting that the key bottle-neck in failed remyelination is the differentiation of OPCs into functional, myelinating oligodendrocytes. Recent advances in glial biology have uncovered a range of cellular and molecular mechanisms that inhibit or promote oligodendrocyte differentiation and these are now being exploited for therapeutic development. The most advanced therapeutic candidate in terms of clinical trial is anti-LINGO-1 (BIIB033), a monoclonal antibody that binds the protein LINGO-1 – an inhibitor of oligodendrocyte differentiation. Anti-LINGO-1 is currently in Phase II trials for relapsing and progressive MS with results expected in 2016. Another reason that remyelination therapies are sought is recent exciting discoveries that myelin does much more than support axonal electrical conductance. Oligodendrocytes deliver metabolites such as lactate through microchannels in myelin to underlying axons which facilitates local ATP production. This metabolic support is key to limiting axonal vulnerability to degeneration and as such, remyelination therapies hold potential to be neuroprotective. If enhancing myelin repair does indeed change disease course and progression it will be a landmark turning point in the treatment of demyelinating diseases such as MS.

Novel rational clinical trial design, particularly for progressive MS is another area of considerable development. As yet there are no clear, definitive measures of neuroprotection or neuroregeneration which render new trials measuring progression, difficult to assess. Validation of the first neuroregenerative therapy (e.g. remyelination enhancing agent) will with it, bring the first validation of clinically relevant readouts of progression inhibition that will serve as a launch-pad for developing more accurate progressive MS clinical trial endpoints.

Exploitation of genetic insights is another key area of opportunity for future advances. The true value of large GWAS investigations is as yet limited. However, understanding genetic susceptibilities incorporated into pathway analyses may yield strategies to personalise therapies for individual patients. Such assemblies of data may also inform selection of cohorts to monitor in predictive clinical studies.

Animal modelling, though extensive, will continue to develop. New models that more accurately capture the progressive phases of MS are needed. While larger mammals such as non-human primates are employed for some of these studies emerging murine models with progressive phenotypes and pathology will provide a more affordable bridge to clinical development of therapies with ample species-specific research reagents.

Overall the future is brighter for MS patients than ever before. Treatment options are expanding for RR-MS, trials are underway for regenerative therapies and we have a greater understanding of the interplay between genetics and environment that ever before. While much work remains, it is the partnership between patients, clinicians, scientists and associated personnel that make these exciting developments possible.

Suggested Reading

Albert M, Antel J, et al. Extensive cortical remyelination in patients with chronic multiple sclerosis. Brain Pathol. 2007;17(2):129–38.

Bartos A, Fialova L, et al. Antibodies against light neurofilaments in multiple sclerosis patients. Acta Neurol Scand. 2007;116(2):100–7.

Beecham AH, Patsopoulos NA, et al. Analysis of immune-related loci identifies 48 new susceptibility variants for multiple sclerosis. Nat Genet. 2013;45(11):1353–60.

Bo L, Vedeler CA, et al. Intracortical multiple sclerosis lesions are not associated with increased lymphocyte infiltration. Mult Scler. 2003a;9(4):323–31.

Bo L, Vedeler CA, et al. Subpial demyelination in the cerebral cortex of multiple sclerosis patients. J Neuropathol Exp Neurol. 2003b;62(7):723–32.

Calabrese M, Filippi M, et al. Cortical lesions in multiple sclerosis. Nat Rev Neurol. 2010;6(8):438–44.

Charcot JM. Lecture VI. Disseminated sclerosis. Pathological anatomy. Lectures on the diseases of the nervous system. London: The New Sydenham Society; 1887. p. 157–81.

Compston A, Confavreux C, Lassmann H, et al. McAlpines multiple sclerosis. 4th ed. Edinburgh: Elsevier, Churchill Livingston; 2006.

Cheng HH, Yi HS, et al. Plasma processing conditions substantially influence circulating microRNA biomarker levels. PLoS One. 2013;8(6):e64795.

Cox MB, Cairns MJ, et al. MicroRNAs miR-17 and miR-20a inhibit T cell activation genes and are under-expressed in MS whole blood. PLoS One. 2010;5(8):e12132.

Crawford AH, Chambers C, et al. Remyelination: the true regeneration of the central nervous system. J Comp Pathol. 2013;149(2-3):242–54.

Danborg PB, Simonsen AH, et al. The potential of microRNAs as biofluid markers of neurodegenerative diseases – a systematic review. Biomarkers. 2014;19(4): 259–68.

De Santis G, Ferracin M, et al. Altered miRNA expression in T regulatory cells in course of multiple sclerosis. J Neuroimmunol. 2010;226(1-2):165–71.

Du C, Liu C, et al. MicroRNA miR-326 regulates TH-17 differentiation and is associated with the pathogenesis of multiple sclerosis. Nat Immunol. 2009;10(12): 1252–9.

Duncan ID, Brower A, et al. Extensive remyelination of the CNS leads to functional recovery. Proc Natl Acad Sci U S A. 2009;106(16):6832–6.

Ehling R, Lutterotti A, et al. Increased frequencies of serum antibodies to neurofilament light in patients with primary chronic progressive multiple sclerosis. Mult Scler. 2004;10(6):601–6.

Eikelenboom MJ, Petzold A, et al. Multiple sclerosis: neurofilament light chain antibodies are correlated to cerebral atrophy. Neurology. 2003;60(2):219–23.

Fenoglio C, Cantoni C, et al. Expression and genetic analysis of miRNAs involved in CD4+ cell activation in patients with multiple sclerosis. Neurosci Lett. 2011; 504(1):9–12.

Fialova L, Bartos A, et al. Serum and cerebrospinal fluid light neurofilaments and antibodies against them in clinically isolated syndrome and multiple sclerosis. J Neuroimmunol. 2013;262(1-2):113–20.

Fillatreau S, Sweenie CH, et al. B cells regulate autoimmunity by provision of IL-10. Nat Immunol. 2002; 3(10):944–50.

Franklin RJ, Ffrench-Constant C. Remyelination in the CNS: from biology to therapy. Nat Rev Neurosci. 2008;9(11):839–55.

Fraussen J, Claes N, et al. Targets of the humoral autoimmune response in multiple sclerosis. Autoimmun Rev. 2014;13(11):1126–37.

Genain CP, Hauser SL. Experimental allergic encephalomyelitis in the New World monkey Callithrix jacchus. Immunol Rev. 2001;183:159–72.

Gandhi R. miRNA in multiple sclerosis: search for novel biomarkers. Mult Scler. 2015;21:1095–1103.

Guerau-de-Arellano M, Smith KM, et al. Micro-RNA dysregulation in multiple sclerosis favours pro-inflammatory T-cell-mediated autoimmunity. Brain. 2011;134(Pt 12):3578–89.

Hafler DA, Compston A, et al. Risk alleles for multiple sclerosis identified by a genomewide study. N Engl J Med. 2007;357(9):851–62.

Haghikia A, Hellwig K, et al. Regulated microRNAs in the CSF of patients with multiple sclerosis: a case-control study. Neurology. 2012;79(22):2166–70.

Hampton DW, Serio A, et al. Neurodegeneration progresses despite complete elimination of clinical relapses in a mouse model of multiple sclerosis. Acta Neuropathol Commun. 2013;1(1):84.

Hauser SL. The Charcot Lecture | beating MS: a story of B cells, with twists and turns. Mult Scler. 2015;21(1):8–21.

Hauser SL, Waubant E, et al. B-cell depletion with rituximab in relapsing-remitting multiple sclerosis. N Engl J Med. 2008;358(7):676–88.

Hauser SL, Chan JR, Oksenberg JR. Multiple sclerosis: prospects and promise. Ann Neurol. 2013;74(3):317–27. doi:10.1002/ana.24009.

Jersild C, Fog T, et al. Histocompatibility determinants in multiple sclerosis, with special reference to clinical course. Lancet. 1973;2(7840):1221–5.

Kappos L, Hartung HP, et al. Atacicept in multiple sclerosis (ATAMS): a randomised, placebo-controlled, double-blind, phase 2 trial. Lancet Neurol. 2014;13(4):353–63.

Keller A, Leidinger P, et al. Multiple sclerosis: microRNA expression profiles accurately differentiate patients with relapsing-remitting disease from healthy controls. PLoS One. 2009;4(10):e7440.

Khalil M, Enzinger C, et al. CSF neurofilament and N-acetylaspartate related brain changes in clinically isolated syndrome. Mult Scler. 2013;19(4):436–42.

Kidd D, Barkhof F, et al. Cortical lesions in multiple sclerosis. Brain. 1999;122(Pt 1):17–26.

Kuhle J, Leppert D, et al. Neurofilament heavy chain in CSF correlates with relapses and disability in multiple sclerosis. Neurology. 2011;76(14):1206–13.

Kuhle J, Malmestrom C, et al. Neurofilament light and heavy subunits compared as therapeutic biomarkers in multiple sclerosis. Acta Neurol Scand. 2013a;128(6):e33–36.

Kuhle J, Plattner K, et al. A comparative study of CSF neurofilament light and heavy chain protein in MS. Mult Scler. 2013b;19(12):1597–603.

Kuhlmann T, Miron V, et al. Differentiation block of oligodendroglial progenitor cells as a cause for remyelination failure in chronic multiple sclerosis. Brain. 2008;131(Pt 7):1749–58.

Magliozzi R, Howell O, et al. Meningeal B-cell follicles in secondary progressive multiple sclerosis associate with early onset of disease and severe cortical pathology. Brain. 2007;130(Pt 4):1089–104.

Magliozzi R, Howell OW, et al. A Gradient of neuronal loss and meningeal inflammation in multiple sclerosis. Ann Neurol. 2010;68(4):477–93.

Martinelli-Boneschi F, Fenoglio C, et al. MicroRNA and mRNA expression profile screening in multiple sclerosis patients to unravel novel pathogenic steps and identify potential biomarkers. Neurosci Lett. 2012; 508(1):4–8.

Oh J, O'Connor PW. Novel and imminently emerging treatments in relapsing-remitting multiple sclerosis. Curr Opin Neurol. 2015;28(3):230–6.

Palanichamy A, Jahn S, et al. Rituximab efficiently depletes increased CD20-expressing T cells in multiple sclerosis patients. J Immunol. 2014;193(2): 580–6.

Paraboschi EM, Solda G, et al. Genetic association and altered gene expression of mir-155 in multiple sclerosis patients. Int J Mol Sci. 2011;12(12):8695–712.

Patsopoulos NA, Esposito F, et al. Genome-wide meta-analysis identifies novel multiple sclerosis susceptibility loci. Ann Neurol. 2011;70(6):897–912.

Peterson JW, Bo L, et al. Transected neurites, apoptotic neurons, and reduced inflammation in cortical multiple sclerosis lesions. Ann Neurol. 2001;50(3):389–400.

Pryce G, O'Neill JK, et al. Autoimmune tolerance eliminates relapses but fails to halt progression in a model of multiple sclerosis. J Neuroimmunol. 2005;165(1–2):41–52.

Richert ND, Ostuni JL, et al. Serial whole-brain magnetization transfer imaging in patients with relapsing-remitting multiple sclerosis at baseline and during treatment with interferon beta-1b. AJNR Am J Neuroradiol. 1998;19(9):1705–13.

Salzer J, Svenningsson A, et al. Neurofilament light as a prognostic marker in multiple sclerosis. Mult Scler. 2010;16(3):287–92.

Sawcer S, Franklin RJ, Ban M. Multiple sclerosis genetics. Lancet Neurol. 2014;13(7):700–9. doi:10.1016/S1474-4422(14)70041-9. Epub 2014 May 19.

Sawcer S, Hellenthal G, et al. Genetic risk and a primary role for cell-mediated immune mechanisms in multiple sclerosis. Nature. 2011;476(7359):214–9.

Sievers C, Meira M, et al. Altered microRNA expression in B lymphocytes in multiple sclerosis: towards a better understanding of treatment effects. Clin Immunol. 2012;144(1):70–9.

Silber E, Semra YK, et al. Patients with progressive multiple sclerosis have elevated antibodies to neurofilament subunit. Neurology. 2002;58(9):1372–81.

Sondergaard HB, Hesse D, et al. Differential microRNA expression in blood in multiple sclerosis. Mult Scler. 2013;19(14):1849–57.

Srivastava R, Aslam M, et al. Potassium channel KIR4.1 as an immune target in multiple sclerosis. N Engl J Med. 2012;367(2):115–23.

Stys PK, Zamponi GW, van Minnen J, Geurts JJ. Will the real multiple sclerosis please stand up? Nat Rev Neurosci. 2012;13(7):507–14.

t Hart BA, van Meurs M, et al. A new primate model for multiple sclerosis in the common marmoset. Immunol Today. 2000;21(6):290–7.

Teunissen CE, Khalil M. Neurofilaments as biomarkers in multiple sclerosis. Mult Scler. 2012;18(5):552–6.

Villar LM, Picon C, et al. Cerebrospinal fluid immunological biomarkers associated with axonal damage in multiple sclerosis. Eur J Neurol. 2015;22: 1169–75.

Vogt MH, Teunissen CE, et al. Cerebrospinal fluid anti-myelin antibodies are related to magnetic resonance measures of disease activity in multiple sclerosis. J Neurol Neurosurg Psychiatry. 2009;80(10):1110–5.

Waschbisch A, Atiya M, et al. Glatiramer acetate treatment normalizes deregulated microRNA expression in relapsing remitting multiple sclerosis. PLoS One. 2011;6(9):e24604.

Clinical Trials in Neurodegeneration

16

Orla Hardiman, Julie A. Kelly, Thomas H. Bak,
Marwa Elamin, Dragos L. Mihaila, Pamela J. Shaw,
Hiroshi Mitsumoto, and Jeremy M. Shefner

16.1 Introduction

Over the past two decades, there have been significant advances in the management and treatment of many neurodegenerative diseases. For example, the development of cholinergic agonists for Alzheimer's Disease (AD) have improved both functional abilities and quality of life, and newer monoamine oxidase inhibitors and transdermal dopaminergic patches improve function in Parkinsons Disease (PD). A combination of dextromethorphan and quinidine reduce pseudobulbar emotional lability in Amyotrophic Lateral Sclerosis (ALS), and the development of atypical

antipsychotics has improved management of the neuropsychiatric features of neurodegeneration. The use of mechanical devices can also improve function and in some cases prolong survival, for example deep brain stimulation is beneficial in PD, while use of non-invasive ventilatory techniques clearly improves symptoms of respiratory dysfunction in ALS.

However the development of agents that can meaningfully impact disease progression has proved elusive. Indeed, a review of the labeling approved by the FDA for all agents thus far approved for use in PD reveals that none are indicated to impact underlying disease. Similarly in AD, 124 Phase 1 trials, 206 Phase 2 trials, and 83 Phase 3 trials were performed between 2002 and 2012. 36.6 % of these trials were of symptomatic agents aimed at improving cognition, followed by trials of disease-modifying small molecules (35.1 %) and trials of disease-modifying immunotherapies (18 %). The overall success rate

O. Hardiman (✉) • M. Elamin
Academic Unit of Neurology,
Trinity Biomedical Sciences Institute,
Dublin, Ireland
e-mail: orla@hardiman.net

J.A. Kelly
The Academic Unit of Neurology,
Trinity Biomedical Sciences Institute,
Trinity College Dublin,
Dublin, Ireland

T.H. Bak
The Anne Rowling Regenerative Neurology Clinic,
Centre for Clinical Brain Sciences (CCBS),
University of Edinburgh, Edinburgh, UK

D.L. Mihaila
Department of Neurology,
SUNY Upstate Medical University,
Syracuse, NY, USA

P.J. Shaw
Sheffield Institute for Translational Neuroscience
(SITraN), University of Sheffield, Sheffield, UK

H. Mitsumoto
Department of Neurology,
Columbia University Medical Center,
New York, NY, USA

J.M. Shefner
Barrow Neurological Institute,
University of Arizona College of Medicine,
Phoenix, AZ, USA

© Springer International Publishing Switzerland 2016
O. Hardiman, C.P. Doherty (eds.), *Neurodegenerative Disorders: A Clinical Guide*,
DOI 10.1007/978-3-319-23309-3_16

during the 2002–2012 period was 0.4 % (99.6 % failure).

At present, the only disease modifying compound for neurodegenerative conditions is Riluzole, which was found in 1993 to prolong survival in amyotrophic lateral sclerosis (ALS), presumably by impacting rate of disease progression. Riluzole treatment does not appear to affect muscle strength but displays small beneficial effects on bulbar and limb function in ALS patients. Subsequent trials of many agents intended to impact disease progression, particularly in ALS and AD, have failed to show efficacy.

Clearly, there are urgent needs for new effective disease modifying drugs to treat CNS disorders. This is especially critical given that the prevalence of these conditions is set to increase dramatically with ageing world populations (with more than 18 million people estimated in the USA alone to be suffering from Alzheimer's or Parkinson's disease by 2050). Crucially, there are historically high rates of attrition in CNS drug development and translation of CNS drugs has one of the lowest success rates. Most notably, many of the failures only emerge in late stage clinical trials.

Many trials in neurodegeneration have been flawed for reasons other than an ineffective drug. Given gaps in our current knowledge about the etiology and pathophysiology of neurodegenerative disease in general, the acknowledged heterogeneity both of clinical presentation and pathobiology and the pitfalls inherent in clinical trial design, the failure to develop efficacious drugs in neurodegeneration is perhaps unsurprising.

This chapter will explore the models by which new drugs are developed, and analyse the reasons why a high proportion of clinical trials fail to demonstrate drug efficacy despite huge financial investments. Improvements in trial design will be discussed in the context of increased understanding of disease heterogeneity, and the development of new generations of targeted "biologic" therapies with potential for enhanced efficacy in defined subcohorts, but with the likelihood of increased cost to healthcare systems.

16.2 Models of Drug Development

Over the years, drug development has been based on three main approaches: (1) Prior knowledge (2) Serendipity and (3) Targeted drug discovery

16.2.1 Prior Knowledge

Examples of drugs that were developed with prior knowledge include opiates, aspirin, digitalis and belladonna alkaloids. The active agents were extracted and purified from plants based on pre-existing knowledge of efficacy from herbal remedies. In most instances the benefits and side effects of the compounds were known prior to any knowledge of the biologic pathway upon which the active agent operates. Indeed, in some cases the action of the compound provided pharmacodynamics insights ("classical pharmacology") – for example the separation of cholinergic receptors into those responsive to muscarine (derived from *Amanita muscaria*) and those responsive to nicotine (derived from *Nicotiana tabacum),* and the use of opiates in development of our understanding of the endorphin pathways. Typically, compounds developed from prior knowledge were in general use prior to the establishment of rigorous regulatory requirements. Doses and untoward effects have accordingly been well characterized and safety and toxicity profiles established through population-based use over time. While drug development through prior knowledge continues (e.g. cannabinoids may play a role in management of spasticity and pain), the newly developed compounds must now progress through the standard process of regulatory approval, with evidence of drug purity and appropriate evidence of safety and efficacy.

16.2.2 Serendipity

It has been estimated that 263 (18.3 %) of the pharmaceuticals in clinical use today are derivatives of the drugs discovered with the aid of serendipity. In some cases the compound was in use for another indication e.g. sildenafil, in others it was identified in the context of a "prepared mind" e.g. penicillin, or as a chance finding e.g. sodium valproate, which was initially used as a solvent. Serendipitous discovery sometimes occurred in the context of an idiosyncratic or unexpected reaction by a small group of patients to a compound designed for a different target population e.g. clozapine in schizophrenia. For these reasons, some drugs discovered though serendipity in the last century often did not progress through the standards required by current regulatory authorities, and efficacy, untoward effects and toxicity profiles were established in the context of widespread use.

There remains space for serendipitous discovery of beneficial pharmacological effects by ensuring that clinicians are alert to apparently idiosyncratic reactions to compounds. This includes close observation and collection of data about the effects of all drugs administered to patients in a clinical trial setting, and the availability of datasets from clinical trials for post-hoc analyses. An example of this is the use of dextramethorphan and quinidine for pseudobulbar affect. Dextramethorphan was initially tested as a disease modifying drug for ALS, with negative results in clinical trial. However when the trial completed, some patients requested that they continue on drug as they had noticed a positive effect on their symptoms of pseudobulbar affect. Dextramethorphan was then combined in clinical trial with quinidine as Nudextra for pseudobulbar affect with positive outcomes and the drug is now licensed in the US.

Notwithstanding, new drug development is best achieved through rational drug design, perhaps with increased emphasis and greater financial incentives towards discovery of compounds that target novel theories or unexplored mechanisms of action

16.2.3 Targeted Drug Discovery

As the complexities of disease pathogenesis are unravelled, modern drug development has focused on targeted drug discovery. This approach to drug design has largely been inspired by Paul Ehrlich's concept of a 'magic bullet' and the idea that a synthetic molecule or ligand can be designed to target and bind to a specific cellular structure to bring about effective treatment of a particular disease. The process begins with identifying a potential therapeutic target, which may be a protein, DNA or RNA, validating that target and developing an assay such that one can identify molecules i.e. ligands that are capable of binding to the target. Libraries of compounds can then be screened for their ability to bind to the target and modulate its action. From such studies a lead compound may be identified that can be optimized and carried forward through preclinical and clinical development.

Identification of potential ligands may be achieved through rational drug design, where the molecular structure is often based on a natural ligand for the target (especially if the 3D structure of the target is not known), or via high-throughput screening. Pharmaceutical drugs include small molecules, naturally occurring peptides or peptide analogs, nucleotide-based compounds, and more recently "biologics" (agents that are produced by biological processes and often involving recombinant DNA technology).

Molecular properties conferring advantageous absorption, distribution, metabolism and excretion in humans of prospective drug compounds were described in 1997 by the medicinal chemist Christopher Lipinski. These are referred to as the "rule of five" (RO5) and predict that oral bioavailability in humans is favored by the presence of no more than 5 hydrogen bond donors; not more than 10 hydrogen bond acceptors; a molecular mass less than 500 daltons and an octanol-water partition coefficient log P not greater than 5. Many biologically-active peptides and newer "biologics" do not comply with Lipinski's RO5 and thus may potentially be less likely to be suitable for oral administration.

Drug development can be divided into "preclinical" and "clinical" phases with a relatively standard and costly progression of a candidate compound from bench to bedside. Failure rates across all aspects of medicine are high, and

Fig. 16.1 Targeted drug
development in
neurodegenerative diseases

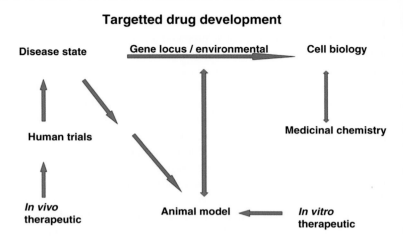

within neuroscience are in the order of 96 % of all candidate compounds in the early pre-clinical phase.

This relates in part to the problems inherent in treating CNS disorders that involve unknown causes, multiple pathological mechanisms and cell types. Indeed, given the complex and multifaceted nature of neurodegenerative conditions, it is likely that agents with multiple potential therapeutic mechanisms may be more effective than a single 'magic bullet' drug that engages a single target. Encouragingly, since several pathological mechanisms are common to a broad range of neurodegenerative disorders, it is conceivable that a drug found to be effective in treating a particular CNS disorder may have application in the treatment of others.

16.3   Pre-Clinical Drug Discovery

Current methods of targeted drug development often use high throughput screening tools including libraries of previously developed small molecules. Potentially efficacious compounds may be identified on the basis of their activity at a biological target that is thought to be important in disease pathogenesis. Assays may evaluate binding affinity, agonist or antagonist actions, and readouts can range from optical probes to gene activation profiles, to changes in protein levels.

Many neurodegenerative diseases are thought to result in similar downstream pathology. The

paucity of specific information about initiating events in many diseases has therefore driven investigation of pathways that lead to neuronal death more generally (Fig. 16.1) (See also Chap. 1). However, as the process of neurodegeneration is complex and poorly understood, appropriate selection of putative pathways of biological and clinical relevance, as well as identification of a specific "read out" from the targeted pathway for biomarker development, remains challenging.

Once identified, candidate compounds are optimized for selectivity and affinity using in vitro models. Subsequently, testing in laboratory animals that model a particular disease is undertaken to establish therapeutic efficacy in vivo.

As a part of the drug development process it is necessary to establish the physicochemical properties of the candidate compound, including its chemical composition, stability, solubility, and the facility by which it can be consistently manufactured with a high degree of purity for use in the clinical trial setting. Preclinical toxicology studies on at least two animal species including one large animal specials is required, with chronic as well as acute dosing being evaluated. Pharmacokinetic studies are also critical, including studies of potentially active metabolites and investigations of potential drug-drug interactions. Regulatory requirements include demonstration that the drug candidate material can be manufactured, stored and delivered according to the highest specifications. The results of such studies provide the basis for submission of an Investigational New Drug (IND) or Clinical Trial Authorization (CTA) application to the appropriate regulatory authority to enable commencement of human clinical trials.

16.3.1 Cellular Based Models

Disease related pathways can be modelled in vitro using cultured cell lines with particular and relevant properties. For example immortalized HEK 293 cells, (derived from human embryonic kidney cells transformed with adenovirus) and the SHSY5Y (derived from human neuroblastoma cells) have many properties of immature neurons and are used for studies of gene expression and protein interactions. Other human cell lines including embryonic teratocarcinomas (NT2, hNT) and human H4 neuroglioma cell lines have been used to study protein misfolding and autophagy.

These immortalised cell lines although useful, are limited to modelling biological pathways that are variably important in both neuronal and non-neuronal structures. For more detailed analysis of specific neuronal functions (e.g. axonal transport), or to evaluate the properties of specific neuronal subpopulations, primary neuronal cultures developed from embryonic animals can be used. As there is now compelling evidence for glial involvement throughout the spectrum of neurodegenerative disease (See Chap. 1), systems that can model neuronal-glial interactions are used such as organotypic slices of brain or spinal cord. These cultures can be generated from both wild type and from transgenic animals expressing alterations in genes associated with neurodegenerative disease.

The advent of stem cell technology, particularly the development of induced pluripotent stem cells, has enabled development of cell lines derived directly from patients. Expansion and differentiation of iPS cells can generate large numbers of functional neurons in vitro, which can then be used to study the disease of the donating patient. iPS systems have been developed from patients with Alzheimer's disease, Parkinson's disease, amyotrophic lateral sclerosis, frontotemporal dementia, Huntington's disease, spinal muscular atrophy and other neurodegenerative diseases. Advancements in reprogramming technology now enable investigators to study patient specific neurons that have been differentiated into specific cell types vulnerable to the disease being studied.

Interpretation the effects of a compound in vitro requires caution, as the information provided relates solely to modulation of specific targeted pathways. Translation to the more complex in vivo *system* is preferable prior to progression of a compound for late pre-clinical and early human studies. Indeed as most neurodegenerations are not cell autonomous, and are most likely due to disruptions at the level of large integrated networks, the extrapolation of findings to the infinitely more complex human system can only be undertaken with extreme caution.

16.3.2 In Vivo Models

Although in vitro models can provide detailed information regarding biochemical pathways, more complex integrated systems are also necessary to dissect the biological effects of candidate compounds. In neurodegenerative diseases, relatively simple organisms can provide an important resource to screen for in vivo modifiers of putative pathogenic processes. Simple organisms such as *Drosophila melanogaster*, *Caenorhabditis elegans* (*C. elegans*) and *zebrafish* have been developed as useful models for AD, PD, ALS, and Huntington's disease. For example, an eye-specific overexpression of human Tau has been developed in *Drosophila melanogaster* that has identified signalling pathways that are dysregulated in models of proteinopathies. Similarly, a range of informative *C. elegans* models of neurodegeneration have been developed manifesting abnormal behavioural or pathological phenotypes that partially recapitulate cellular, molecular and pathological aspects of several distinct human neurodegenerative processes. Zebrafish are useful as vertebrate models. Because they are suitable for large scale phenotypic screening, zebrafish have been used for mutagenesis studies, facilitating both selection of possible new targets, in addition to target validation and large scale drug screening.

Analysis of larger and more complex organisms are also required for pre-clinical drug development. Genetically modified animals with uniform genetic background can provide standardised controlled environments that permit molecular analysis of neurodegenerative pathways.

Transgenic rodents have been developed using human pathogenic mutations including the SOD1 mouse for ALS; AD mouse models including human mutations in amyloid precursor protein (APP) presenilin and tau; PD models including mutations in LRRK2 and HD models containing trinucleotide repeat expansions in huntingtin. To a greater or lesser extent, these models can be shown to imitate diverse neurodegeneration related pathologies, and are used for both basic and therapeutic investigations. A very wide variety of preclinical trials of potential therapeutic agents have been undertaken using these models including over 140 substances in AD between 2001 and 2011, and up to 250 in ALS during the same period.

However, translation of effective therapies in transgenic mouse models to human neurodegenerative disease has been singularly unsuccessful to date. Likely reasons for this failure include issues related to drug availability, lack of information regarding specific targets, and lack of pharmacodynamics markers in either models or humans that reflect adequate target engagement.

16.4   Clinical Phase of Drug Discovery

Following successful completion of the requirements for Investigative New Drug (IND) in the US or a Clinical Trial Authorisation (CTA) in Europe, clinical trials of a lead compound can be initiated.

Clinical trials have been traditionally divided into four main phases i.e. phases I–IV (see

Table 16.1 Standard phases for clinical trials

Clinical trials
Phase 1: safety (controls- unaffected by disease)
Phase 2: proof of concept (small numbers with disease)
Phase 3: pivotal (large numbers, *required for regulatory approval*)
Phase 4: post marketing

Table 16.1). However, Phase 0 first in human microdosing studies may also be undertaken as a means to identify promising candidates for further evaluation in Phase I–II trials. In Phase 0 trials, a small number of healthy volunteers are treated with single sub-therapeutic doses to ensure that pharmacokinetics of the drug in humans recapitulates those of the pre-clinical studies.

Phase 1 Phase 1 studies are conducted either in healthy individuals or in patient populations for whom the drug is being developed. The purpose is to evaluate safety, tolerability, pharmacokinetics and pharmacodynamics, and identification of side effects of the new compound in humans. Depending on the delivery method, a small placebo group may be included to provide information about adverse events not specific to the therapeutic agent. In general, small numbers of patients are exposed to single or multiple doses of the experimental agent, with small doses evaluated first and doses escalating toward a maximum tolerated dose. More recently, the continuous reassessment method (CRM) has been developed, which assigns patient dose levels according to a Bayesian statistical model. CRM models have the dual advantages of potentially reducing the number of patients exposed to drug in Phase 1, and ensuring that patients are dosed at levels more likely to be clinically relevant.

Phase 2 Phase 2 studies are usually placebo controlled and doubled blinded and are conducted in the target patient population. The purpose is dose finding, tolerability and early evidence of activity. Phase 2 trials can also be undertaken to search for better outcomes or to test biomarkers that can be used for more pivotal

Phase 3 studies. While clinical efficacy is evaluated, a primary focus of Phase 2 trials is most often on assessment of pharmacodynamic markers. A pharmacodynamic marker is usually an objective measure of a drug's ability to engage a specific target and to modulate it in some way. Thus, a pharmacodynamic marker may be a change in gene activation profile, evidence of up or down regulation of an enzymatic pathway, or excitation or blocking of a specific receptor. Such markers may not have a direct impact on the disease state being studied; determining whether such a relationship exists is a question for phase 3. Phase 2 studies can be sometimes divided into Phase 2A and Phase 2B, with the former designed for dosing and the latter for PD activity. The majority of new therapeutic agents fail at the Phase 2 stage.

Phase 3 This is the pivotal phase of a new drug and is designed to prove efficacy. The design is double blinded and placebo controlled and takes place in a number of different centres. The drug is administered to larger groups of people to confirm effectiveness and characterize side effects. Comparisons may be against placebo, or best available care. For example, in ALS, the only drug proven to affect disease progression is Riluzole, so that most studies compare patients taking riluzole plus the new agent versus patients taking riluzole alone. Phase 3 trials are generally expensive, costing upwards of €60 million. The outcome of Phase 3 trials are presented to the regulatory authorities for approval of the compound as a new therapeutic agent.

Phase 4 This phase is undertaken post-marketing to generate detailed datasets relating to the effect of the drug on different populations, and to collect side effects following longer term use.

16.5 Clinical Trial Design

Clinical trials are designed with a primary end point, which most often is a measure of drug safety in phase 1, pharmacodynamic activity in phase 2, and efficacy in phase 3. The number of patients recruited is based on power calculations, in which the expected effect of the drug is estimated and the number of patients needed to be treated accordingly calculated to reach a statistically significant threshold. The duration of the trial is generally pre-defined, and following completion of assessment of the final enrolled patient, the database is locked for analysis.

As clinical trials are extremely expensive, and patient recruitment can be challenging, a number of different types of trial design have been proposed, primarily for phase 2 studies (Table 16.2). The goal of a Phase 2 study is not necessarily to produce conclusive evidence of efficacy, and a suggestion of drug activity may be sufficient for a sponsor or investigator to decide that further studies are warranted.

Futility Design One possible approach is to apply what is called a "futility design". Rather than stating that the goal of the study is to show evidence of efficacy or pharmacodynamic activity, the purpose of a futility study is to determine whether it is worthwhile going forward. It may be very important to determine whether further investigation of a drug would be considered unwise either for clear lack of efficacy or for safety. For example, if all treated subjects did worse on all measures than all placebo subjects in a small study, it would be unlikely that the drug would be efficacious if more subjects were studied; ie futility would have been demonstrated. Futility designs require that the traditional null hypothesis used in statistical comparisons be changed; the null hypothesis in a futility study is that it is not futile to go forward. If the null hypothesis is rejected, futility is concluded. Demonstration of non futility requires far fewer subjects than demonstration of efficacy; however, depending on the measure used, non futility may be demonstrated even when two comparison groups are identical.

16.5.1 Pick the Winner Design

Another approach is to use what has been called a "pick the winner" design' to make decisions

Table 16.2 Different types of trial design, aimed at reducing required sample size

Trial designs
Futility
Lead in
Adaptive
Sequential
Combined assessment of function and survival (CAFS) (In Amyotrophic Lateral Sclerosis)

regarding which drug or dose level should be progressed to a phase 3 study. Such designs may or may not involve a placebo group. Some compare several groups that may either be given different doses of the same drug or different drugs over a defined time period. At the end of the study, the best performing group is declared the "winner," and further studies are then performed using that drug or dose and comparing it to placebo in a phase 3 study. The potential advantages of such a design are that many doses or drugs can be tested concurrently; however, there are several limitations. First, there will always be a winner, so that even if chance dictates the best performing group, going forward with further testing will always be the recommended outcome. Second, especially if multiple drugs are compared together, it is possible that in fact more than one active compound is among the agents tested. In that situation, only one drug will be chosen for further testing even though two or more are active and potentially important. A pick the winner design was recently employed in a phase II clinical trial of coenzyme Q in ALS

16.5.2 Crossover Design

Lead-in or crossover designs have also been suggested for phase 2 studies. Crossover studies have not been deemed appropriate for disease modification, as ALS is a progressive disease with clinical features that are likely to vary over time. Thus, a therapeutic agent that is neuroprotective is likely to have a more beneficial effect if given early in the disease than late, so that the effects of therapy after a crossover may not be the same as the effect noted before the crossover. However, for drugs that may exert a symptomatic

benefit, crossover designs can be very efficient. Recent crossover studies in ALS include evaluations of nuedexta for pseudbulbar affect and bulbar function, as well as a phase 2A study of tirasemtiv to improve motor function.

16.5.3 Lead-In Design

Lead-in studies involve enrolling patients into a trial, then following them with assessment of outcome measures for a period of time before starting active treatment. If the outcome measure chosen changes in a linear fashion,

one can estimate the rate of change before active treatment, and use that rate of change as a covariate in the efficacy analysis, potentially reducing the sample size required to detect a given effect. However, most outcomes in neurodegeneration trials do not decline linearly throughout the disease course, so that behaviour before active treatment does always predict the behaviour of that outcome measure later in the study. Lead in designs also require that subjects receive treatment later than other designs, as all subjects have to be followed off treatment for a period of usually 3–6 months. Thus, if a drug is neuroprotective, administration later in the disease course may reduce the sensitivity of the study. For example, a lead-in design was employed in a dose ranging study of TCH346 for ALS, all groups declined more rapidly during active treatment than during lead-in, even the placebo group.

16.5.4 Delayed Start Design

When a drug with a well-known symptomatic effect is studied for putative neuroprotection, providing an adequate washout period may not be practical due to excessive burden on patient, and could lead to an increase in number of patients dropping out during this phase.

To overcome these shortcomings, a delayed-start design can be used in trials when the potential neuroprotective drug is also known to have symptomatic effects. In these trials, after a randomized placebo-control phase, subjects receiving placebo are switched to active treatment (delayed-start group) while the active treatment group continues on the study drug. Both groups are then evaluated after an additional predetermined duration of time. The underlying reasoning is that, to the extent that the active treatment is disease modifying, those receiving it later should experience less benefit than those receiving it earlier.

16.5.5 Historical Controls

Most studies used matched placebo groups with whom to compare the effects of treatments. However, some studies have included historical controls rather than a placebo group in phase II studies. If historical controls are used, the natural history of the rate of change of the outcome measure chosen must be well known, and shown to not significantly change over time or from study to study. For example, in ALS, this is clearly not true for survival studies, as the 1-year survival of ALS patients participating in studies from 1994 to 2007 has varied greatly.

16.5.6 Patient Stratification

There is strong evidence for disease heterogeneity in the neurodegenerative diseases. For example, In ALS, 11 % of those of European extraction carry a repeat expansion in C9orf72, and exhibit a distinctive clinical, imaging and pathologic signature.

Clinical trial design requires appropriate stratification of subphenotypes across treatment and placebo groups. A significant challenge in neurodegenerative disease is to identify the appropriate clinical and genetic markers to facilitate appropriate stratification and to limit the confounding effects of disease heterogeneity.

16.6 Publication of Clinical Trial Data

It is essential that the outcomes of all clinical trials are published in peer reviewed journals in a timely manner, and that data from studies funded by industry are made available in complete format to lead clinical investigators for review prior to publication. Failure to publish negative studies leads to the risk of publication bias, and confounds the existing literature. While this is currently not of concern in the neurodegenerative diseases as there is a current dearth of clinically efficacious compounds, the problems with selective publication of positive findings and suppression of negative studies by failing to publish have been recognized in other disciplines including cardiology and psychiatry.

16.7 Defining Outcomes in Neurodegeneration: Rating Scales and Outcome Measures in Clinical Trials

Clinical trials are designed with an a priori primary outcome measure, with the optional inclusion of secondary and tertiary measures. Power calculations are generally based on the primary measure – usually with knowledge of known rates of decline within a validated disease specific clinical measurement scale.

Depending on the disease and the cardinal symptom associated with the specific neurodegenerative disease, a variety of clinical rating scales and quality of life measures are employed. As the purpose of clinical trials is to obtain regulatory approval of a new therapeutic entity, clinical trial sponsors will often engage with regulatory authorities prior to finalization of the clinical trial design to agree an acceptable primary outcome measure for approval purposes, particularly if the outcome measure is novel.

For example, in PD, several rating scales have been useful. The Hoehn and Yahr scale, developed in the pre-levodopa era, is a five-point simple descriptive scale (stage 1 – unilateral involvement with minimal or no functional impairment; stage 2 – bilateral or midline involvement without impairment of balance; stage 3 – bilateral involvement with impaired righting reflexes, mild to moderate disability and independent physically; stage 4 – severely disabling disease, able to walk and stand unassisted, markedly incapacitated; stage 5 – confinement to bed or chair unless assisted). The scale is a broad assessment of motor dysfunction and its progression has been shown to correlate with other measures of motor deterioration. More recently, the Unified Parkinson Disease Rating Scale (UPDRS) has become the most extensively utilized clinical rating scale to measure the severity of motor impairment and associated disability in PD in clinical practice and clinical research. The UPDRS is organized in four subsections containing both impairment and disability sections: UPDRS 1 Mentation, screening for the presence of cognitive and mood dysfunction; UPDRS 2 ADL addressing primarily but not entirely the disability that results from the motor dysfunction; (UPDRS 3 measuring the motor function; UPDRS 4 assessing complications of therapy). The scale has been shown to have good validity and reliability for the severity and disability of motor symptoms in both early and advanced PD, although a potential ceiling effect of the test to detect changes is suspected. The annual changes in UPDRS scores of patients with early PD enrolled in the placebo arm of randomized controlled intervention trials have been very consistent across multiple studies and shown to be a reliable tool to estimate the natural progression of motor symptoms in untreated PD and change due to pharmacologic intervention.

For ALS, recent trials have employed functional rating scales (either the Appel ALS Rating Scale (AALSRS), the ALS Functional Rating Scale (ALSFRS) or the ALS Functional Rating Scale- Revised (ALSFRS-R), which was originally developed from the UPDRS. In addition, measures of muscle strength (MRC qualitative strength grading or Isometric Strength testing) pulmonary function (primarily vital capacity, but more recently including sniff nasal inspiratory pressure (SNIP) and maximum voluntary ventilation (MVV)), and quality of life measures have been employed as secondary outcomes. All of these involve subject cooperation; effort independent measures including Motor Unit Number Estimation (MUNE) and Electrical Impedance Myography (EIM) have been more recently introduced, also as secondary measures.

For conditions that are rapidly progressive and invariably fatal, survival can be an endpoint that should reflect underlying disease progression, and indeed the single approved ALS therapy impacts survival and is generally presumed to alter underlying disease processes. However, this can be problematic as the increased use of non invasive ventilatory assistance in patients with early respiratory failure likely prolongs survival as well. Additionally, interventions such as nutritional support also likely impact survival, again without a direct disease modifying mechanism.

While outcome measures for clinical trials involving neurodegenerative dementia syndromes are not specified by regulatory bodies such as the FDA, it is recommended that such trials include a combination of cognitive measures and as well as measures of clinical meaningfulness. For example, most AD trials to date have included measures of global function (e.g. the Clinical Dementia Rating or CDR, the Clinicians' Interview-Based Impression of Change or CIBIC), a measure of functioning during everyday activities (e.g. the Alzheimer's Disease Cooperative Study Activities of Daily Living scale or the Disability Assessment for Dementia, DAD), in addition to tests of cognitive function such as the Mini-Mental State Examination (MMSE) or the Alzheimer's Disease Assessment Scale – Cognitive Portion (ADAS-Cog). Some trials have also included economic measures (e.g. resource utilization and cost analyses) and estimates of quality of life. Moreover, as behavioural decline is the most salient symptom in behavioural variant FTD, clinical trials involving this dementia sub-group usually include informant-based behavioural questionnaires (e.g. Neuro-Psychiatric Inventory or NPI, Cambridge Behavioural Inventory or CBI).

One of the major limitations of published dementia trials is the use of crude tests such as the MMSE as the only measure of cognition. This particularly problematic in disorders in which executive dysfunction, which is not assessed by MMSE, play an important role, e.g. FTD. Two strategies can be used to address this problem. One is to combine MMSE with a specific test of frontal function e.g. Trail Making test, verbal fluency, or Frontal Assessment Battery. The other is the use of screening tools which include as assessment of executive function such Montreal Cognitive Assessment (MoCA). An emerging area not previously assessed is the use of tasks social cognitive skills. A recent FTD clinical trial included tests of social cognitive skills (emotional processing and theory of mind) as outcome measure in an attempt to improve sensitivity to subtle changes in this population. The use of such measures might become more common in future trials.

Other criticisms of used outcome measures include lack of standardization of tests used and scoring techniques across trials prohibiting robust meta-analyses.

16.7.1 Biomarkers

In design of clinical trials in the neurodegenerative diseases, the incorporation of a biomarker for both diagnostic purposes, and to provide a "read out" of the likely pharmacodynamic effects of the compound is highly desirable. The National Institutes of Health defines a biomarker as "a characteristic that is objectively measured and evaluated as an indicator of normal biologic processes, pathogenic processes, or pharmacologic responses to a therapeutic intervention" This is such a broad definition as to be not terribly useful. In practical terms, a biomarker usually refers to a potential surrogate endpoint, which is a laboratory value, image, or objective assessment intended to substitute for or predict a clinically relevant outcome, a pharmacodynamic endpoint, which has been defined previously, or a diagnostic test that can be both sensitive and specific for the disease being studied.

The availability of a reliable diagnostic marker could permit early enrollment into clinical trials of homogeneous groups of patients. In AD, Aβ and tau-related biomarkers in CSF are considered reliable for early diagnostic purposes. In PD the most promising tools to probe disease relevant pathways are functional magnetic resonance imaging (fMRI), positron emission tomography (PET) and single-photon emission computed

tomography (SPECT). No reliable diagnostic markers are as yet available for ALS, although diagnostic certainty in clinical practice is higher than for PD or AD, as clinic-pathological concordance in ALS is close to 100 %, and in the order of approximately 80 % for PD and AD.

Surrogate or pharmacodynamic markers have been employed with increasing frequency in neurodegenerative disease, most prominently in Parkinsons Disease. Specific neuroimaging modalities, including multimodal MRI and PET, can contribute to understanding of pathways involved in neurodegeneration, and how these pathways might progressively deteriorate over time. However, when these tools have been applied to clinical trials, results have been quite variable. In some studies of PD, functional imaging studies have suggested benefit where clinical measures have not. For example, Fluorodopa PET was used to study progression of PD in patients treated with ropinirole or levodopa, using the percentage reduction of putamen flurodopa uptake between baseline and 2-year studies as the primary end point and UPDRS as a secondary endpoint. A difference in favor of ropinirole (less significant drop in uptake) was observed. However, the UPDRS showed the opposite effect, with better motor UPDRS scores in levodopa group compared to ropinirole group at 2 years.

In general, markers of drug activity in clinical trials should be predicated on the proposed mechanism of action – for example a drug that purports to reduce oxidative stress should incorporate a markers of oxidative stress in blood (gene expression), plasma or CSF. To date, no effective pharmacodynamic markers have been available for incorporation into clinical trials in ALS. However, surrogate markers, while not completely validated, have been commonly employed, mostly as secondary endpoints. Although not directly clinically relevant, vital capacity and quantitative strength measurements are endpoints that have been used as surrogates for disease status. Motor unit number estimates are a more direct probe of neuronal status, and showed a clear signal in a recent study of olesoxime in spinal muscular atrophy. Another promising marker of changes in muscle structure is electrical impedance myography, which has been shown to be very reproducible and to change monotonically with disease progression. These markers are not specific, and do not query underlying mechanisms. However, to the extent that the variability of measurement is low and change over time is predictable, they may be more sensitive to therapeutic intervention than rating scales or survival. Evidence of change in disease state can be shown using rating scales such as ALSFRS-R, UPDRS and a variety of Alzheimer rating scales. In general these scales are highly reproducible, but their sensitivity to subtle changes in function have been questioned.

16.8   Reasons for Failure of Clinical Trials

With the exception of riluzole in ALS, there have been no trials demonstrating efficacy of disease modifying drugs for neurodegenerative diseases. This is despite many Phase 2 and Phase 3 clinical trials of candidate drugs that had shown efficacy in animal models. While it is likely that lack of efficacy is the primary reason for some drugs, the translational disconnect in CNS drug discovery is also likely to include the limitations of current models, and faulty trial design and interpretation in the clinical phase. Factors potentially undermining efficacy in human clinical trials are differences in the affinity of a particular drug candidate for its target between animals and humans or poor passage of the drug candidate across the blood brain barrier (BBB). Thus, for a candidate compound it is important to establish its affinity for its pharmacological target in human tissue if possible, and its ability to cross the BBB.

16.8.1 Limitations of Current Models

The limitations in the predictive validity of the animal models for CNS disorders has been highlighted by numerous failures in clinical trials of compounds that were robustly active in a variety

of preclinical models. It is now appreciated that in most cases no single animal model can faithfully and fully represent the human condition, especially given the complexities of CNS disorders. Thus, demonstration of efficacy in more than one clinically-relevant model, preferably a non-transgenic and a transgenic model, as well as evidence of disease-relevant mechanism of action, is needed to build confidence in the translation potential of a drug candidate. While the utility of transgenic animals cannot and should not be disputed as models by which pathobiological processes can be dissected and understood, it cannot be assumed that favourable findings of a candidate compound in a single model at pre-clinical level will predict clinical efficacy in humans. This is because transgenic animals are generated using over-expressed human mutations on a homogeneous genetic background. Low copy number transgenic animals have less severe phenotypes, and considerable variation in phenotype can be also demonstrated across diverse genetic murine genetic backgrounds. Some aggressive human mutations, such as the A4V variant in human SOD1 related ALS, do not produce a phenotype in mice. Additionally the human mutations account for a very small proportion of neurodegeneration – for example familial AD accounts for only 5 % of all forms of AD and generally has a younger age of onset and different phenotype to the more typical age-related form of AD. Moreover, the individual animal models of AD do not fully recapitulate the human disease. Similarly, in ALS mutations in SOD1 account for only approximately 2 % of all patients with the disease, and the neuropathologic signature of SOD1 differs from that of other types of familial and sporadic ALS.

A further reason for failure to translate may partly relate to problems in early mouse studies. These include failure to adequately replicate positive findings in a second laboratory and using a different genetic background prior to progression of a candidate compound to clinical studies. Additionally, many of the earlier pre-clinical trials were inadequately powered, and confounded by failure to control for differential effects on gender and copy number variation. Differences in animal husbandry and mouse strain genetic backgrounds can also confound data and lead to potentially erroneous conclusions. A further difficulty has been the use of therapeutic agents prior to symptom onset in animal models, rather than after disease onset, as is the case in human disease.

16.8.2 Failures at Phase 2

There is an evolving recognition that CNS disorders are more likely to due in part imbalances of network, and that targeting single biochemical processes in isolation may not provide sufficient clinical advantage. This may account for some of the failures of Phase 2 trials. However, other problems arising at the level of Phase 2 can include faulty trial design, poor patient stratification due to patient heterogeneity, absence of early diagnostic markers and consequent recruitment to clinical studies later in the stage of disease, incomplete early dosing studies, poor studies of pharmacokinetics, poor access of drugs to the CNS, and absence of adequate pharmacodynamic biomarkers.

16.8.3 Failures at Phase 3

Drugs that succeed at Phase 2 can also fail at Phase 3. Pivotal Phase 3 trials requires large numbers of patients for proof of efficacy and regulatory approval. Errors in trial design are extremely costly. Recent spectacular failures in Phase 3 trials include Dexpramipexole as a disease modifying agent in ALS. The Phase 2 study of this compound demonstrated a strong safety profile, an apparent dose response, and a trend toward efficacy in the primary end point of a combination of survival and attenuation in decline of the ALS-FRS-R. Over 800 patients were enrolled in the Phase 3 study, The was no difference between those treated with active drug and those with placebo in any of the primary or secondary endpoints, and the overall cost of development of Dexpramipexole has been estimated at approximately $100,000,000.

Reasons for failure of the Phase 3 can include over-interpretation of positive trends in efficacy measures from phase 2 studies. Other factors that can contribute to failure of Phase 3 studies include the selection of more than one primary end point; an excessively short study period that does not capture possible longer term benefits of the study drug, and an imbalance of enrolled patients with incorrect stratification parameters.

For compounds that are currently available but not indicated as treatment modalities for neurodegeneration, there is a risk of off-label use by patients, thus potentially confounding the analysis. There is also a risk of interaction with existing drugs, attenuating the effect of the study drug. And as is the case for errors in Phase 2 design, drugs can fail in Phase 3 because of incomplete data regarding pharmacokinetics, poor penetration to the CNS, and the absence of a reliable pharmacodynamics biomarker.

16.9 Lessons from Previous Trials

Despite the disappointing results of clinical trials of disease modifying agents in neurodegeneration to date, much can be learned from negative studies. At a pre-clinical level, animal studies are now conducted in accordance with standardised guidelines. Ideally, such trials should also incorporate a "human RCT" design with clinical pharmacology expertise in trial design and methodology. Positive findings should be replicated in independent laboratories. Negative studies should be published to avoid publication bias.

Findings from animal models should be interpreted at a scientific level, and extrapolation to humans should be undertaken with caution. The validity of pre-clinical studies should be evaluated rigorously by evidence-based analyses, and translation should be undertaken only if findings are robust and reproducible.

As the neurodegenerative disorders are essentially human diseases and may relate in part to failure of complex networks, there is a reasonable case to be made for undertaking proof of concept studies of selected plausible candidate compounds without prior testing in animal models.

In such instances, or in the context of translation from pre-clinical to clinical trials, careful phase I and 2 studies are required prior to moving to more costly and high risk Phase 3 trials. These early trials should include detailed pharmacokinetic studies with extensive dose-finding and toxicity studies. Detailed correlative analysis of drug levels in serum and CSF are necessary and all trials should include a biomarker readout of target engagement.

With respect to clinical cohorts, the heterogeneous nature of the neurodegenerative conditions is well recognized at a clinical level, but has not been adequately addressed in clinical trial settings. Deep phenotyping studies of clinical cohorts, coupled with genetic, and possibly transcriptomic and metabolomics clustering are likely to assist in subcategorization of cohorts in the future. These subcohorts should be randomised accordingly. Pre-specified (a priori), post-hoc analyses should be determined to identify potential responder groups and reasons for study failures, and nested studies should be included in all future designs to obtain maximal information.

16.10 "Biologics", New Drugs and Personalized Medicine

There is strong evidence that neurodegenerative conditions are heterogeneous and it is therefore likely that treatments will be targeted to subcohorts that share pathogenic mechanisms. While the pathobiology of most forms of neurodegeneration remains to be fully elucidated, there is a rich pipeline in new therapeutics that target known mutations and pathogenic pathways. Pre-clinical data using anti-sense oligonucleotides are promising in the treatment of Huntingtons Disease, and early Phase I trials are underway using anti-sense oligonucleotides in SOD1 related ALS. Much as has happened in cancer therapeutics, future treatments are likely to be targeted at specific and biomarkers, personalized to the individual disease subtype. As technologies develop and our understanding of the spectrum of neurodegenerative diseases improves, It is likely that future clinical trials will be in patient subcohorts that have been extensively phenotyped and sub-stratified using genomics, transcriptomics, metabolomics and advanced imaging.

Selected Reading

Ban TA. The role of serendipity in drug discovery. Dialogues Clin Neurosci. 2006;8(3):335–44.

Beach TG. Alzheimer's disease and the "Valley Of Death": not enough guidance from human brain tissue? J Alzheimers Dis. 2013;33 Suppl 1:S219–33. doi:10.3233/JAD-2012-129020. Review. PubMed.

Carlsson CM. Lessons learned from failed and discontinued clinical trials for the treatment of Alzheimer's disease: future directions. J Alzheimers Dis. 2008;15(2):327–38. Review.

Cheung K, Kaufmann P. Efficiency perspectives on adaptive designs in stroke clinical trials. Stroke. 2011;42(10):2990–4.

Cummings J, Morstorf T, Zhong K. Alzheimer's disease drug-development pipeline: few candidates, frequent failures. Alzheimers Res Ther. 2014;6:37.

Ferretti MT, Partridge V, Leon WC, Canneva F, Allard S, Arvanitis DN, Vercauteren F, Houle D, Ducatenzeiler A, Klein WL, Glabe CG, Szyf M, Cuello AC. Transgenic mice as a model of pre-clinical Alzheimer's disease. Curr Alzheimer Res. 2011;8(1):4–23.

Geldenhuys WJ, Van der Schyf CJ. Designing drugs with multi-target activity: the next step in the treatment of neurodegenerative disorders. Expert Opin Drug Discov. 2013;8(2):115–29.

Gladman M, Cudkowicz M, Zinman L. Enhancing clinical trials in neurodegenerative disorders: lessons from amyotrophic lateral sclerosis. Curr Opin Neurol. 2012;25(6):735–42.

Goldacre B. Bad Pharma Harper Collins. 2012. pp 172–224.

Höglund K, Salter H. Molecular biomarkers of neurodegeneration. Expert Rev Mol Diagn. 2013;13(8):845–61.

Li C, Ebrahimia A, Hermann S. Drug pipeline in neurodegeneration based on transgenic mice models of Alzheimer's disease. Ageing Res Rev. 2013;12:116–40.

Mitsumoto H, Brooks BR, Silani V. Clinical trials in amyotrophic lateral sclerosis: why so many negative trials and how can trials be improved? Lancet Neurol. 2014;13:1127–38.

Nicholson KA, Cudkowicz ME, Berry JD. Clinical trial designs in amyotrophic lateral sclerosis: does one design fit all? Neurotherapeutics. 2015;12(2):376–83. PubMed PMID: 25700798.

Palesch YY, Tilley BC, Sackett DL, et al. Applying a phase II futility study design to therapeutic stroke trials. Stroke. 2005;36:2410–4.

Pollastri MP. Overview on the rule of five. Curr Protoc Pharmacol. 2010;Chapter 9:Unit 9.12.

Schapira AH, Olanow CW, Greenamyre JT, Bezard E. Slowing of neurodegeneration in Parkinson's disease and Huntington's disease: future therapeutic perspectives. Lancet. 2014;384(9942):545–55.

Schneider LS, Mangialasche F, Andreasen N, Feldman H, Giacobini E, Jones R, Mantua V, Mecocci P, Pani L, Winblad B, Kivipelto M. Clinical trials and late-stage drug development for Alzheimer's disease: an appraisal from 1984 to 2014. J Intern Med. 2014; 275(3):251–83.

Southwell AL, Skotte NH, Bennett CF, Hayden MR. Antisense oligonucleotide therapeutics for inherited neurodegenerative diseases. Trends Mol Med. 2012;18(11):634–43.

Palliative Care and End of Life Care

17

David Oliver, Sinead Maguire, Orla Hardiman, and Peter Bede

17.1 Introduction

End of life care relies heavily on a dynamic partnership between the patient, carers and the multidisciplinary palliative care team. Palliative care provides symptomatic management of late stage conditions focussing on relief of suffering, dignity and respect for patient autonomy, regardless of the underlying diagnosis. .

In addition to medical management, palliative care seeks to address individual psychological, social and spiritual needs. While specialist palliative care has been traditionally associated with the symptomatic management of advanced neoplastic disorders, in recent years palliative care has gradually expanded into the management of progressive non-malignant conditions such as neurodegenerative conditions, chronic obstructive pulmonary disease, HIV, renal and cardiac failure.

In the absence of effective disease modifying therapies in most neurodegenerative conditions, specialist palliative care has a major role in improving the quality of life of patients. The effectiveness of palliative care intervention has been demonstrated by multiple studies in progressive neurological conditions.

17.2 The Definition of Palliative Care

Palliative care is defined by the WHO as "an approach that improves the quality of life of patients and their families facing problems associated with life-threatening illness, through the prevention and relief of suffering, early identification and impeccable assessment and treatment of pain and other problems, physical, psychosocial and spiritual".

This definition has been expanded to include, that palliative care:

- Provides relief from pain and other distressing symptoms
- Affirms life and regards dying as a normal process
- Intends neither to hasten or postpone death
- Integrates the psychological and spiritual aspects of patient care
- Offers a support system to help patients live as actively as possible until death
- Offers a support system to help the family cope during the patient's illness and in their bereavement

D. Oliver
Wisdom Hospice, Consultant in Palliative Medicine, High Bank, Rochester, UK

University of Kent, Kent, UK

S. Maguire • O. Hardiman • P. Bede (✉)
Academic Unit of Neurology,
Trinity Biomedical Sciences Institute,
Dublin, Ireland
e-mail: orla@hardiman.net

© Springer International Publishing Switzerland 2016
O. Hardiman, C.P. Doherty (eds.), *Neurodegenerative Disorders: A Clinical Guide*,
DOI 10.1007/978-3-319-23309-3_17

Fig. 17.1 The multidisciplinary team in neurodegeneration. Evidence suggest improved quality of life as well as survival benefit if patients are cared for by an integrated multidisciplinary team (Rooney et al. 2014)

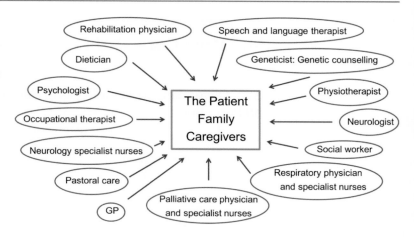

- Uses a team approach to address the needs of patients and their families, including bereavement counselling
- Will enhance quality of life, and may also positively influence the course of illness
- Is applicable early in the course of illness, in conjunction with other therapies that are to prolong life, such as chemotherapy or radiation therapy, and includes those investigations to better understand and manage distressing clinical complications.

17.3 The Definition of End of Life Care

End of life care is more complex to define and there is often uncertainty. This period is often considered to be the last 6–12 months of life, when there is increasing deterioration and the prospect of recovery has been abandoned. Within neurology there is increasing awareness of the need to consider both palliative and end of life care in patients with progressive disuse. This has been emphasised in the various guidelines on the care of people with neurological disease – including the Practice Parameters from the American Association for Neurology, the European Federation of Neurological Societies Guidelines on ALS (Andersen et al. 2012).

17.4 Palliative Care in Neurology

There is considerable evidence that palliative care intervention is beneficial in neurological conditions. A randomised controlled trial in multiple sclerosis, using a waiting list delayed service protocol, demonstrated superior symptom management, in particular nausea, as well as improved patient and caregiver satisfaction. Using a similar randomised waiting list for patients with ALS/MND, MS, progressive supranuclear palsy (PSP) and Parkinson's disease (PD), improvement in a variety of symptoms – pain, breathlessness, sleep disturbance and bowel symptoms- and overall quality of life was observed.

Thus there is robust evidence that palliative care may help people with progressive neurological conditions and that this will extend to end of life care. It is also recognised that multidisciplinary care for people with progressive neurodegenerative conditions enhances quality of life (Van den Berg et al. 2005; Rooney et al. 2014) (Fig. 17.1).

Given the complex nature of the illness, with inexorable decline and death as the inevitable outcome, a significant proportion of evidence of palliative care intervention in neurology comes from ALS/MND. It has been elegantly demonstrated by several authors that overall quality of life is not directly dependent on physical function (Neudert et al. 2004; Simmons et al. 2000). In fact, health

Table 17.1 International frameworks for palliative care in neurology

Palliative care initiatives for non malignant conditions			
Name of the program	Country	Year	Focus
Gold Standards Framework	UK	2000	Community based service, Carer Support
PEACE – Palliative Excellence in Alzheimer's Care Efforts	US	2003	Patients with dementia, Advance planning, Death at desired location
Liverpool Care Pathway (Version 12)	UK	2009	Holistic approach to physical, psychological, social and spiritual care
Preferred Priorities for Care	UK	2004	Discussion and respect of patient preferences
Neurological Care Pathway	UK	2007	Management algorithm with indicators to advance care planning and specialist palliative care referral
Neurology Taskforce of the EAPC	EU	2009	Palliative Guidelines for ALS, HD, AD, PD
Guidelines for a Palliative approach in Residential Aged Care	Australia	2006	Evidence based palliative guidelines for elderly patients in residential units
Respecting Patient Choices Program	Australia	2005	A comprehensive advance care planning program
My Home Life	UK	2007	Support for staff working in care homes

related quality of life is only a minor contributor to overall quality of life. This provides an important rationale for specialist palliative care intervention in neurological conditions. Indeed, with the expansion of specialist palliative care provision to non-malignant conditions, a number of national frameworks have recently been developed to enable the optimal timing of palliative intervention and coordination of care between primary care physicians, neurologists, the multidisciplinary team, and palliative care specialists (Table 17.1).

17.5 Aims of Palliative Care

Palliative care aims to carefully address to physical, psychological, social, and spiritual needs of patients in an integrative approach.

17.5.1 Physical

These aspects of care involve consideration of

- Symptoms – such as pain, dyspnoea, dysphagia, communication issues
- Mobility and comfort issues

- Positioning and provision of help to aid daily living – small aids to help with limb/arm weakness, mobility aids such as frames and wheelchairs, and adaptions to housing and work environment

17.5.2 Psychological

This aspect of palliative care monitors reactions to the diagnosis, disability, dependency and dying and attempts to foresee and address psychological distress, such as anxiety, depression.

17.5.3 Social

Most patients will be part of local communities or wider social circles – whether family, friends or carers (both informal and professional). It is important to recognize and evaluate the personal reaction to the disease process.

17.5.4 Spiritual

Existential questions and spirituality are unique aspects of palliative care which require attentive consideration of individual cultural and religious needs. In a multi-cultural society an open-minded, empathetic, and sensitive approach is needed to address individual existential concerns about the deeper issues of life. There may be concerns about the meaning of life, about facing the changes that may occur with progressive disease, and about specific religious issues. Pastoral care or the involvement of the patients own support group, religious or otherwise, can be highly beneficial in reducing anxiety and improve quality of life.

17.5.4.1 Assessment Scales

Underreporting of pain and discomfort and inability to recall symptoms is a well-known problem of treating patients with long term conditions and in particular for those with impaired cognition. A comprehensive assessment and review of symptoms is the initial step following referral to specialist palliative services. It is clear the generic quality of life (QoL) instruments such as the Sickness Impact Profile(SIP), SF-36 Health Survey, or EuroQol EQ-5D are not directly applicable to neurological conditions. Disease specific instruments are superior in neurodegeneration, such as individualized QoL scales based on patients own QoL priorities, instruments optimised for patients with cognitive impairment or dementia, visual analogue scales or observer rated instruments taking the caregivers perspective into account. A number of validated tools are available for QoL evaluation in neurology. Some of them had been optimised for elderly people and have a role in neuropalliative assessments. Validated assessment scales also enable the measurement of the efficacy of palliative interventions.

The **Memorial Symptom Assessment Scale (MSAS)** is a scale used to assess 32 physical and psychological symptoms in three different dimensions: intensity, frequency, and distress.

The **Rotterdam Symptom Checklist (RSCL)** is another tool that measures both psychological and physical aspects of quality of life. These instruments, despite being recognised as highly sensitive, are too lengthy to be administered routinely in progressive neurological conditions.

The **Edmonton Symptom Assessment Scale (ESAS)** is patient-rated symptom visual analogue scale that may be particularly useful in patients with neurodegeneration. It is based on the assessment of 15 domains; activity, fatigue, physical discomfort, dyspnoea, pain, lack of well-being, appetite, depression, anxiety, nausea, difficulty sleeping, weakness, dizziness, cognition, and constipation.

The **Disability Distress Assessment Tool** (DisDAT, Regnard et al.) was developed in 2001 to identify distress in people with severe communication difficulties. The assessment tool uses a so-called "Distress Passport" a summary of signs and behaviours when patient is content and when distressed. Assessment takes Appearance, Vocal signs, Habits, Mannerisms and Posture into consideration.

Additionally, a number disease-specific of Quality of life assessment tools have been developed and used both in clinical practice and in the assessment of palliative interventions (Table 17.2).

17.6 The Timing and Triggers of Palliative Care Interventions

More recently a Consensus document produced by the European Association for Palliative Care (EAPC) and the European Federation of Neurological Societies (EFNS)/European Academy of Neurology (EAN) has recommended that: "Palliative care should be considered early in the disease trajectory, depending on the underlying diagnosis" (Oliver 2014).

This is based on the evidence that for cancer care the earlier involvement of palliative care can increase survival of patients with lung cancer, reduces the cost of hospital care (Bakitas et al. 2009) and may improve symptom management and family satisfaction.

The initiation of specialist palliative care involvement will depend on the specific disease process – with involvement for patient with ALS/MND suggested from the time of diagnosis in many cases (Bede et al. 2011; Oliver 2014) whereas in MS involvement may only towards the end of life. In traditional care

Table 17.2 A selection of Quality of Life assessment instruments in neurodegenerative conditions

Alzheimer's Disease-Related Quality of Life – ADRQL	Optimised for AD, 47 items in 5 domains: Social Interaction, Awareness of Self, Feelings and Mood, Enjoyment of Activities, Response to Surroundings
The Cornell-Brown Scale for Quality of Life in Dementia – CBS	Incorporation of caregivers perspective
Dementia Care Mapping -DCM	Observational assessment tool developed to be used in residential care for patients with moderate to severe disability
Parkinson's Disease Quality of Life – PDQL questionnaire	37 item questionnaire; four subscales: parkinsonian symptoms, systemic symptoms, emotional functioning, and social functioning
Quality of Life in Late-Stage Dementia -QUALID Scale	Observational scale for late stage dementia, brief, used in residential care
Psychological Well-Being in Cognitively Impaired Persons PWB-CIP	11 item, observer rated assessment instrument
Dementia Quality of Life questionnaire D-QOL	29 item scale in 5 domains: Positive Affect, Negative Affect, Feelings of Belonging, Self-esteem, Sense of Aesthetics
Quality of Life-Alzheimer's Disease (QOL-AD)	Composite scores from patient and caregiver responses on a 13 item scale
Schedule for the Evaluation of Individualized Quality of Life-Direct Weighting SEIQoL-DW	A brief instrument used extensively in ALS research. Respondents identify the areas of life which are most important to their QoL, then rate their level of functioning or satisfaction with each.
McGill QoL Questionnaire – MQOL	A 20 item scale frequently used in ALS, 5 domains: physical well-being, physical symptoms, existential well-being, psychological symptoms and support

models, palliative input is sought at the relatively later stages of a progressive condition, resulting in patients potentially missing out on the expertise of palliative physicians in controlling distressing symptoms. More flexible models advocate early, and episodic involvement based on specific triggers – for instance for a person with ALS/MND this may be at diagnosis, consideration of gastrostomy, consideration and commencement of ventilatory support and in the final stages of life. The model of intermittent, symptom-based involvement has been proposed in neurodegenerative conditions where palliative involvement may overlap with active neurological care (Fig. 17.2).

17.7 Specific Symptoms Requiring Specialist Palliative Input

While the underlying pathophysiology may be different in various neurodegenerative conditions, there are a number of symptoms that may be common to most progressive neurological diseases.

17.7.1 Pain

Many patients will experience pain during the course of the disease progression – varying from 76 % for ALS/MND, 86 % in MS, and 85 % in PD. The aetiology of pain may be different in these conditions and should be managed accordingly:

Musculoskeletal pain – due to abnormal tone around joints which may respond to physiotherapy, positioning and non-steroidal anti-inflammatory medication.

Muscle spasm from increased tone, such as in primary lateral sclerosis, which may be helped by physiotherapy, positioning or muscle relaxant medication such as baclofen or tizanidine.

Skin pressure pain, due to immobility, particularly in ALS/MND where there is normal sensation may require regular analgesics, starting at

A, A traditional model of late involvement of specialist palliative services

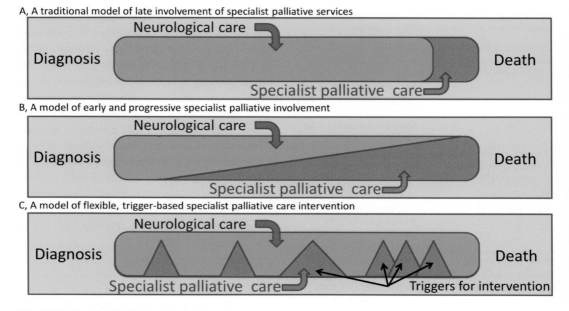

Fig. 17.2 Models of palliative care intervenetion in neurology

simple analgesics but opioids may be necessary. These may need to be given transcutaneously or subcutaneously if swallowing is poor or at the end of life.

If there is cognitive change and dementia, the assessment of pain may be more challenging. Caregivers who know the patient well may be in a better position to judge requirement for analgesia in this situation, as well as assessing the response to pain medications. A number of instruments have been developed to assess pain in cognitive impairment., there may be particularly helpful in these circumstances.

17.7.2 Dyspnoea

Dyspnoea may occur in any progressive neurological disease and may be related to poor posture, immobility, diaphragmatic weakness or due to infection. Aspiration pneumonia and infections are common in patients with dysphagia and should be treated with antibiotics when appropriate

ALS/MND leads to increasing respiratory muscle weakness. This may cause progressive breathlessness. Initial symptoms may present with orthopnea when lying down, disordered

sleep, vivid dreams, multiple arousals through the night, morning fatigue and headache and more general symptoms such as anorexia, fatigue, and even cognitive change. Regular assessment of respiratory function is therefore essential in ALS and if there is evidence of respiratory muscle weakness more detailed respiratory assessment is necessary. Early morning ABGs, sniff nasal inspiratory pressure (SNIP) and overnight pulse-oxymetry are the most commonly used respiratory instruments in ALS. Non-invasive ventilation has been shown to both improve the quality of life, and survival. However, the disease continues to progress and some patients may wish to withdraw NIV as they become increasingly dependent and eventually totally NIV dependent. Although this is a clear ethical choice for someone with capacity, or who has expressed their wishes clearly before loss of capacity, there are many practical issues to cope with. There are specific guidelines on the withdrawal of NIV but there is evidence that the all involved – patient, family and professionals – find the process very stressful (Faull et al. 2014; Oliver and Tumer 2010).

Rarely, patients with ALS/MND may undergo tracheostomy and invasive ventilation.

This may increase the stress on all involved, particularly the carers (Oliver and Tumer 2010; Veronese et al. 2014). It is possible to maintain life with a tracheostomy and gastrostomy but with increasing dependency and at the risk of becoming "locked in" with no voluntary movement or communication. The withdrawal of ventilation is again a complex and difficult decision but may become necessary, at the request of the patient.

Breathlessness may be effectively eased by physiotherapy. Positioning, and newer techniques such as "cough-assist" machines and "Breath stacking" technique proved particularly effective both for symptomatic relief and in enhancing quality of life. The education of patients and their family members on these techniques have become an important part of integrated multidisciplinary clinics. Support of both patient and carers is essential, as breathlessness leads to anxiety, which may worsen the symptom. Opioids have been found to be helpful although there is a limited evidence base. Benzodiazepines can be helpful, particularly reducing the concomitant anxiety.

17.7.3 Dysphagia

Swallowing may be affected in most neurodegenerative conditions and careful assessment by a speech and language therapist is helpful. Specific issues may be helped by positioning, modification or fortification of diet, education and support of carers who provide food or help with feeding. Food supplements may be tolerated more easily but palatability must be considered and it is important to allow patients to be involved in the social aspects of eating.

If swallowing becomes more difficult, and nutrition is compromised, with an increased risk of aspiration, consideration of enteral feeding may be necessary. This should involve a wider multidisciplinary assessment, to ensure that respiratory function and other factors, such as cognition are carefully considered. Various forms of gastrostomy, such as percutaneous endoscopic gastrostomy (PEG), radiologically

inserted gastrostomy (IRG) or per-oral radiologically inserted gastrostomy (PIG) may allow medication to be continued until the end of life and allow continued hydration even if the patient cannot swallow at all. There is evidence in ALS/MND that the use of a gastrostomy may improve quality of life, by reducing the risks and stress around oral feeding with compromised swallowing, but the evidence for improved survival remains poor. On occasions, a nasogastric tube may be passed as a short term intervention – this may be helpful in PD as it allows medication to be continued even in the final stages of life.

17.7.4 Sialorrhoea

As swallowing becomes gradually affected, drooling of saliva becomes increasingly problematic, as the normal daily saliva production of 1–1.5 l cannot be swallowed effectively. This is common in ALS/MND – 50–70 % – and in PD – 65 % and may have significant impact on the quality of life of patients. An assessment by a speech and language therapist is helpful and ensuring that the person has good oral hygiene and an upright position may help. In PD there is evidence that swallowing frequency is reduced and it has been suggested that a metronome may help remind people to swallow. The use of suction can be helpful on occasions, but the continual use of suction may cause an increased saliva production and be counterproductive.

A number of pharmaceutical options exist to control sialorrhoea effectively. Transdermal hyoscine (scopolamine) patch, sublingual hyoscine hydrobromide, PO glycopyrrolate or tricyclic antidepressant may all be beneficial depending on the co-existing symptoms and preferred route of administration. Alternatively, Botulinum toxin injection into the salivary glands or in selected cases salivary gland irradiation may also be considered. At the end of life a continuous subcutaneous infusion of gycopyrrolate or hyoscine hydrobromide may be helpful.

17.7.5 Dysarthria

Speech may be directly affected by weakness, incoordination or spasticity of the muscles involved in speech, or indirectly by fatigue, respiratory weakness, or medications . Hypophonia is a common symptom of Parkinson's disease and speech is invariably affected by movement disorders. Depending on the phenotype up to 77 % of ALS/MND patients and 69 % of PD patients experience dysarthria.

Speech and communication are essential components of quality of life especially in the presence of significant physical disability. Therefore careful multidisciplinary assessment, including in particular the speech and language therapist, is important. In certain neurodegenerative conditions, such as ALS or PD, extra time is often needed for the person to express their thoughts and wishes and careful listening is essential. Augmentative communication devices may be important, such as voice amplifiers, alphabet boards, laptops or touch sensitive devices such as tablets or smart-phones. In some cases, more sophisticated equipment, such as eye gaze systems are required to enable communication when other movements are restricted or unreliable. Augmentative systems should be able to be used not only for day to day communication but increasingly for the internet and email. However, some individuals may prefer simpler systems, such as pad and paper or a simple board with representation of basic needs.

17.7.6 Fatigue

Fatigue is commonly described by people with progressive neurological disease – for instance in MS reports suggest fatigue affecting 39–78 % of patients. The cause may be caused directly by the disease itself, or indirectly by disease progression, such as respiratory failure in ALS/MND, medications, depression, or anaemia. It is crucial to explore potential causative factors and address them appropriately as fatigue has a major impact on quality of life. Treatment of depression or revision of medications, such as reducing

benzodiazepines or opiates may be needed. In PD the optimisation of dopaminergic medication can be helpful and in MS explanation of pacing and making the most of available energy can enable patients to remain more active. Finally, modafinil has been off-label in some health system in Multiple Sclerosis and Parkinson's disease.

17.7.7 Sleep Disorders

Sleep disturbance may be affected directly by the disease process. REM sleep behaviour disorder in multiple systems atrophy (MSA) and PD may manifest with dreams and extreme limb movements at night and may be helped by clonazepam.

Additionally, sleep in MSA may be affected by stridor due to vocal cord dysfunction. These symptoms can be helped by non-invasive ventilation and (NIV) or continuous positive airway pressure (CPAP). Restless legs syndrome (RLS) is a common complaint across the spectrum of neurodegenerative disorders. The irresistible urge to move the limbs, with only temporary relief from moving them may cause significant discomfort. Oral iron supplementation should be considered if low ferritin levels are demonstrated. Dopamine agonists, such as Pramipexole, Ropinirole, or Rotigotine taken 2 h before bedtime are often the first line of therapy. Pregabalin and gabapentin have also been used successfully. Poor sleep may be a symptom of respiratory failure due to respiratory muscle weakness in ALS/MND.

Sleep may be affected indirectly by pain, depression or anxiety – such as anxiety about calling for help due to poor speech and generalised weakness.

General advice on sleep hygiene, such as regular rituals before going to bed, avoiding day time naps and ensuring the environment is favourable for sleep, is important for all patients.

17.7.8 Mobility

Most people with progressive neurological disease face changes in mobility due progressive pyramidal, extrapyramidal and cerebellar dysfunction.

This may be difficulties in initiation of movement, such as in PD, or increasing limb weakness in MS and ALS/MND reducing the ability to walk safely. There are increased risks of falling, and possible fracture, and loss of independence, ranging from problems in feeding, toileting or getting around in their home environment. There are often concomitant psychological sequelae, such as isolation, fear, loss of confidence and loss of purpose and meaning in life.

A multidisciplinary assessment is essential, including particularly the physiotherapist and occupational therapist, but often including the wider team. There is often resistance to the use of aids, from sticks and frames to wheelchairs. It may be necessary to encourage the patient, family and carers to use these aids that may improve their quality of life by maintaining their independence and prevent falls. It is important that there is clear explanation and education in the use of any equipment so that is it used correctly and safely. If at all possible, equipment should be able to be adapted as the disease progresses, so that it can be used as the person's abilities deteriorate and the stress of having to cope with new equipment is minimised.

17.7.9 Other Physical Issues

There are many symptoms that are unique to a specific disease process. For instance, in PD dyskinesia and rigidity may become a major physical problem and require optimisation of medication and, on occasions, more invasive treatment such as deep brain stimulation. There is a need for close collaboration between all teams involved – neurology, rehabilitation and palliative care – to ensure that all treatments regimes are maximised, avoiding treatment related side effects, and appropriate to the patient's needs and wishes.

17.7.10 Psychological Issues

Patients with neurodegenerative conditions face an ever evolving constellation of symptoms. Patients frequently perceive their disease as a series of losses – from loss of mobility, to loss of speech or swallowing, loss of cognition – leading to changes in their relationships. Fear and anxiety Fear and existential distress are two of the most important psychological stressors in neurodegeneration. Fear of the disease itself, as this may be a new diagnosis with which the person has never had contact before and there are often myths of the disease which can lead to fear and anxiety – for instance many people with ALS/MND fear choking to death, but with good symptom management this is extremely rare.

Fear of deterioration and dependency. Many people are very concerned about becoming dependent to others for their care – particularly very personal care such as bathing, toileting or feeding.

Fears of dying and death. These may be very different as some people may fear the process of dying – fearing choking, breathlessness, pain or a distressing death – whereas others may fear death itself – of oblivion or of heaven/hell (see Spiritual issues below).

Fear of loss of control over activity and day to day living. This is related to dependency but is often used as a reason for considering assisted dying. In Oregon 75 % of the people asking for physician assisted suicide speak of their fear of loss of control over their lives and seek control over their death (Ganzini et al. 2002). Fear of loss of identity – particularly for people facing cognitive loss and dementia, such as in PD and often in MS and ALS/MND.

17.7.11 Cognitive Change

Cognitive change may vary from subtle impairment in selected functions through multi-domain impairment to dementia. The most commonly assessed cognitive domains include memory, executive function, language, visuospatial skills and social cognition. Behavioural change is often more distressing for the caregivers than selected cognitive impairment and may cause considerable distress until a formal diagnosis is established. Deficits in all of these domains are very distressing for both the patient and family and have implications on the management of the condition, adherence to therapy, safety awareness, decision making, formulating care preferences and making end-of-life decisions. Cognitive change is a feature of most neurodegenerative conditions.

In multiple sclerosis up to 65 % of patients have evidence of impairment, often problems in learning new facts, altered information processing and verbal fluency. In 25 % of patients the cognitive change may be very obvious whereas in others the changes may be more subtle and only found on careful neuropsychological assessment.

Fifteen percent of patients with ALS/MND have fronto-temporal dementia. Frontotemporal dysfunction may precede motor symptoms, which may lead to misdiagnoses. Up to 50 % of ALS patients have evidence of cognitive change – often impaired executive function, language deficits or behavioural changes .

PD patients may have problems with executive functioning, difficulties in planning, apathy and hallucinations. Up to 30 % develop dementia, with memory and attention problems.

PSP may have changes leading to forgetfulness and slowing of information processing and executive dysfunction may occur later in the disease progression

Huntington's Disease (HD) is associated with cognitive decline, including executive dysfunction, problems initiating and organising thoughts. Behavioural changes such as aggression, impulsivity, distractibility are also commonly observed.

All of these changes impact on management as the patient may be less able to make decisions and may need to be helped and supported "in their best interest". For instance, it may be necessary to make decisions for the person, in consultation with their family and carers, and even restrict their liberty and activities if these could lead to harm. Removing the car or house keys are frequently considered in these patient cohorts, so that they are not able to drive or leave the house when this may be a risk to themselves and others. This can lead to disagreements and conflict not only with the patient, but within families and professional caring teams.

17.7.12 Social Issues

Most patients identify closely with their communities and wider families. These people may have similar concerns about the disease progression, such as fears of the disease, progressive dependency and of dying and death. The patient's social circles and family experience similar series of losses, shifting of roles and relationships as the disease progresses. Cognitive impairment may lead to a spouse losing the partner with whom they could previously share their experiences and feelings. Caring for a person with behavioural or cognitive impairment leads to considerable additional emotional strain.

There may be additional social stressors, such as financial concerns. The patient may need to give up employment because of disease progression but the partner, and sometimes other family members, may need to stop work in order to care for them. This may lead to severe financial difficulties and advice and support in ensuring that they claim the necessary benefits and entitlements is paramount. There is frequently need for house adaptions, such as the installation of a stair lift, wheel chair ramps, downstairs bathrooms or other specialist equipment for lifting, transfers or hygiene. There is often a sudden need to organise additional home help. . These issues need to be anticipated in advance, carefully planned for, the appropriate applications and supporting documents need to be provided on time in order to address these pertinent social issues.

Most multidisciplinary neurology teams work with an experienced social worker which is of considerable benefit in addressing these problems. Often with severe progression admission for temporary respite care or longer term residential care may be necessary and this also need to be anticipated and organised effectively.

The involvement of children and young people in the patient's care can be a difficult and sometimes disheartening experience. It is important to ensure that children, of any age, are able to talk about their concerns and be involved in the care. However the support of social workers or counsellors may be helpful in supporting parents in these discussions of these difficult issues with the children or grandchildren of the patient. The involvement of school and college support systems and counsellors may be helpful

For many couples there may be major changes in their life together, and a change in how they express their feelings to each other. It may be more difficult to cuddle and kiss when someone is in a wheelchair or has developed behavioural changes. Sexual activity may change and couples often need the opportunity to express and share their concerns. Advice on the alternative ways to express their feelings and intimacy together should be offered sensitively.

17.7.13 Spiritual Issues

Spiritual issues may be religious – such as the wish to see a religious leader or be involved in certain ceremonies or worship – but may also be related to the deeper meaning of life. This may include feelings of guilt or concerns about the future, either of dying itself or of an afterlife. For a person with a progressive neurological disease these issues may be particularly prominent as the loss of abilities and feelings of dependency may lead to questioning of life and their previous beliefs (Lambert 2014).

There are no easy answers to many of these issues. If there are specific religious questions or concerns, the involvement of the appropriate faith leader may be helpful. For many patients it may be important to have the opportunity to express some of these concerns and fears, to an empathetic member of the multidisciplinary team, such as a specialist nurse or social worker. Some multidisciplinary teams include a non-denominational pastoral care worker.

17.8 End of Life Care

As the disease progresses there is a need to plan future care and to consider the end of life Connolly et al. (2015). The varying prognosis in neurological disease – from an average of 2–5 years in ALS/MND to possibly over 30 years in MS makes planning particularly difficult (Oliver and Silber 2013). Even within a single condition there is considerably variation in survival and

prognosis. In ALS/MND the mean time from the first symptom to death is 2–5 years, patients presenting with bulbar symptoms have a shorter prognosis of 18 months but 25 % are alive at 5 years and 10 % at 10 years. Thus the end of life may be difficult to recognise.

17.8.1 Advance Care Planning

It is strongly recommended that planning for future care takes place early in the disease course. The development of language and communication deficits together with cognitive change may mean that patients are unable to make decisions about their care preferences in late-stage disease. Advance care planning is often necessary – so that the patient can express their wishes while they are able to do so and these are definite and clearly stated so that they can be respected later, even if the patient can no longer express their view themselves.

17.8.1.1 Advance Care Planning Can Include

An Advance Statement – outlining the person's views about treatment options, but without specific details of any particular treatment that they did not wish. Such a statement would have no legal status as such but would be very helpful in planning care if the person did lose capacity

An Advance Decision to Refuse Treatment – specific statements are made refusing specific treatments, such as tracheostomy ventilation, cardiopulmonary resuscitation or admission to hospital. In England and Wales if this includes a statement that the person realized that this refusal could shorten their life it is legally binding.

A Power of Attorney – where the person defines other people to make the decision in their stead if they are not able to do so themselves. This may be for Property and Affairs or Health and Welfare.

Expression of the patient's wishes as to the place of care and death

A **Do Not Attempt Cardio-pulmonary Resuscitation Order** (DNACPR) may be completed, with discussion with the patient (if possible/appropriate) and the family/carers can ensure that the patient is spared futile resuscitation attempts when they die.

While the exact format of such advance care planning may vary from country to country, the overall aim is to allow the clear expression of a person to refuse specific treatments or ensure that a proxy is appointed to do so. Such documents would only be used if the person loses capacity and in specifically defined situations. If there is a lack of clarity in the person's views any information may be helpful in aiding the multidisciplinary team, and in particular the lead clinician, to make a decision in the patient's "best interests", integrating all the available information and taking the views of the family into consideration.

17.8.2 Recognition of the End of Life Phase

The recognition that the person is deteriorating and end of life is nearer may be challenging, particularly when there has been a long illness with relatively slow progression, such as in MS. Moreover, there may be periods of increased symptoms followed by a plateau of no progression, which can be confusing for all involved. The patient, family and carers may all be unsure if there will be a continued deterioration or whether this is another period of stabilisation, even if this is to a lower level than before. This can be particularly so when there is a period of sepsis – urinary tract infection, chest infection or aspiration pneumonia - when recovery may occur, but this may also be a sign of the person reaching the final stages of the illness and death approaching.

The end of life period may be signaled by the constellation of certain symptoms which appear to be commoner nearer to death. The National End of Life Care Programme 2010 (UK) highlighted the following symptoms and factors that may herald the end-of-life period in neurological conditions and should trigger specialist palliative care intervention.

- patient request
- family request

- dysphagia
- cognitive decline
- dyspnea
- recurrent infections – in particular aspiration pneumonia
- weight loss
- marked decline in condition
- complex symptoms – such as pain, spasticity, nausea or psychosocial or spiritual issues (End of life care in long term neurological conditions: a framework for implementation 2010; Oliver and Silber 2013)

In addition, there are disease-specific triggers which warrant palliative care intervention:

ALS/MND: respiratory failure or increased breathlessness, reduced mobility, dysphagia

MS: dysphagia, choking attacks, poor hydration and nutrition, frequent infections, cognitive decline, reduced communication, fatigue, profound, reduced response to the environment

PD: rigidity, pain, agitation/confusion from sepsis, neuropsychiatric decline

PSP: dysphagia, speech poor, weight loss, severe pressure sores, psychiatric symptoms, medication no longer effective (Oliver and Silber 2013).

A recent retrospective study has shown that the incidence of the above symptoms increased progressively in the 6 months preceding death. Aspiration was frequently observed in the last 6 months of life, and was particularly common in the last 2 months of life and would seem to be particularly indicative of end of life (Hussain et al. 2014). Further studies are currently being undertaken to identify these triggers and allow a clearer method of anticipating the end of life phase.

17.8.3 Symptom Management at the End of Life

As the person's health deteriorates it is even more important to ensure that the symptoms are managed as effectively as possible. This particularly applies to pain, sialorrhoea, dysphagia and dyspnoea as these symptoms may cause particular distress to both the patient and their family. The principles outlined should be followed, with careful multidisciplinary assessment and appropriate management.

Although it may not always be clear when end of life care may be required it is important to ensure that the patient, family and professional carers become aware of the deterioration and have a realistic understanding of the prognosis. This will allow increasing discussion and consideration of the patient's wishes for their future care, the consideration of advance care planning and consideration of preferred place of care and later of death.

A candid discussion of these areas may be necessary long before the last few months of life, especially if there are increasing communication or cognitive issues. There is an imperative to ensure that plans and preferences are discussed and the wishes of the patient ascertained while they can be clearly communicated. This can be difficult in the earlier stages of disease, as the patient, their families, caregivers and professionals may be reluctant to discuss advance planning. A clear explanation of the necessity for earlier discussion is essential so that patients are given the best opportunity to express their wishes and preferences. It is also imperative to recognise that the attitudes, culture and personal beliefs of patients, caregivers and health care providers all influence the decision-making process and ultimately acceptance or refusal of various interventions. The timing and pace of these discussions should be set by the patient and not by the professional.

As the person deteriorates it may be necessary to look at the methods of administration of medications. If swallowing is impaired, due to dysphagia or drowsiness, alternative non-oral routes of administration may be needed. For instance in PD, transdermal preparations, such as rotigotine, may be helpful if swallowing is difficult. It is important to ensure that medication that is necessary for symptom control, including those related to the disease progression, are maintained if at all possible, even if oral medication can no longer be taken.

The symptoms that may need targeted assessment and specific management at the end of life for people with progressive neurological disease include pain, dyspnoea, respiratory secretions, and restlessness.

Pain – as described above – needs careful assessment and the use of analgesics is essential. Opioids are very helpful but may need to be given as a transdermal patch (such as fentanyl), parenterally by injection, or by a continuous subcutaneous infusion by syringe driver.

Respiratory secretions and "noisy" breathing at the end of life, as the patient is unable to clear secretions or cough effectively, can be distressing for the family and carers, often more than for the patient. The use of anticholinergic medication, such as glycopyrronium bromide or hyoscine hydrobromide (scopolamine) by injection or subcutaneous infusion can be helpful in reducing both secretions and caregiver distress.

Restlessness may reflect confusion or agitation, but may be due to treatable causes such as a full bladder, faecal loading or hypoxia, all of which can be helped. However, often there is a need to ensure that the symptom is treated effectively by providing sedative medications, such as midazolam or levomepromazine (although this is contraindicated in PD, MSA and PSP) by injection or a subcutaneous infusion. Levomepromazine also has antiemetic properties.

Dyspnoea may respond to both opioids and benzodiazepines. There may be concerns that giving such medication could shorten life. Ethically however, it is appropriate to reduce the distress of the patient, even if there is the risk of causing a shortening of life, under the doctrine of double effect – as long as it is clear that the doctor's intention of using the medication was to reduce the distress and not to shorten life.

The use of non-invasive ventilation (NIV) for the management of respiratory weakness in ALS/MND has increased significantly over the last 15 years, and there is good evidence that this both improves quality of life and extends life. However, while the symptoms of respiratory weakness are eased, the disease itself continues to progress and the patient becomes more disabled. This may lead to the patient asking for the NIV to be withdrawn or discontinued. If the patients have the capacity to make this decision it should be respected. Similarly, many patients will complete an ADRT stating that they would wish withdrawal in certain circumstances – such as if communication is lost- if they do lose capacity to make the decision at the time. It is paramount that medication is given to prevent distress when the NIV is removed, and opioids with midazolam are usually needed to sedate the patient and prevent breathlessness. This can lead to complex ethical debates. Although the ethics of removing an unwanted treatment from a patient at their request is clear, it may seem to all involved that this is euthanasia. Wider discussions, involving the wider multidisciplinary team and the family and carers are essential.

The provision of anticipatory medication – such as injections of morphine sulphate for pain and dyspnoea, midazolam for agitation or stiffness, glycopyrronium bromide for chest secretions and levomepromazine or ondansetron for nausea and vomiting can be helpful a so that they are readily available if needed. These medications are then ready "just in case" and the Motor Neurone Disease Association in the UK has produced a "Just in case" box for the storage of such medication, together with instructions as to when/how to administer so that the medications are readily available for use if there is increasing distress or severe symptoms (MND Association website).

17.8.4 Moral Distress and Compassion Fatigue Among Health Professionals

Compassionate engagement with distressed patients and their families can exert a considerable emotional toll, and moral and ethical distress, even among experienced professionals. Moral distress refers to a response to a situation in which the person is aware of a moral problem, acknowledges moral responsibility, and makes a moral judgment about the correct action, but as a result of real or perceived constraints, participates in what is perceived as moral wrongdoing (Rushton et al. 2013).

Moral distress is an under-recognized feature of the clinical landscape, and is associated with a high risk of burnout. Formal structures to protect against moral distress, compassion fatigue and burnout are not well developed, although frameworks for understanding and addressing moral distress have been recently proposed within the palliative care literature. These frameworks describe four dimensions that contribute to the moral compass, – namely: empathy (emotional attunement), perspective taking (cognitive attunement), memory (personal experience), and moral sensitivity. Frameworks that seek the alignment of these dimensions can provide the clinician with the equipment to address distressing conflicts with compassion and resilience, and could be easily adapted to terminal neurological disease.

Conclusion

The provision of palliative care is important to help people with progressive neurological disease and their families as the disease progresses. Careful assessment and management will allow the patient to remain as active as possible, maintain a quality of life, dignity, autonomy and to die peacefully.

References

Andersen PM, Abrahams S, Borasio GD, de Carvalho M, Chio A, Van Damme P, Hardiman O, Kollewe K, Morrison KE, Petri S, Pradat PF, Silani V, Tomik B, Wasner M, Weber M, The EFNS Task Force on Diagnosis and Management of Amyotrophic Lateral Sclerosis. EFNS guidelines on the Clinical Management of Amyotrophic Lateral Sclerosis (MALS) – revised report of an EFNS task force. Eur J Neurol. 2012;19:360–75.
Bakitas M, Lyons KD, Hegel MT, et al. Effects of a palliative care intervention on clinical outcomes in patients with advanced cancer; the Project ENABLE II randomised controlled trial. JAMA. 2009;19:741–9.
Bede P, Oliver D, Stodart J, van den Berg L, Simmons Z, O Brannagáin D, Borasio GD, Hardiman O. Palliative care in amyotrophic lateral sclerosis: a review of current international guidelines and initiatives. J Neurol Neurosurg Psychiatry. 2011;82(4):413–8.

Connolly S, Galvin M, Hardiman O. End-of-life management in patients with amyotrophic lateral sclerosis.
Lancet Neurol. 2015;14(4):435–42.

Faull C, Rowe Haynes C, Oliver D. Issues for palliative
medicine doctors surrounding the withdrawal of non-
invasive ventilation at the request of a patient with
motor neurone disease: a scoping study. BMJ Support
Palliat Care. 2014;4:43–9.

Ganzini L, Harvath TA, Jackson A, et al. Experiences of
Oregon nurses and social workers with hospice
patients who requested assistance with suicide. N Engl
J Med. 2002;347(8):582–8.

Hussain J, Adams D, Allgar V, Campbell C. Triggers in
advanced neurological conditions: prediction and
management of the terminal phase. BMJ Support
Palliat Care. 2014;4:30–7.

Lambert R. Spiritual care. In: Oliver D, Borasio GD,
Johnston W, editors. Palliative care in amyotrophic lat-
eral sclerosis- from diagnosis to brereavement. 3rd ed.
Oxford: Oxford University Press; 2014.

Neudert C, Wasner M, Borasio GD. Individual quality of
life is not correlated with health-related quality of life
or physical function in patients with amyotrophic lateral sclerosis. J Palliat Med. 2004;7(4):551–7.

Oliver D. Palliative care. In: Oliver D, Borasio GD,
Johnston W, editors. Palliative care in amyotrophic lat-
eral sclerosis- from diagnosis to brereavement. 3rd ed.
Oxford: Oxford University Press; 2014.

Oliver D, Silber E. End of life care in neurological disease. In: Oliver D, editor. End of life care in neurological disease. London: Springer; 2013.

Oliver DJ, Tumer MR. Some difficult decisions in ALS/
MND. Amyotroph Lateral Scler. 2010;11:339–43.

Rooney J, Byrne S, Heverin M, Tobin K, Dick A, Donaghy
C, Hardiman O. A multidisciplinary clinic approach
improves survival in ALS: a comparative study of
ALS in Ireland and Northern Ireland. J Neurol
Neurosurg Psychiatry. 2014. pii: jnnp-2014-309601.
doi:10.1136/jnnp-2014-309601. [Epub ahead of print]
PMID: 25550416.

Rushton CH, Kaszniak AW, Halifax JS. A framework for
understanding moral distress among palliative care
clinicians. J Palliat Med. 2013;16(9):1074–9.

Simmons Z, Bremer BA, Robbins RA, Walsh SM, Fischer S.
Quality of life in ALS depends on factors other than strength
and physical function. Neurology. 2000;55:p388–92.

Veronese S, Valle A, Chio A, Calvo A, Oliver D. The last
months of life of people with amyotrophic lateral sclerosis in mechanical invasive ventilation: a qualitative
study. Amyotroph Lateral Scler Frontotemporal
Degener. 2014. doi:10.3109/21678421.2014.913637.

Additional Reading

Connolly S, Galvin M, Hardiman O. End-of-life management
in patients with amyotrophic lateral sclerosis. Lancet
Neurol. 2015;14(4):435–42.

End of life care in long term neurological conditions: a
framework for implementation. National End of Life
Care Programme. 2010.

Index

© Springer International Publishing Switzerland 2016
O. Hardiman, C.P. Doherty (eds.), *Neurodegenerative Disorders: A Clinical Guide*,
DOI 10.1007/978-3-319-23309-3

Printed in the United States
By Bookmasters